Register Now for Online Access to Your Book!

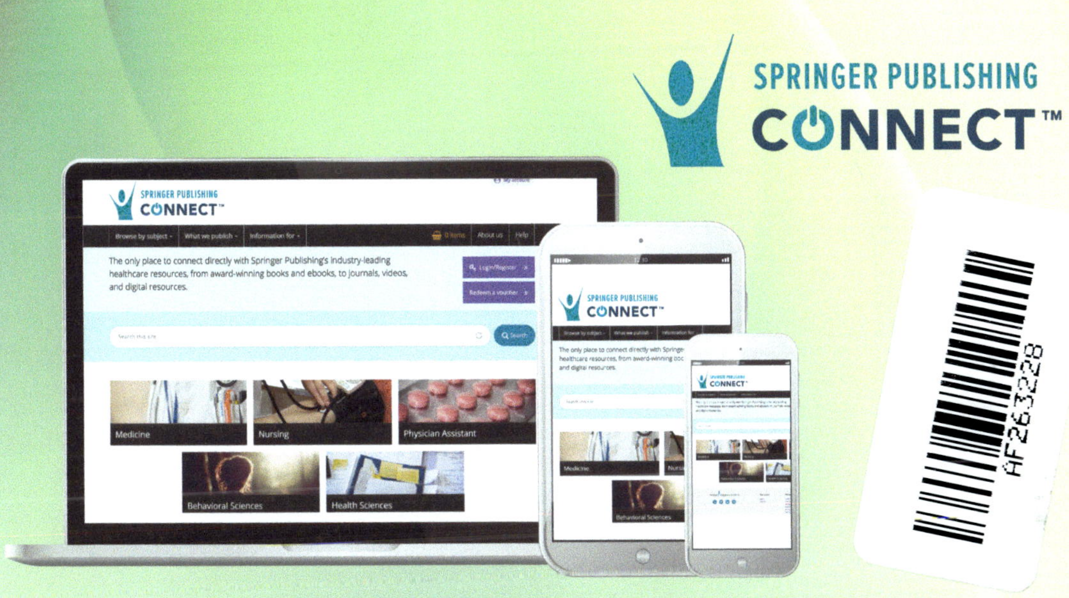

Your print purchase of *Bone Stress Injuries: Diagnosis, Treatment, and Prevention* **includes online access to the contents of your book**—increasing accessibility, portability, and searchability!

Access today at:
http://connect.springerpub.com/content/book/978-0-8261-4424-9
or scan the QR code at the right with your smartphone. Log in or register, then click "Redeem a voucher" and use the code below.

8E282SSA

Scan here for
quick access.

Having trouble redeeming a voucher code?
Go to https://connect.springerpub.com/redeeming-voucher-code

If you are experiencing problems accessing the digital component of this product, please contact our customer service department at cs@springerpub.com

The online access with your print purchase is available at the publisher's discretion and may be removed at any time without notice.

Publisher's Note: New and used products purchased from third-party sellers are not guaranteed for quality, authenticity, or access to any included digital components.

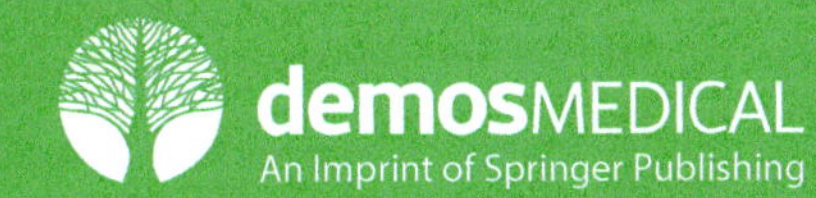

View all our products at springerpub.com/demosmedical

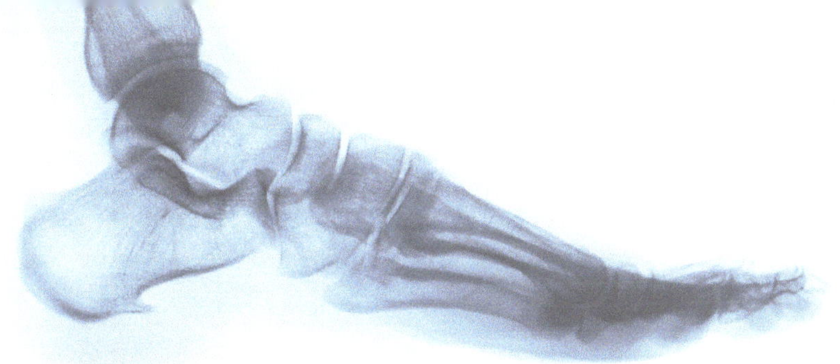

Bone Stress Injuries

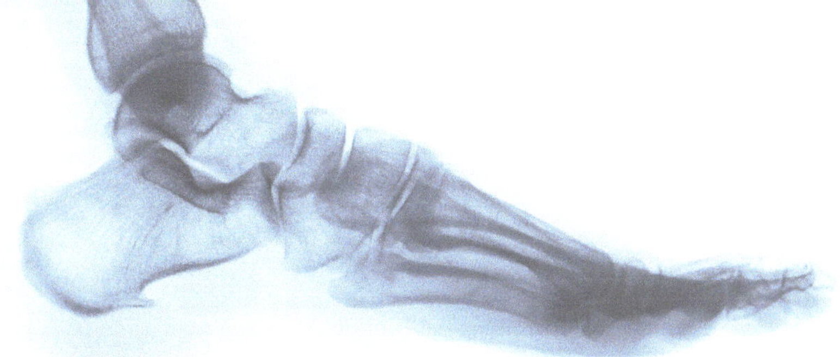

Bone Stress Injuries

Diagnosis, Treatment, and Prevention

Editors

Adam S. Tenforde, MD, FACSM

Director of Running Medicine
Spaulding Rehabilitation Hospital;
Associate Professor
Department of Physical Medicine and Rehabilitation
Harvard Medical School
Boston, Massachusetts

Michael Fredericson, MD, FACSM

Professor and Director, PM&R Sports Medicine
Fellowship Director, Primary Care Sports Medicine
Team Physician, Stanford Intercollegiate Athletics
Department of Orthopaedic Surgery
Stanford University
Palo Alto, CA

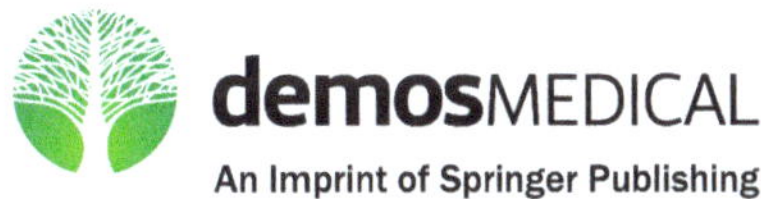

Springer Publishing Company, LLC
11 West 42nd Street
New York, NY 10036
www.springerpub.com
connect.springerpub.com/

Acquisitions Editor: Beth Barry
Compositor: Transforma

ISBN: 978-0-8261-4423-2
ebook ISBN: 978-0-8261-4424-9
DOI: 10.1891/9780826144249

21 22 23 24 25 / 5 4 3 2 1

Medicine is an ever-changing science. Research and clinical experience are continually expanding our knowledge, in particular our understanding of proper treatment and drug therapy. The authors, editors, and publisher have made every effort to ensure that all information in this book is in accordance with the state of knowledge at the time of production of the book. Nevertheless, the authors, editors, and publisher are not responsible for any errors or omissions or for any consequence from application of the information in this book and make no warranty, expressed or implied, with respect to the content of this publication. Every reader should examine carefully the package inserts accompanying each drug and should carefully check whether the dosage schedules therein or the contraindications stated by the manufacturer differ from the statements made in this book. Such examination is particularly important with drugs that are either rarely used or have been newly released on the market.

Library of Congress Cataloging-in-Publication Data
Names: Tenforde, Adam S., editor. | Fredericson, Michael, editor.
Title: Bone stress injuries : diagnosis, treatment, and prevention /
    editors, Adam S. Tenforde, Michael Fredericson.
Description: New York, NY : Springer Publishing Company, LLC, [2022] | Includes bibliographical references and index. | Summary: "This book is organized to address aspects of clinical diagnosis, rehabilitation, and prevention. We invited experts across a range of topics to provide a more complete understanding of the full spectrum in BSI treatment. Initial chapters focus on evaluating injury, including the role of the clinical examination and imaging to guide treatment. Recognition of risk factors for BSI are separated into biological and biomechanical risk factors, including gender, age, and anatomical location. Methods to optimize treatment are reviewed in each section by anatomical location, and strategies for refractory injuries are reviewed in designated chapters on medications, emerging technologies, and interventions. Further, we identify what is known about future injury prevention and methods to optimize bone strength"-- Provided by publisher.
Identifiers: LCCN 2021012261 | ISBN 9780826144232 (paperback) | ISBN
    9780826144249 (ebook)
Subjects: MESH: Fractures, Stress
Classification: LCC RD101 | NLM WE 180 | DDC 617.1/5--dc23
LC record available at https://lccn.loc.gov/2021012261

Contact sales@springerpub.com to receive discount rates on bulk purchases.

Publisher's Note: **New and used products purchased from third-party sellers are not guaranteed for quality, authenticity, or access to any included digital components.**

Printed in the United States of America.

Contents

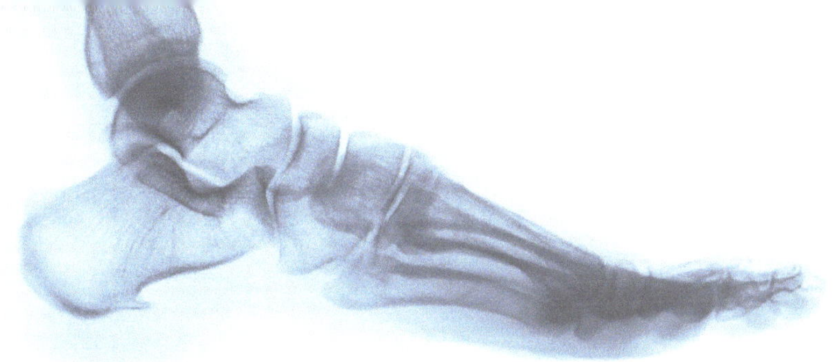

Part III. Special Populations

Part IV. Special Considerations

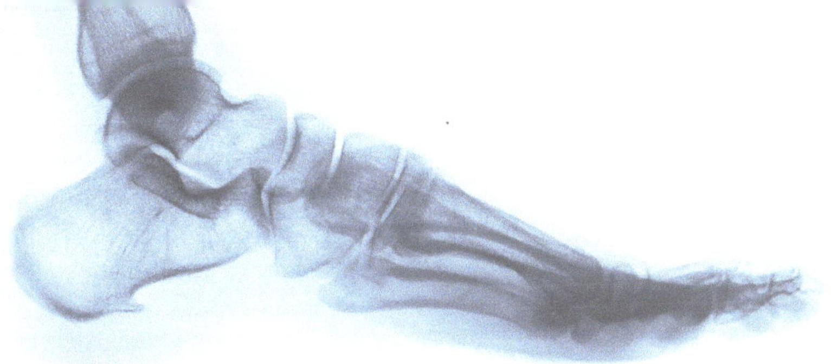

Haylee Borgstrom, MD, MS   Staff Physiatrist, Department of Physical Medicine and Rehabilitation, Spaulding Rehabilitation Hospital, Charlestown, Massachusetts; Staff Physiatrist, Sports Medicine Division, Massachusetts General Hospital; Instructor, Harvard Medical School, Boston, Massachusetts

Irene S. Davis, PhD, PT, FACSM, FAPTA, FASB   Professor, Department of Physical Medicine and Rehabilitation, Harvard Medical School; Director, Spaulding National Running Center, Boston, Massachusetts

Stephanie DeLuca, MD   Resident, Department of Physical Medicine and Rehabilitation, Spaulding Rehabilitation Hospital, Harvard Medical School, Charlestown, Massachusetts

Aleksei Dingel   Medical Student, University of Washington School of Medicine – Idaho, Moscow, Idaho

Stephanie R. Douglas, MD   Research Assistant, Boston, Massachusetts

Nicole M. Farnsworth, MS, RD, CSSD, LDN, CPT   Clinical Nutrition Specialist, Orthopedics/Sports Medicine Division, Boston Children's Hospital, Boston, Massachusetts

Katherine Fahy, MD   Primary Care Sports Medicine Fellow, Division of Sports Medicine, UCLA Department of Family Medicine, UCLA Family Health Center, Los Angeles, California

Michael Fredericson, MD, FACSM   Professor and Director, PM&R Sports Medicine, Fellowship Director, Primary Care Sports Medicine, Team Physician, Stanford Intercollegiate Athletics, Department of Orthopaedic Surgery, Stanford University, Palo Alto, California

Brian W. Fullem, DPM   Podiatric Surgery Specialist, Elite Sports Podiatry, Clearwater, Florida

Rahul Kapur, MD CAQSM Assistant Professor, Family Medicine and Sports Medicine, St John's Family Medicine Residency Program, University of Minnesota Sports Medicine; Team Physician, US Lacrosse and Minnesota Twins, Minneapolis, Minnesota

Kristine Karlson, MD Associate Professor, Departments of Community and Family Medicine, Orthopaedics and Pediatrics, Geisel School of Medicine at Dartmouth, Hanover, New Hampshire

Emily Kraus, MD Assistant Clinical Professor, Division of Physical Medicine and Rehabilitation and Sports Medicine, Department of Pediatric Orthopaedic Surgery, Stanford University School of Medicine, Palo Alto, California

Andrea Kussman, MD Clinical Assistant Professor, Department of Orthopaedics, Stanford University, Palo Alto, California

Alexander Lloyd, MD Sports Medicine Fellow, Swedish Medical Center, Seattle, Washington

Charles Milgrom, MD Professor Emeritus of Orthopedic Surgery, Hebrew University Medical School, Jerusalem, Israel

Emily Miller Olson, MD Primary Care Sports Medicine Fellow, Department of Orthopaedic Surgery, Stanford University, Palo Alto, California

Madhusmita Misra, MD, MPH Fritz Bradley Talbot and Nathan Bill Talbot Professor of Pediatrics, Department of Pediatrics, Harvard Medical School; Chief, Division of Pediatric Endocrinology, Massachusetts General Hospital, Boston, Massachusetts

Erin Moix Grieb, MD Clinical Assistant Professor, Department of Orthopaedic Surgery, Stanford University, Palo Alto, California

Laura J. Moretti, MS, RD, CSSD, LDN Clinical Nutrition Specialist, Orthopedics/Sports Medicine Division, Boston Children's Hospital, Boston, Massachusetts

Kevin M. Mullins, MD Assistant Clinical Professor, Department of Physical Medicine & Rehabilitation, UC Davis Health, Sacramento, California

Aurelia Nattiv, MD Professor, Division of Sports Medicine and Non-Operative Orthopaedics, Departments of Family Medicine and Orthopaedic Surgery, UCLA Family Health Center; Director, Bone Health Practice, David Geffen School of Medicine at UCLA; Associate Team Physician, UCLA Athletics, Los Angeles, California

David E. Oji, MD Clinical Assistant Professor, Department of Orthopaedic Surgery, Stanford University School of Medicine, Palo Alto, California

Kentaro Onishi, DO Assistant Professor, Departments of Physical Medicine and Rehabilitation and Orthopedic Surgery, University of Pittsburgh Medical Center, Pittsburgh, Pennsylvania

James Policy, MD Clinical Assistant Professor, Department of Orthopaedic Surgery, Stanford University, Palo Alto, California

Megan Roche, MD   Clinical Researcher, Department of Orthopaedic Surgery, Stanford University, Palo Alto, California

Amol Saxena, DPM   Podiatrist, Department of Sports Medicine, Palo Alto Medical Foundation, Palo Alto, California

Kevin G. Shea, MD   Professor, Department of Orthopaedic Surgery, Stanford University, Palo Alto, California

Matthew C. Sherrier, MD   Resident Physician, Department of Physical Medicine and Rehabilitation, University of Pittsburgh Medical Center, Pittsburgh, Pennsylvania

Kate Temme, MD, CAQSM   Assistant Professor, Departments of Physical Medicine and Rehabilitation and Orthopaedics, University of Pennsylvania; Director, Penn Center for the Female Athlete; Associate Director, Primary Care Sports Medicine Fellowship, Philadelphia, Pennsylvania

Adam S. Tenforde, MD, FACSM   Director of Running Medicine, Spaulding Rehabilitation Hospital; Associate Professor, Department of Physical Medicine and Rehabilitation, Harvard Medical School, Boston, Massachusetts

Karen L. Troy, PhD   Associate Professor, Department of Biomedical Engineering, Worcester Polytechnic Institute, Worcester, Massachusetts

Kenneth Vitale, MD, FACSM, FAAPMR, CAQSM   Associate Professor, Division of Sports Medicine, Department of Orthopedic Surgery, University of California San Diego, La Jolla, California

Stuart J. Warden, BPhysio (Hons), PhD, FACSM, FASBMR   Associate Dean for Research and Professor, Department of Physical Therapy, School of Health & Human Sciences, Indiana University, Indianapolis, Indiana; Research Professor, La Trobe Sport and Exercise Medicine Research Centre, La Trobe University, Bundoora, Victoria, Australia

Richard W. Willy, PT, PhD   Chair and Assistant Professor, School of Physical Therapy and Rehabilitation Science, University of Montana, Missoula, Montana

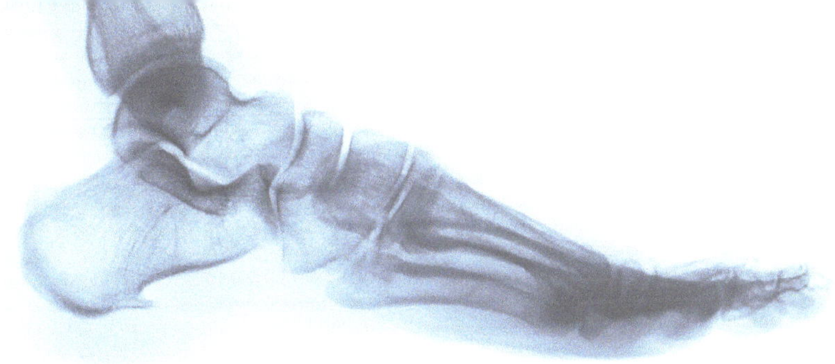

Preface

Bone stress injury (BSI) represents an overuse injury to bone seen in athletes and active individuals. Despite being a common injury seen in clinical practice, there exists confusion on multiple aspects of this injury, including appropriate terminology. For example, "stress fracture" is often used interchangeably with "stress reaction" or "stress response." Our understanding of the pathophysiology of this injury has advanced communication of bone stress injury using grading scales that reflect the severity of the injury and set expectations for rehabilitation and return to play.

Recent scientific discoveries on the topic of BSI have advanced our understanding of risk factors for injury. Rarely can the injury be attributed solely to training errors. While training volume, intensity, and frequency do influence bone remodeling, most BSI is multifactorial and involve a combination of biological, anatomical, and biomechanical risk factors for injury. Recognizing risk factors for BSI may help to develop a comprehensive treatment plan to address each injury. Further, the goal of treating the injury should focus on methods to optimize bone health and develop strategies for future injury prevention.

Our book is organized to address aspects of clinical diagnosis, rehabilitation, and prevention. We invited experts across a range of topics to provide a more complete understanding of the full spectrum in BSI treatment. Initial chapters focus on evaluating the injury, including the role of the clinical examination and imaging to guide treatment. Recognition of risk factors for BSI are separated into biological and biomechanical risk factors, including gender, age, and anatomical location. We also provide considerations for management unique to military personnel and youth athletes. Methods to optimize treatment are reviewed in each section by anatomical location, and strategies for refractory injuries are reviewed in designated chapters on medications, emerging technologies, and interventions. Further, we identify what is known about future injury prevention and methods to optimize bone strength.

Our goal of this book is to provide a comprehensive understanding of BSI that improves clinical outcomes and provides a patient-centered treatment program. We are grateful to the content experts who served as authors for book chapters and to the scientific community for developing the foundational knowledge that contributes to our evolving understanding of BSI. Special acknowledgment to Kate Tenforde for her editorial expertise and support of this project. We hope that everyone will enjoy reading this book and applying the principles to clinical practice.

Adam S. Tenforde, MD, FACSM
Michael Fredericson, MD, FACSM

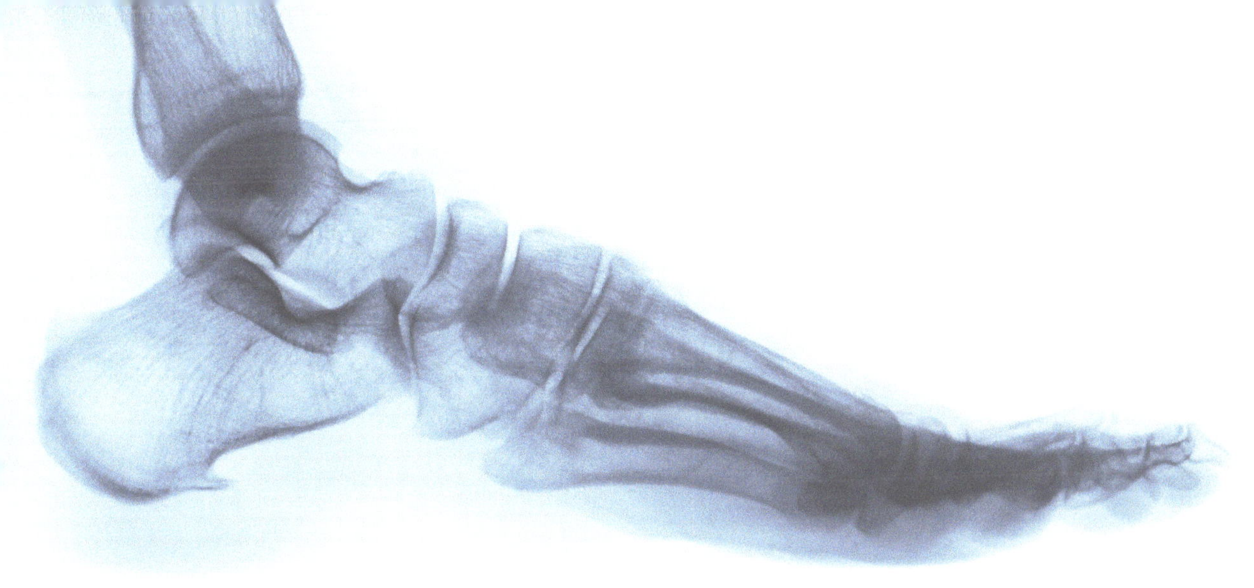

PART I

GENERAL TOPICS

CHAPTER 1

History and Evaluation

Stuart J. Warden

INTRODUCTION

Bone stress injuries (BSIs) occur along a pathology continuum. The continuum begins with the accumulation of load-induced microdamage that can progress to the generation of a stress reaction, stress fracture and, ultimately, complete fracture.[1-3] The earlier bone tissue is considered a potential source of an individual's symptoms, the earlier within the continuum the pathology can be identified, and the quicker the individual may be able to return to activity.[4,5] Importantly, the earlier a diagnosis is made, the less likely the pathology will progress to a catastrophic complete fracture.

Suspicion of a potential BSI should be heightened in active populations, such as athletes and military personnel. These populations frequently "push the envelope" in an attempt to induce maximal physiological adaptation and improve performance. However, the possibility of a BSI should not be discounted in individuals who are not regularly active, particularly if they report recent performance of a strenuous unaccustomed activity and present with appropriate signs and symptoms.[6-8]

Within active populations, BSI risk varies according to sex and type of physical activity. Females have more than double the risk of suffering a BSI compared to males.[9,10] However, the potential of a BSI should be equally considered across sexes as over one third of BSIs occur in males.[9] In terms of physical activity, some activities place individuals at greater risk than others. For instance, BSI risk in collegiate-level female and male athletes is greatest in those participating in cross country, followed by gymnastics (in females), outdoor track, basketball, and indoor track (Figure 1.1).[9] Suspicion of a BSI is heightened when individuals participating in these activities present with injury; however, BSIs do occur and should not be missed in individuals participating in activities less commonly associated with BSIs.

The physical activity an individual participates in not only influences their overall risk of a BSI but also influences where within their skeleton a BSI is most likely to occur. The lower extremities are most frequently exposed to repetitive high-magnitude loads introduced at high rates of loading and, thus, most BSIs occur at weight-bearing sites such as the tibia, fibula, metatarsals, and tarsals.[9] Therefore, the potential presence of a BSI should be high on the list of differential diagnoses for individuals who participate in weight-bearing physical activities and present with lower leg and/or foot symptoms. However, site-specific risk varies between activities. Cross-country athletes have a

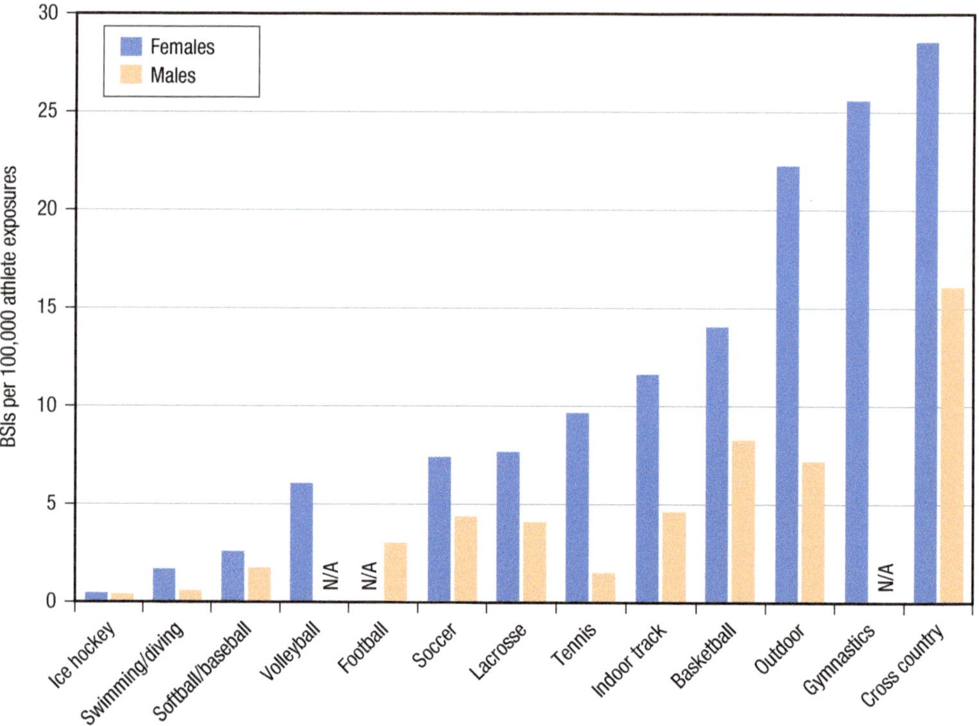

FIGURE 1.1 BSI risk varies according to sport and sex. Data indicate BSI rates per 100,000 athlete-exposures in select National Collegiate Athletic Association sports from 2004-2014. BSI rates were greatest in females, and those competing in cross country, gymnastics (in females), outdoor track and basketball. N/A indicates data not available for this sex for this sport. Data from Rizzone et al.[9]

BSI, bone stress injuries.

higher proportion of BSIs in the femur compared to athletes competing in other high BSI-risk activities, whereas gymnasts and basketball players have a higher proportion of BSIs in the spine and metatarsals compared to other athletes, respectively (Figure 1.2).[9]

Although BSIs most commonly occur in the lower legs and feet, they can occur in virtually any bone in the body under suitable loading conditions (Figure 1.3).[11] This includes sites considered non–weight bearing. For instance, rowers repetitively load their rib cage during the drive phase of the rowing stroke and, consequently, are at risk of generating rib BSIs.[12] Similarly, overhead throwing athletes expose the humerus to high-magnitude loads at high rates of loading[13] and, subsequently, have a heightened risk of BSIs within the humeral diaphysis (see Chapter 5).[14] Additionally, athletes with disabilities who participate in adaptive sports often have increased reliance on the upper body and noted to have a high prevalence of upper extremity BSIs.[15] By knowing the activity that an individual participates in and the associated regional skeletal loading, risk for a BSI at a particular site can be estimated. This knowledge will increase clinical suspicion and hopefully lead to an earlier diagnosis when an individual presents with symptoms at an "at risk" site for their particular activity. However, the potential for a BSI to occur at a less common or more unusual site should not be discounted.

Ultimately, bone tissue and the potential presence of a BSI should be considered in the differential diagnosis of every individual presenting with an overuse-related injury.

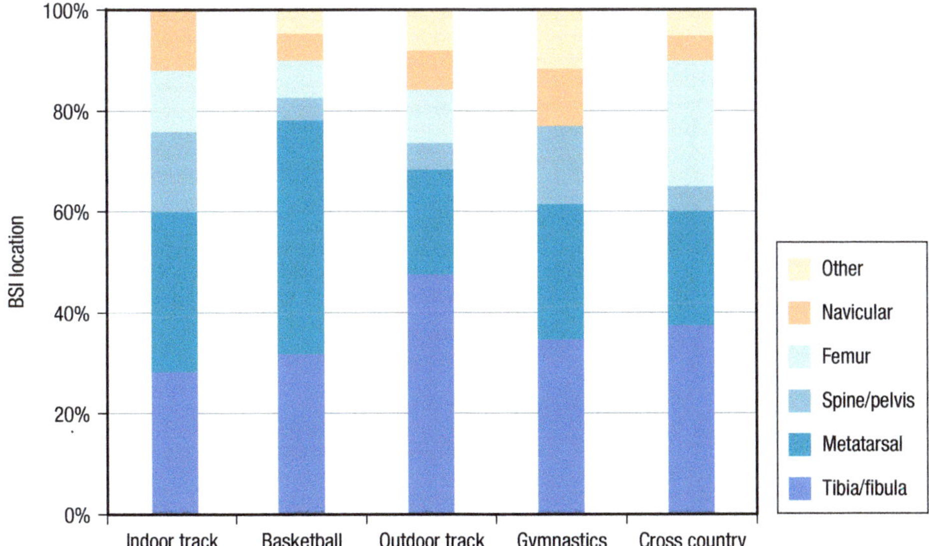

FIGURE 1.2 The location of BSIs varies according to sport. Data indicate the relative distribution of BSIs in females competing in high-risk sports. Cross-country athletes have a higher proportion of BSIs in the femur compared to those competing in other high-risk sports, whereas gymnasts and basketball players have a higher proportion of BSIs in the spine and metatarsals, respectively. Data from Rizzone et al.[9]

BSIs, bone stress injuries.

HISTORY

Pain

Individuals with a BSI most commonly present with a consistent and predictable history that usually centers on pain. Some individuals may initially present with stiffness or tightness, such as those with a BSI in the pars interarticularis region of the lumbar spine (a so-called pars defect). The description of BSI pain can vary from a mild diffuse ache to very localized sharp pain or a combination of both. The variation in pain presentation results from the innervation pattern of bone and the relative involvement of mechanical versus chemical stimuli.

Bone tissue is innervated by thinly or non-myelinated A-delta and C sensory nerve fibers, both of which detect and signal noxious mechanical and chemical signals.[16] The relative density of sensory fibers has a ratio of 100:2:0.1 in the outer bone covering (periosteum), bone marrow, and cortical bone, respectively.[17] The heterogeneous density distribution has implications for how a BSI is perceived by an individual and how they present with symptoms.

Intracortical bone changes in isolation, that is, in the absence of any changes on the outer periosteal or inner endosteal bone surfaces, typically do not generate symptoms. Sensory nerve fibers in cortical bone are sparse relative to those on the bone surfaces and co-localize with blood vessels to run through some of the canals (e.g., Haversian and Volkmann canals) residing at the center of cortical bone osteons.[16] The type of microdamage (i.e., linear microcracks) that is thought to proceed generation of a BSI principally develops in the interstitial bone tissue between osteons,[18] which is at a

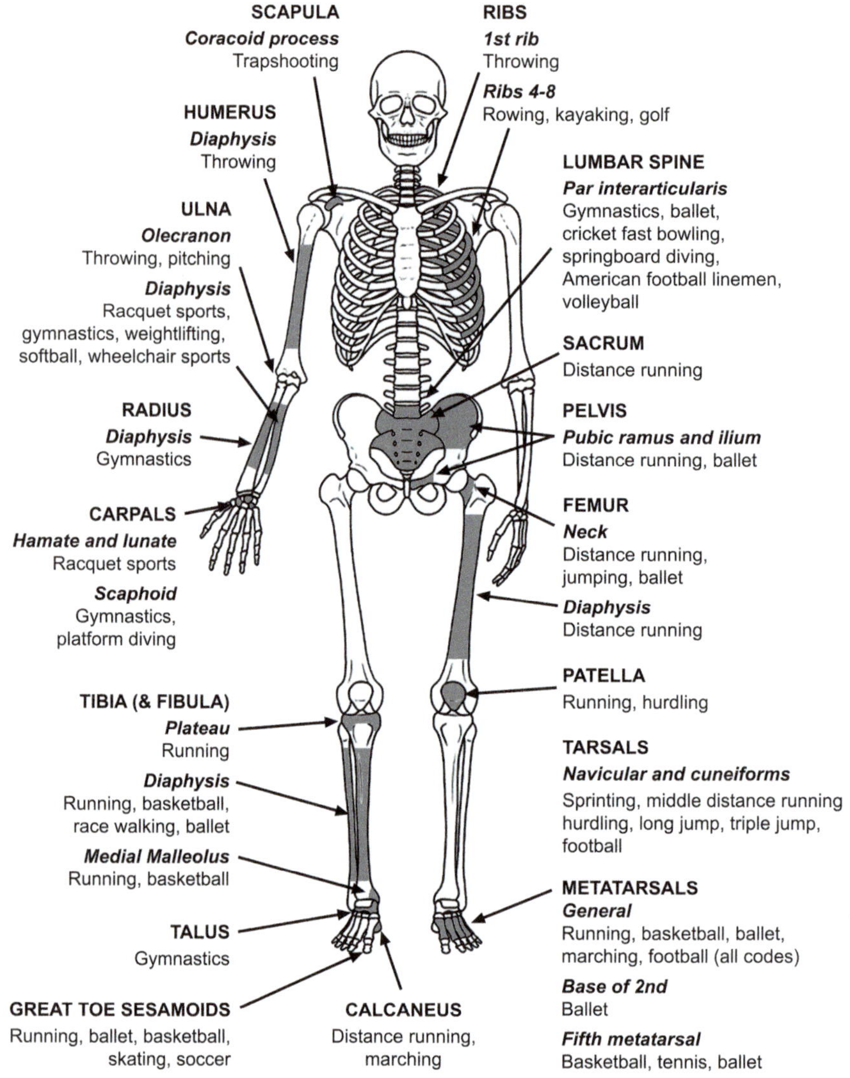

FIGURE 1.3 Sites for bone stress injuries and representative associated sports/activities.

distance from cortical bone sensory fibers. Also, microdamage is usually efficiently removed and replaced by targeted remodeling.[19] Thus, normal levels of microdamage do not generate symptoms; otherwise, we would all be in a constant state of pain.

Progressive accumulation of microdamage resulting from an imbalance in loading-induced damage formation and its removal has the potential to generate pain, particularly if it begins to involve and/or triggers a reaction on the bone surfaces or a reaction within the bone marrow/medullary cavity. The pathology at this stage is usually visible on imaging, where it is often referred to as a stress reaction on the BSI pathology continuum (Grades 1–3 on BSI imaging grading scales [see Chapter 2]). The pain associated with these lower grade BSIs is often initially described as a mild, diffuse ache that occurs after an activity bout or specific amount of activity. It may also only develop hours after loading completion or on the following day and is often initially passed off as a typical ache or pain associated with physical activity. When the pain does occur during activity, it does not tend to resolve during "warm-up" with continued activity and only abates once activity (i.e., bone loading) is ceased. The absence of loading-related bone pain (warming-up) is a characteristic diagnostic feature for a BSI when compared to overuse-related soft tissue injuries, which often initially warm up, at least in the early stages of pathology.

The initial stress reaction pain is thought to result from chemical stimulation of sensory fibers by inflammatory mediators within the stress reaction combined with mechanical stimulation of the chemically sensitized nerve fibers. The pain may not initially be reproducible during discrete, specific bone-loading activities (such as hopping) as the mechanical integrity of the bone remains relatively intact. This non-reproduction of symptoms during initial clinical loading tests is often falsely believed to indicate that bone tissue and a BSI are not the source. However, as activity and loading continue over days and weeks, the pathology progresses and so do the symptoms.

Stress reactions predominantly impacting the medullary cavity and/or trabecular bone generally produce more vague and difficult-to-localize symptoms due to the deep location of these areas, the diffuse nature of the stress reaction, and a relatively low number of intramedullary sensory fibers which limits spatial localization. In contrast, a stress reaction involving the periosteal surface physically deforms the periosteum to produce more localized site-specific pain. The improved localization results from the large density of sensory fibers in the periosteum, which are organized in a dense net-like mesh to produce high nociceptive spatial resolution.

An astute clinician may be able to suspect the presence of a BSI at the early stress reaction stage and consider imaging to confirm the diagnosis (see Chapter 2). However, some patients may not present until symptoms have progressed to being present earlier during activity and during specific bone-loading activities. Reproducible mechanically induced bone pain indicates that the pathology has progressed to a level where the mechanical properties of the bone have been compromised. This particularly occurs at the stage of a true stress fracture where a cortical defect is present (Grade 4 on BSI imaging grading scales [see Chapter 2]). The localized reduced bone strength at the site of the BSI results in the concentration of stresses during loading, stretching of the periosteum, and an increase in intramedullary pressure. The latter mechanically stimulates the sensory fibers within the medullary cavity, which are pressure sensitive, while stretching of the periosteum and its high-density mesh of sensory fibers produces very site-specific acute sharp pain. The sharp pain quickly subsides once the loading is removed, but the more constant diffuse aching pain associated with any coexisting stress reaction persists and may contribute to resting and/or night pain.

Beyond Pain

Pain is the predominant presenting symptom of a BSI, and a comprehensive assessment of an individual's pain profile is the first step in the diagnosis of a BSI. It is important to ask the usual questions with regard to pain location, its behavior over a 24-hour period, and its relationship to physical activity (i.e., bone loading). In addition, mapping the historical trajectory of the pain is informative. For example, it is informative to ask when the pain was first noticed in relation to activity (e.g., at the beginning vs. during vs. at the end vs. after an activity bout) and how the pain has progressed or changed over time and whether the pain fails to warm up with activity

However, pain alone is often not enough to suspect bone as the source of symptoms in the early stages of the BSI pathology continuum because of its initial vague nature and sometimes inconsistent relationship with mechanical loading. Also, BSIs in some locations (e.g., femoral neck or pelvis) do not always produce a predictable pattern both in terms of pain location and in terms of its behavior in relationship to activity.

A complete picture of the presenting individual beyond pain may lead to bone being suspected as the potential source of symptoms. As discussed earlier, it is

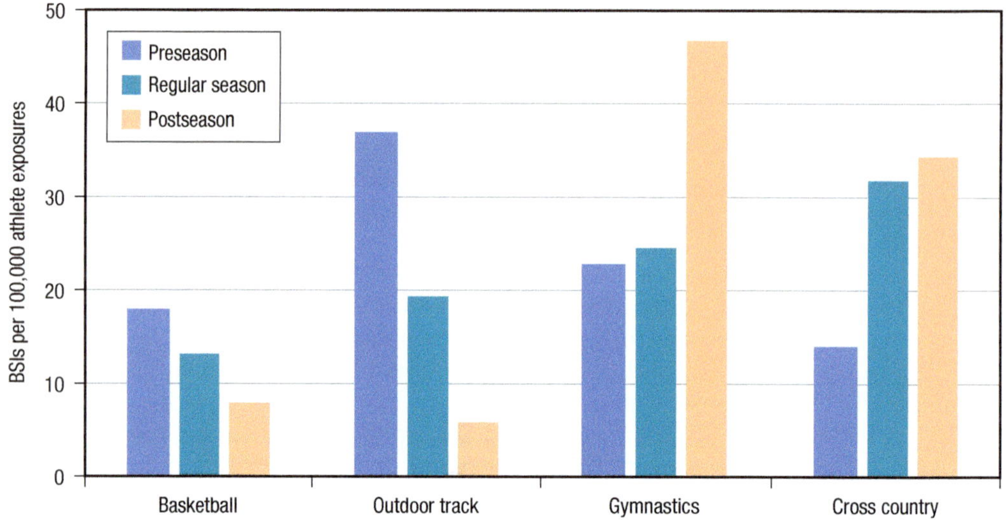

FIGURE 1.4 **BSI risk varies across the competitive season. In seasonal sports (e.g. basketball and outdoor track), BSI risk is greatest during preseason and early regular season where loading ramps up following the off-season. In contrast, in more year round sports (e.g. gymnastics and cross country), BSI risk progressively increases as the competitive season progresses. Data from Rizzone et al.[9]**

BSI, bone stress injuries.

important to consider the activity that the individual participates in and the location of symptoms in relation to the common BSI sites for the activity (Figure 1.2). Whether the individual has a history of a previous BSI is easy and important to ask as a past history of a BSI is one of the strongest risk factors for a BSI, increasing risk over fivefold.[20]

Many BSIs result from a "training error," whereby greater load is introduced than can be tolerated. However, attention should be paid to documenting the individual's recent (acute) and usual (chronic) activity workload. Particular attention should be paid to changes in activity in the past 4 to 6 weeks as there is usually a delay between a change in workload and the development of BSI symptoms. Changes in workload may have been in the form of a large change in a single training feature, such as training duration, frequency, intensity, or type. Or the change may be in the form of small but simultaneous changes in multiple training features.

It is important to consider the stage of the competitive season as most BSI injuries occur in the preseason or early in the season, particularly in seasonal physical activities, where there is frequently a large change in loading from the off-season to preseason and from preseason to the rigors of the competitive season (Figure 1.4). For example, the risk of a BSI was 43% greater during preseason than the competitive season across a range of collegiate-level sports,[9] and half of BSIs occurred in the first 6 weeks of the season in professional basketball players.[21] In year-round sports, such as gymnastics and cross-country, where training is more constant, BSI risk is actually lower during the preseason when compared to the competitive season (cross country) and postseason/ championship period (gymnastics).[9]

Questions should be asked in relation to the potential presence of other BSI risk factors, including the female athlete triad and relative energy deficiency in sport (RED-S; see Chapter 3). In the presence of 2 to 3 risk factors for RED-S (e.g., menstrual dysfunction, elevated dietary restraint, participation in a leanness sport/activity), female athletes who perform purposeful physical activity for >12 hours per week have a more than threefold increased risk of a BSI independent of bone health.[22] The risk balloons out to a 14.6-fold increase when 3 to 4 risk factors are combined with compromised bone health.[22] Thus, questioning on the potential presence of the female athlete triad and RED-S risk factors is required, particularly with regard to prevention of future BSIs. The questioning should not be limited to females as males are not immune to the BSI consequences of RED-S.[23,24]

EVALUATION

On physical evaluation, the most important diagnostic feature is localized bony tenderness.[3] BSI tenderness can be palpated at subcutaneous bones with minimal overlying soft tissue, such as the fibula, tibia, metatarsals, and tarsal bones. In these locations, an inflammatory periosteal reaction may include associated features of warmth, redness, and/or swelling. Advanced BSIs may include periosteal thickening and palpable callus formation. When these features are present along with a pain history consistent with a BSI, imaging may not be performed and a clinical diagnosis of a BSI made. However, imaging confirmation can be useful in grading the pathology and indicating prognosis as BSI grade can influence length of recovery (see Chapter 2).[4,5] Also, imaging is indicated when a BSI is potentially located in a high-risk location, such as the femoral neck or pelvis (see Chapter 7), anterior cortex of the tibia (see Chapter 6), or navicular (see Chapter 10).

BSIs at some sites have specific areas of tenderness. For instance, clinical suspicion of a navicular BSI is raised when tenderness is elicited over the so-called N-spot (Figure 1.5).[25,26] Although the diagnostic accuracy of N-spot palpation has not been formally explored, it appears to be specific whereby a positive test (increased focal tenderness compared to the contralateral side) is generally found in those with a BSI. However, it should be remembered that navicular BSIs can occur bilaterally, reducing the ability to use the contralateral side as a comparative site; the site remains tender in some even well after management and return to activity,[27] and some individuals participating in kicking sports can have tenderness in this region. However, the kicking usually produces more diffuse symptoms across the dorsum of the foot as opposed to very localized tenderness at the N-spot.

Direct palpation is obviously not possible at deeper sites (such as the femoral neck and shaft and the pars interarticularis region of the spine), with symptoms at these sites producing less localized pain and more complex symptomology. For example, femoral neck BSIs can present heterogeneously, with symptoms being felt in the hip, groin, gluteal, thigh, and/or knee regions.[28,29] Similarly, BSIs at the femoral shaft may present as a vague ache or tightness in the anterior thigh.

Beyond the history of the individual's pattern of pain in relation to loading and its trajectory and the presence of risk factors for generation of a BSI (e.g., rapid change in workload, participation in a high-risk activity, etc.), clinical diagnosis of a BSI at a deeper skeletal site may be facilitated by specific bone-loading tests.

One of the first specific bone loading tests was the one-legged "hop test" reported by Matheson and colleagues.[30] Initially simply described as having an individual hop on one leg in an attempt to reproduce BSI symptoms, variations of the test include having the individual land with a straighter leg to increase shock propagation proximally through the lower extremity long bones and hopping in multiple directions to increase shear forces and load the bone in different directions. Other specific bone-loading tests include the fulcrum test for diagnosing BSIs at the femoral shaft,[31] one-legged hyperextension test for a pars defect within the spine,[32] and the calcaneal squeeze test for differentiating calcaneal bone pain from local soft tissue pathologies (Figure 1.6).[33,34]

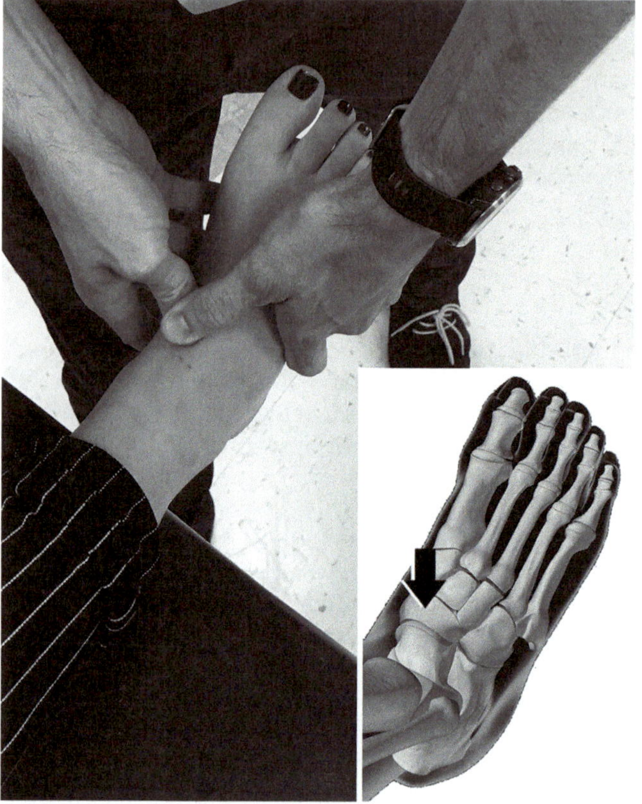

FIGURE 1.5. Palpation of the "N-spot" for aiding in the diagnosis of a navicular BSI. The N-spot is located lateral to the tibialis anterior tendon and medial to the extensor hallicus longus tendon over the proximal dorsal portion of the navicular close to its articulation with the talus.

BSI, bone stress injuries.

Specific bone-loading tests are widely used clinically; however, their sensitivity and specificity in diagnosing BSIs either are not completely known or have been questioned. The fulcrum test for femoral shaft BSIs has been reported as being very sensitive, as it has been found to be positive in 38 out of 40 (95%) cases.[31,35–37] However, the ability of the test to elicit symptoms in early femoral shaft BSIs has not been confirmed, with one report describing a case where the fulcrum test only became positive once loading continued and symptoms (and the underlying pathology) had progressed.[37] It is more likely the test is specific whereby it is only positive in those who have a femoral shaft BSI. In comparison, the one-legged hyperextension test for a pars defect was reported to be neither sensitive nor specific when compared to bone scintigraphy with single photon emission computed tomography (SPECT) in individuals with low back pain.[38] False negative and false positive findings were observed in approximately half of tested individuals, which casts doubt on the utility of the one-legged hyperextension test in the differential diagnosis of a pars defect.

Other techniques reported in the clinical diagnosis of BSIs have included the application of a vibrating tuning fork or therapeutic ultrasound, but their use has not been fully supported.[39] Tuning fork tests (looking for pain induction and/or reduced sound conduction) have relatively good sensitivity (≥75%) but are heterogenous and of generally

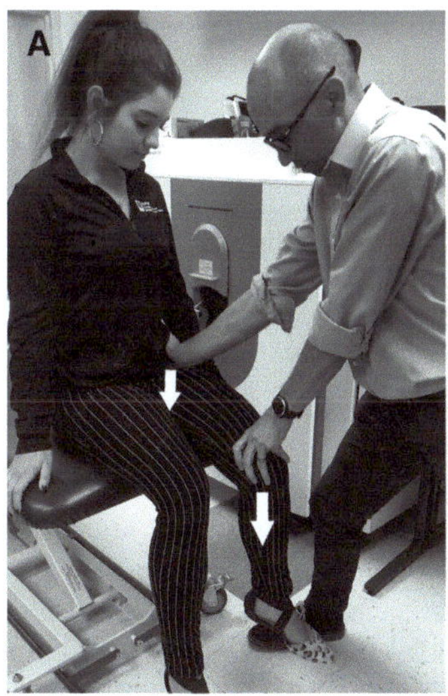

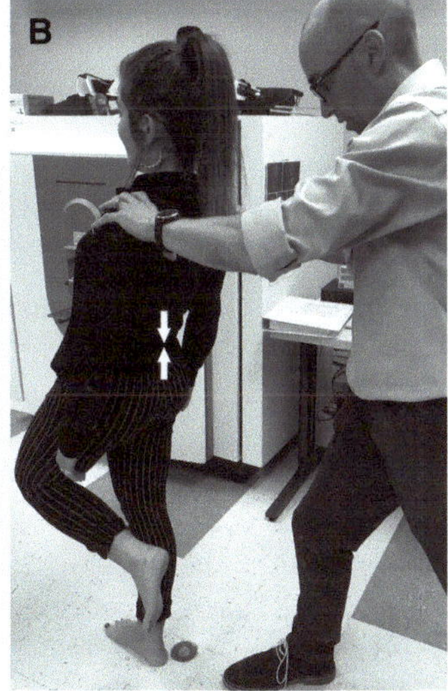

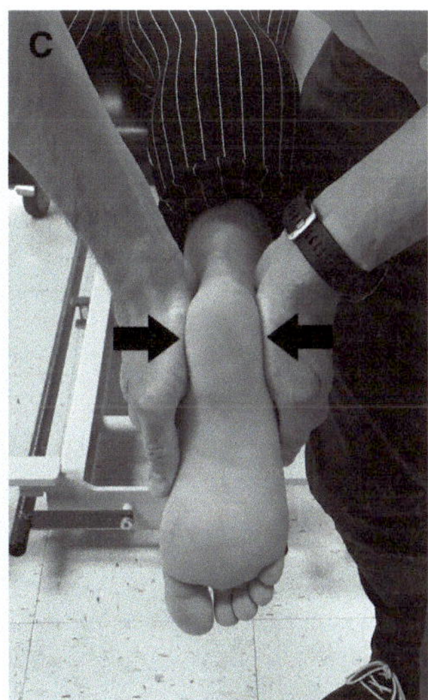

FIGURE 1.6. Bone-loading tests to aid diagnosis of BSIs at specific sites. (A) Fulcrum test to elicit symptoms of a femoral shaft BSI. The patient is positioned with the edge of the plinth positioned underneath the thigh at the level of their symptoms. The examiner stabilizes the pelvis with one hand and applies downward pressure over the distal femur to bow the femur (i.e. tension the anterior cortex of the diaphysis). (B) One-legged hyperextension test to reproduce symptoms of a low back BSI. The patient stands facing away from the examiner, lifts the leg on the side opposite their symptoms, and extends their lumbar spine to increase compressive forces through the symptomatic side of the low back. To increase compression, side bend and/or rotation toward the stance leg can be added. (C) Squeeze test for reproduction of calcaneal BSI symptoms. The patient is placed in prone. The examiner cups and compresses the sides of the calcaneus between the heels of their hands.

BSIs, bone stress injuries.

low specificity.[40] The implication is that tuning fork tests are positive in the majority of individuals, and only a negative test has some diagnostic potential in ruling out the presence of a BSI. In terms of pain induction using therapeutic ultrasound, sensitivity and specificity values from seven pooled studies were both in the range of 63% to 64%, indicating relatively poor discriminative ability.[39]

In addition to differential diagnosis of an individual's symptoms, clinical evaluation should be used to explore potential contributing risk factors from the standpoint of developing an intervention plan to reduce risk of reoccurrence. Biological and biomechanical risk factors are presented in detail in Chapters 3 and 4, respectively.

CONCLUSION

BSIs remain a frustrating problem, particularly for athletes and military personnel. They invariably require some period of training and/or competition interruption as the risk for progression to complete bone fracture is real. The earlier a BSI is identified, the quicker the individual may be able to return to activity. This chapter revealed the clinical features of BSIs with the goal of identifying BSIs at their earliest stages. Cardinal signs of a BSI include the presence of localized bone tenderness that is aggravated by loading and that does not warm up as participation continues. When these signs are coupled with a history of BSI development, imaging should be considered to confirm the diagnosis, grade the injury, and guide management.

KEY REFERENCES

Only key references appear in the print edition. The full reference list appears in the digital product found on http://connect.springerpub.com/content/book/978-0-8261-4424-9/part/sec01/chapter/ch01

3. Warden SJ, Davis IS, Fredericson M. Management and prevention of bone stress injuries in long-distance runners. *J Orthop Sports Phys Ther*. 2014;44:749–765.

9. Rizzone KH, Ackerman KE, Roos KG, et al. The epidemiology of stress fractures in collegiate student-athletes, 2004-2005 through 2013-2014 academic years. *J Athl Train*. 2017;52:966–975.

20. Wright AA, Taylor JB, Ford KR, et al. Risk factors associated with lower extremity stress fractures in runners: a systematic review with meta-analysis. *Br J Sports Med*. 2015;49:1517–1523.

22. Barrack MT, Gibbs JC, De Souza MJ, et al. Higher incidence of bone stress injuries with increasing female athlete triad-related risk factors: a prospective multisite study of exercising girls and women. *Am J Sports Med*. 2014;42:949–958.

39. Schneiders AG, Sullivan SJ, Hendrick PA, et al. The ability of clinical tests to diagnose stress fractures: a systematic review and meta-analysis. *J Orthop Sports Phys Ther*. 2012;42:760–771.

CHAPTER 2

Diagnostic Imaging

Katherine Fahy, Aurelia Nattiv, and Michael Fredericson

INTRODUCTION

Bone stress injuries (BSIs) happen in the setting of repetitive force on bone and occur on a continuum with stress fractures as part of that spectrum of injury. Stress fractures were first described in 1855 before the invention of radiographs.[1] The first radiograph of a BSI occurred in 1897, just 2 years after the invention of radiographs, when fractures of the metatarsal shaft were named "march fractures" as they were common in military personnel. Radiographs served as the primary imaging tool for over a century, with the addition of bone scintigraphy in the 1970s to aid with the low sensitivity of radiographs.[2] Since the 1980s, MRI has become the gold standard for imaging BSIs with an emerging role for ultrasound as a possible point-of-care method of assessing for BSI.[3]

RADIOGRAPHS

Radiographs have served as the imaging modality for stress fractures for over 100 years. Within 2 to 8 weeks of the start of a patient's symptoms, evidence of a BSI may be seen on radiographs.[4] However, initial radiographs are commonly normal, which is expected due to the remodeling happening on a microscopic basis in the early stages of a BSI.[5] Imaging early on can have a sensitivity as low as 10%, with an increase to 30% to 70% at later intervals.[2,6] Many athletes may decrease their activity at the start of symptoms, which would allow the injury to heal before visualization on radiographs and contribute to the low sensitivity.[2] Yet another limitation of radiographs for evaluating BSIs is the inadequate ability to assess the extent of bone involvement and any damage to surrounding soft tissue.[7] As radiographs are not adept at detecting early signs of stress reaction, further imaging should be pursued if there is a high clinical suspicion based on the patient's history and physical exam.

The initial finding in cortical bone on a radiograph is "the gray cortex" or a cortical area of hypodensity.[8] This subtle change is often overlooked until there is new periosteal bone formation or thickening of the endosteal bone to strengthen the area of weakened cortex.[5] If the BSI progresses, then a fracture line will appear. The earliest finding in cancellous bone is subtle blurring of the trabecular margins with possible sclerosis due to peritrabecular callus formation. In cancellous bone, this would progress to a

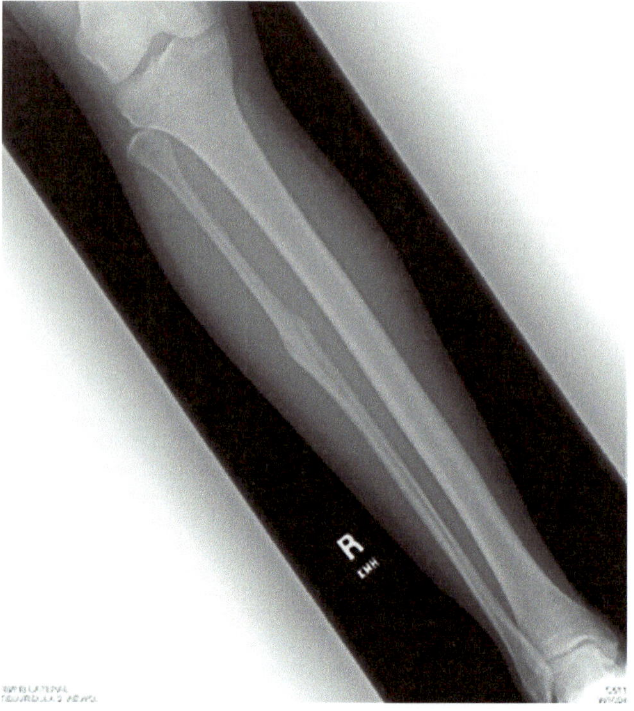

FIGURE 2.1 Radiograph showing healing fibular stress fracture.

sclerotic band as the injury worsens.[2] A 50% difference in bone opacity at the site of injury is needed to detect the difference on radiographs,[1] which partly accounts for the low sensitivity (Figure 2.1).

BONE SCINTIGRAPHY

While bone scintigraphy has primarily been used for malignancy, there is a role for the modality in sports medicine. The technetium phosphate uptake is related to blood flow and osteoblast activity, meaning it highlights areas of bone repair due to bone tumors, metastases, fractures, and infections. With regard to BSIs, scintigraphy is able to pick up injuries in 20% to 40% of symptomatic patients with normal radiographs. The radiation dose is 3 to 5 mSv compared to 0.1 mSv in a radiograph, so one bone scan is equivalent to 2 years of background radiation.[9]

In areas where a BSI has occurred, there will be a fusiform area of uptake. Bone scans can detect BSIs as early as 2 to 8 days after the start of symptoms.[7] One advantage of bone scintigraphy is that it can be performed in a three-phase manner: The perfusion phase refers to sequential images taken over the first 30 seconds, the blood pool phase is obtained at 1 minute, and the uptake phase is captured at 2 to 6 hours. These phases are helpful in evaluating chronicity and severity of the injury and the extent of soft tissue inflammation. If acute BSIs have uptake in all three phases, then the increased perfusion seen in the first phase will resolve followed by resolution of the blood pool seen in the second phase. The last finding to resolve is the focal uptake seen in the delayed third phase of the scintigraph (Figure 2.2).[4]

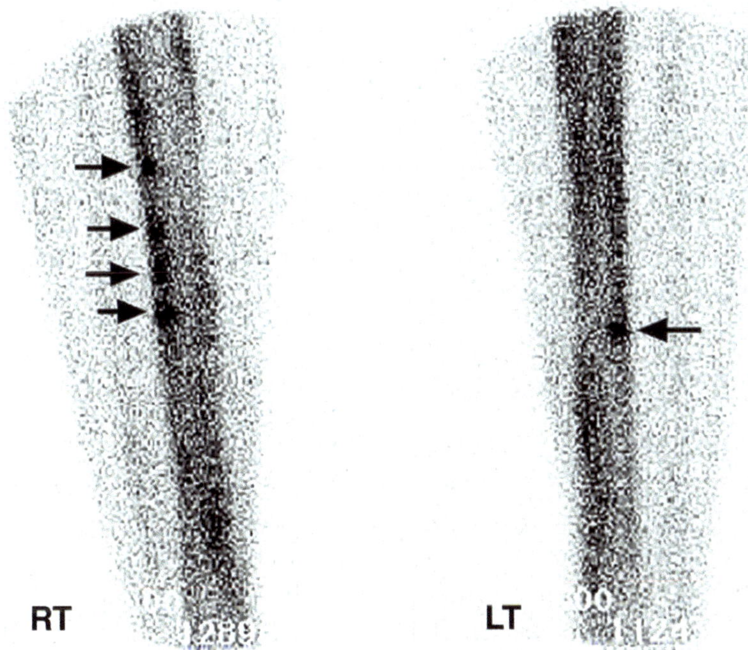

FIGURE 2.2 Bone scan showing multiple bilateral anterior tibial diaphyseal bone stress injury.

Classifications for BSIs were suggested by Roub et al.[7] and then by Greaney,[1] Chisin et al.,[10] and Matin,[11] where more uptake was noted in cortical breaks. Zwas et al. recommended a four-stage model that correlates the increased intake at cortical breaks with recovery time.[12] These models of classifying the degree of injury are helpful clinically in determining the duration of rest needed for recovery. However, MRI has been recommended above bone scan as it more accurately determines the degree of injury and aids in the treatment and return to activity planning.[13] Bone scintigraphy has been shown to be particularly useful in fractures of the scaphoid bone and other carpal bones.[9] However, bone scans as an independent diagnostic tool are limited by low specificity and inability to visualize the actual fracture line.[6]

MRI

MRI remains the gold standard in the imaging of BSIs. Gaeta et al. found the sensitivity of MRI to be 88% with a specificity of 100% in detecting BSIs.[14] Even early in the disease process, this combination of sensitivity and specificity makes MRI the single best imaging modality for BSIs.[13–16]

The first indication of a BSI on MRI is periosteal edema followed by bone marrow edema and then progression to a fracture line.[17] However, periosteal edema is not a necessary criterion for a grade 1 or any MRI-graded BSI though periosteal edema or bone marrow edema needs to be present.[18] Gaeta et al.[14] and Bergman et al.[19] have also shown that bone marrow edema can be present in patients with no symptoms and may also be an asymptomatic stress response. Fredericson et al. graded tibial stress fractures from 0 to 4, with 0 being a normal MRI. Grade 1 injuries involve mild to moderate periosteal edema on T2-weighted images, while grade 2 injuries show moderate to severe periosteal edema and increased signal in the bone marrow or endosteal surface on T2-weighted images. The progression continues to grade 3 injuries, which entail moderate to severe periosteal edema and bone marrow edema on T1- and T2-weighted images. Grade 4, the most severe, shows the same findings as grade 3 though with the addition of a clearly visible fracture line.[13] Fredericson et al. based their grading system of images of the tibia[13] though Arendt and Griffiths[20] and later Nattiv et al.[8] adapted the system to encompass all BSIs. A summary of the grading systems can be seen in Table 2.1 from Nattiv et al.'s study.[18]

BSIs can also be classified as high or low risk on the basis of their location. Locations that are less vascular and/or with more tensile forces are at higher risk of poor healing and require aggressive therapy. These locations include the tension side of the femoral neck, the anterior cortex of the tibia, the medial malleolus, the patella, the tarsal navicular, the fifth metatarsal, the base of the second metatarsal, and the sesamoids of the great toe.[21,22] Other higher risk fractures include insufficiency fractures in the pelvis due to osteoporosis, subchondral insufficiency fractures in the hip or knee, and atypical subtrochanteric femoral fractures due to bisphosphonate therapy.[23]

When imaging patients for BSIs, it is important to understand the difference between cortical and cancellous bones. Cortical bone is the outer layer of bone, while the cancellous or trabecular bone is the spongy inner layer of bone. A cortical stress fracture entails a break in the outer surface of the bone, which commonly occurs in long bones such as the

TABLE 2.1

MRI GRADING SCALES FOR BONE STRESS INJURIES[a]

MRI GRADE	FREDERICSON ET AL.[13]	ARENDT ET AL.[20]	NATTIV ET AL.[18]
1	Mild to moderate periosteal edema on T2; normal marrow on T2 and T1	Positive signal change on STIR	Mild marrow or periosteal edema on T2[b]; T1 normal[c]
2	Moderate to severe periosteal edema on T2; marrow edema on T2 but not T1	Positive STIR plus positive T2	Moderate marrow or periosteal edema plus positive T2; T1 normal
3	Moderate to severe periosteal edema on T2; marrow edema on T2 and T1	Positive STIR plus positive T2 and T1	Severe marrow or periosteal edema on T2 and T1
4	Moderate to severe periosteal edema on T2; marrow edema on T2 and T1; fracture line present	Positive fracture line on T2 or T1	Severe marrow or periosteal edema on T2 and T1 plus fracture line on T2 or T1

[a]Adapted from Table 1 of Fredericson et al.[13] and Table 3 of Arendt et al.[20]

[b]Note that periosteal edema is not a necessary criterion for grade 1 or any MRI grade bone stress injury.

[c]Radiograph results are often negative at all grades; they may be normal, or a periosteal reaction may be evident.

STIR, short T1 inversion recovery.

Source: Reproduced with permission from Nattiv A, Kennedy G, Barrack M, et al. Correlation of MRI grading of bone stress injuries with clinical risk factors and return to play. *Am J Sports Med.* 2013;41(8):1930–1941.

tibia. A trabecular or cancellous stress fracture occurs when stress creates microfractures in the cancellous bone, which leads to sclerosis seen on imaging.[5] Areas commonly affected include the calcaneus, pelvis, and femoral neck.[24] MRI is the best single modality for evaluating BSIs in cancellous bone (examples in Figure 2.3 and Figure 2.4). While cancellous bone stress fractures can be visualized as a full cortical break, they can also be seen as increased T2-weighted signal in the bone marrow. MRI is able to evaluate for

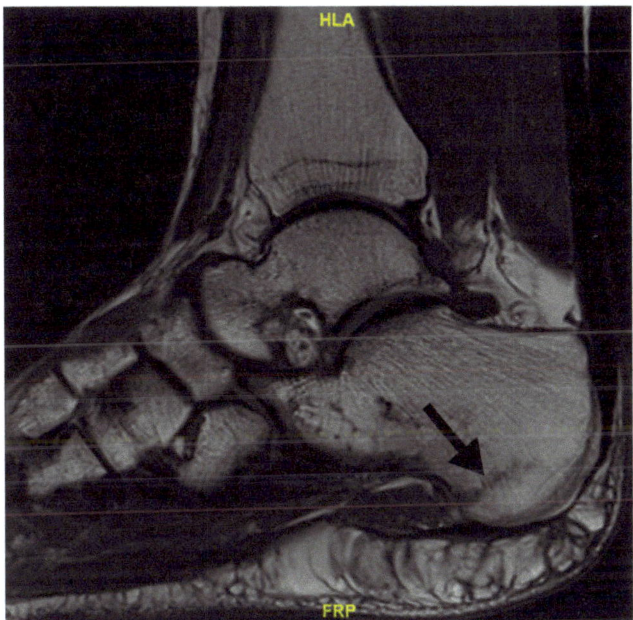

FIGURE 2.3 T1-weighted MRI showing a grade 4 calcaneal bone stress injury.

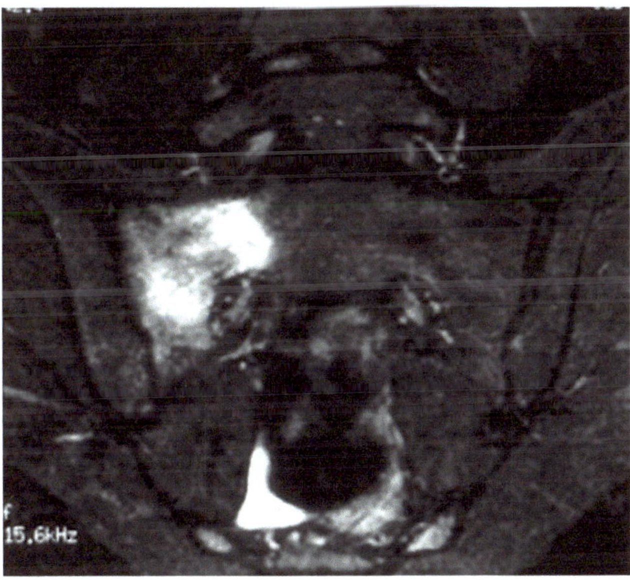

FIGURE 2.4 T2-weighted MRI showing a grade 4 sacral stress injury.

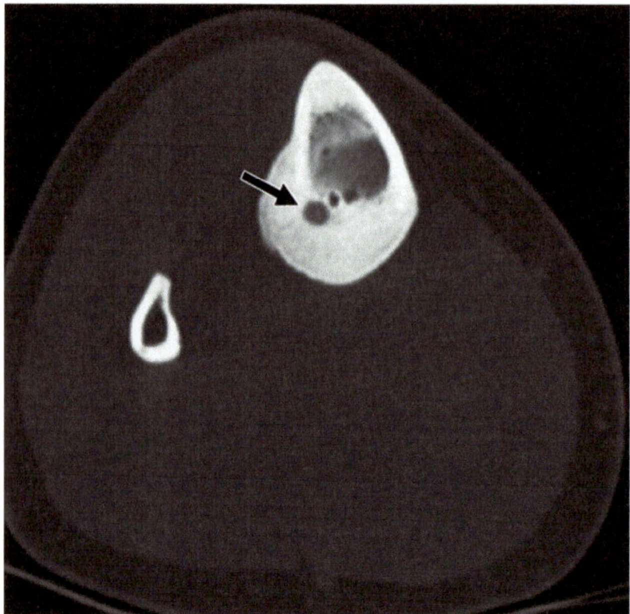

FIGURE 2.5 CT scan showing osteoid osteoma.

cancellous BSIs, while CT, ultrasound, and radiographs are not able to identify those alterations in the bone marrow.[14]

The grade of injury seen on MRI mostly relates to clinical severity when compared to radiography, scintigraphy, and CT.[15] While Deutsch et al. found no association with healing time for radiograph, bone scan, or CT, there was an association between MRI imaging severity and healing time.[15] The presence of an abnormal cortical signal intensity or a discrete fracture line correlates with longer return to activity.[16] Previous research had showed no significant correlation between MRI grade and return to activity[25,26] until a large prospective study by Nattiv et al. found that higher-graded injuries based on the Fredericson model were correlated with longer recovery times.[18] Ramey et al. later had similar findings that grades 2 to 4 on the Arendt grading system had longer return-to-play times than grade 1 injuries.[27]

CT

CT has limited utility in the early evaluation of BSIs,[28] with a sensitivity of 44% and specificity of 100%, though it does prove superior for detecting cortical injury.[14] While it can be helpful in imaging bone once a fracture line is present, this does not occur until late in the process of BSIs.[13] CT is helpful to evaluate for osteopenia, resorption cavities, or striation that precede the development of the cortical fracture.[29] The modality can also be used when there is an equivocal finding on another form of imaging such as MRI, scintigraphy, or radiography yet BSI is suspected (such as in the tarsal navicular, longitudinal tibia, or pars interarticularis) or in distinguishing between BSIs and osteoid osteomas (Figure 2.5).[30] However, the ability to detect BSIs on CT is statistically inferior to both MRI and bone scintigraphy.[14] CT scan has not been clinically adopted due to the low sensitivity, lack of utility early in the disease process, and exposure to ionizing radiation.

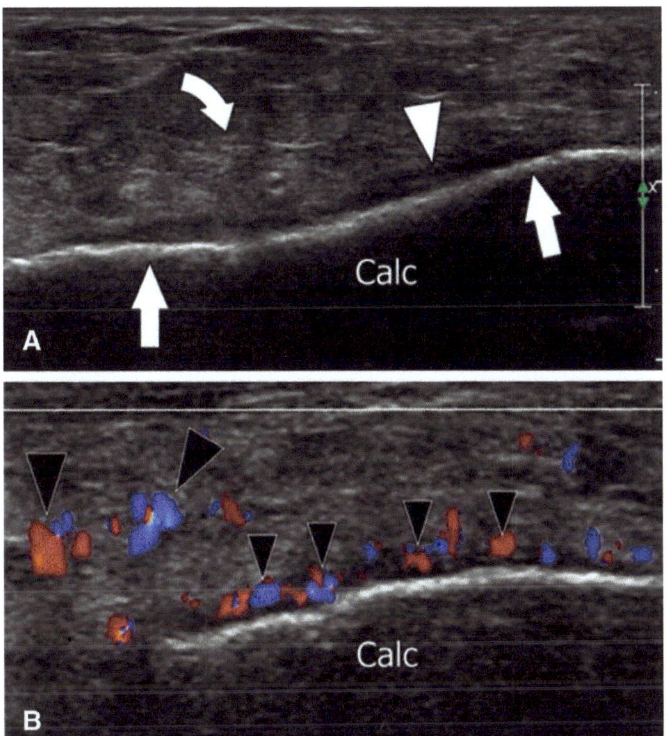

FIGURE 2.6 Grayscale and color Doppler coronal sonograms obtained over the calcaneal medial face.

Source: Reproduced with permission from Bianchi S, Luong D. Stress fractures of the calcaneus diagnosed by sonography: report of 8 cases. *J Ultrasound Med.* 2017;37(2):521–529.

ULTRASOUND

Although there has been recent interest in the use of ultrasound for evaluating BSIs, therapeutic ultrasound was actually used in the early 1980s to detect BSIs before evidence was seen on radiographs.[29] The method is noninvasive, safe, and cost effective. Papalada et al. found that, compared to MRI, the sensitivity and specificity of ultrasound for BSIs was 91.9% and 66.6%, respectively. This study did not compare sensitivity and specificity between different injury sites though it included injuries in the fibula, tibia, navicular, cuboid, talus, calcaneus, metatarsals, and sesamoid bones of the great toe.[29] Previous studies had shown the sensitivity of ultrasound to range from 32% to 49%.[30–33] These studies included fractures of the scaphoid,[31] tibia,[30,32,33] fibula,[33] and distal femur.[3] While there is currently not enough evidence for ultrasound to grade BSIs on a 1-to-4 system, findings of periosteal thickening, callus formation, cortical irregularities, subcutaneous edema, or hypervascularity can help gauge the presence and potentially the severity of injury (Figure 2.6).[34] However, based on current knowledge, if ultrasound shows an injury, then MRI may still need to be done to further evaluate the extent of the BSI. Ultrasound is also not a good option for proximal or deeper injuries to bone such as the pelvis, spine, femoral neck, and posterior tibia.[3] This suggests that ultrasound may be used as a first-line approach to patients with possible BSIs to aid in early diagnosis, though further evaluation with MRI is currently recommended.

CONCLUSION

BSIs account for up to 20% of visits in a sports medicine practice.[6] Early detection of BSIs leads to quicker return to activity,[35] making appropriate choice of imaging clinically significant. While there may be a role for ultrasound as an imaging tool for earlier detection of BSIs, more research and specific ultrasound training for providers are needed.[3] Radiographs are less sensitive at detecting early stages of BSIs, although they are a reasonable imaging modality to start, with possible detection of findings 2 to 8 weeks after symptom onset.[2,4,6] CT has utility in assessing cortical injuries, although it has poor detection of early findings in BSIs.[13,14,30] Bone scintigraphy has a role in sports medicine and in the detection of BSIs as it can show areas of bone repair. However, the modality's shortcomings include difficulty assessing the degree of bone involvement, no information regarding surrounding soft tissue injury, and a dose of radiation equal to 2 years of background radiation.[9] MRI remains the single best tool for imaging of BSIs.[3,13–16,36] Grading systems exist that correlate with clinical symptoms[13,20] and with return to activity.[16,18,27] MRI is able to evaluate the extent of bone involvement along with surrounding soft tissue damage and is more equipped to assess cancellous bone injuries when compared to CT, bone scintigraphy, or ultrasound.[14] While initial imaging with a radiograph, bone scan, or ultrasound can be considered, MRI should be used in cases where more information about the injury is needed, such as grading, and for guiding management and return to play.

KEY REFERENCES

Only key references appear in the print edition. The full reference list appears in the digital product found on http://connect.springerpub.com/content/book/978-0-8261-4424-9/part/sec01/chapter/ch02

3. Fukushima Y, Ray J, Kraus E, et al. A review and proposed rationale for the use of ultrasonography as a diagnostic modality in the identification of bone stress injuries. *J Ultrasound Med.* 2018;37(10):2297–2307.

5. Anderson M, Greenspan A. Stress fractures. *Radiology.* 1996;199(1):1–12.

7. Roub L, Gumerman L, Hanley E, et al. Bone stress: A radionuclide imaging perspective. *Radiology.* 1979;132(2):431–438.

13. Fredericson M, Bergman A, Hoffman K, et al. Tibial stress reaction in runners. *Am J Sports Med.* 1995;23(4):472–481.

14. Gaeta M, Minutoli F, Scribano E, et al. CT and MR imaging findings in athletes with early tibial stress injuries: comparison with bone scintigraphy findings and emphasis on cortical abnormalities. *Radiology.* 2005;235(2):553–561.

18. Nattiv A, Kennedy G, Barrack M, et al. Correlation of MRI grading of bone stress injuries with clinical risk factors and return to play. *Am J Sports Med.* 2013;41(8):1930–1941.

19. Bergman A, Fredericson M, Ho C, et al. Asymptomatic tibial stress reactions: MRI detection and clinical follow-up in distance runners. *Am J Roentgenol.* 2004;183(3):635–638.

CHAPTER 3

Biological Risk Factors

Haylee Borgstrom and Adam S. Tenforde

INTRODUCTION

Bone is a dynamic tissue with an intricate homeostasis affected by many metabolic and biochemical factors. Alterations in any of these biologic pathways can disrupt bone remodeling patterns through an uncoupling of osteoblast and osteoclast activity,[1] ultimately resulting in impaired bone health. While risk factors for bone stress injury (BSI) are often multifactorial, recognizing biological risk factors for impaired bone health can aid in prevention and management of injury (Table 3.1).

The most widely described biological risk factor for impaired bone health and BSI is low energy availability (EA). While the first formal report was published in 1993,[2] the female athlete triad is currently defined as a spectrum of health to disease.[3,4] At the extreme, low EA with or without disordered eating contributes to menstrual dysfunction, and both may contribute to low bone mineral density (BMD).[3,4] The International Olympic Committee (IOC) introduced the terminology of relative energy deficiency in sport (RED-S) in 2014.[5] RED-S expands on the triad to describe the influence of low EA on potential adverse health and performance consequences in both male and female athletes, including BSI. Furthermore, the 2018 IOC update on RED-S stresses the recognition of low EA in athletes with disabilities[6]—a population in which triad/RED-S risk factors are quite prevalent, with BSIs described in nearly 10% of elite adaptive competitors.[7–9] Both the triad and RED-S serve as important clinical constructs to conceptualize the effect of biological risk factors on development of BSIs. Other contributing factors, including dietary requirements and biomechanics, are presented in other chapters.

LOW ENERGY AVAILABILITY

EA is defined as the difference between energy intake and exercise energy expenditure standardized to fat free mass per day (kcal/kg FFM/day).[10] This value represents the energy remaining for metabolic and hormonal processes outside of the demands of exercise. For active girls and women, 45 kcal/kg FFM/day or above is typically defined as adequate EA, while low EA is commonly defined as below 30 kcal/kg FFM/day. These values are based on studies that reflect alterations in reproductive and metabolic hormones, including those that regulate bone turnover.[11] Thresholds for adequate EA in

TABLE 3.1

BIOLOGICAL RISK FACTORS FOR BONE STRESS INJURY

Low EA
   Peripubertal occurrence
   Long duration

Neurohormonal axis dysregulation
   Hypopituitarism
   Hypogonadotropic hypogonadism
   Functional hypothalamic amenorrhea

Low body mass index
Low BMD
History of prior bone stress injury   Trabecular-rich site
Micronutrient deficiency

BMD, bone mineral density; EA, energy availability.

male and adaptive sport athletes have not yet been well defined, and the importance of establishing these values is increasingly recognized and emphasized in the sports medicine community.[6,7,12,13]

Low EA results in alterations of the neurohormonal pathways, which may contribute to impaired bone quality and risk for BSI. A dose-dependent uncoupling of biochemical markers of bone formation and resorption has been described in active women with EA of 10, 20, and 30 kcal/kg FFM/day compared to seen in those with adequate EA of 45 kcal/kg FFM/day.[11] The specific mechanisms by which bone metabolism is affected by low EA are wide ranging and likely differ for male and female athletes. Leptin, an anorexigenic hormone, appears to be suppressed in the low EA states for both men and women[14,15]; however, the effect of other dietary regulatory hormones is variable and counterintuitive in some cases.[13] Low EA states beyond a threshold of 30 kcal/kg FFM/day have been shown to decrease plasma glucose and insulin levels, as well as insulin growth factor (IGF)-I levels, in both male and female athletes.[14,15] Triiodothyronine (T3) levels have been demonstrated to be lower in female athletes with low EA[14,16,17]; while this also appears to be the case for male athletes,[16] this has not yet been well established. Because exercise itself is a stress-inducing activity, cortisol levels are variable regardless of EA state. Functional hypothalamic amenorrhea occurs in female athletes with severe energy restriction, resulting in alterations in luteinizing hormone (LH) pulsatility and reduced estradiol levels[14] with subsequent negative impact on bone health. The effect of low EA on testosterone levels is not consistent in female athletes but is suspected to generally result in reduced testosterone levels in male athletes.[16,18]

Taken in combination, low EA results in significant yet variable alterations in the hypothalamus–pituitary–adrenal and hypothalamus–pituitary–gonadal (HPG) axes, which in turn affect bone health and metabolism. The relationships between EA and insulin, T3, and IGF-I most closely resemble the dose-dependent changes in bone metabolism in female athletes,[11] potentially suggesting these hormones as markers for women who may be at risk for impaired bone health. Metabolic markers of low EA in male and adaptive athletes are less well defined. Among adaptive athletes already at increased risk for low BMD due to altered mobility and reduced weight bearing, the prevalence of triad risk factors is quite high,[9] likely further predisposing this group of athletes to BSI. However, triad risk factors, as well as type and duration of disability, have not been associated with BSI in adaptive sport athletes,[8] underscoring the importance of establishing metabolic markers of low EA in this population.

Additionally, the timing and duration of a low EA state are important factors to consider related to impaired bone health. Previously discussed alterations in metabolic substrate and neurohormonal axes occur with both short- and long-term exposure to low EA, resulting in reduced bone mass and density and increased risk for BSI.[19,20] A "window of vulnerability" for bone injury has been described given the differential speeds at which bone resorption occurs compared to bone formation: 7 to 10 days versus up to 3 months, respectively.[21] Furthermore, the occurrence of low EA state during peripubertal stages with longer duration of menstrual irregularity appears to have the greatest negative effect on development of peak BMD.[21,22]

Independent of—yet often occurring in parallel with—low EA state, specific micronutrient deficiencies can further increase metabolic risk for BSI, particularly vitamin D deficiency and its adverse effect on calcium metabolism. These factors are discussed in detail in other chapters.

SEX-SPECIFIC RISK FACTORS IN FEMALE ATHLETES

Historically, the effect of reproductive hormone dysregulation on impaired bone health was focused on the female athlete due to observed menstrual dysfunction in female athletes. At the extreme, neurohormonal axis disruptions may result in functional hypothalamic amenorrhea.[23] It is important to note that even in normally menstruating women, exposure to only short duration low EA state can cause abnormalities in LH pulsatility and hypoestrogenic state.[14]

The Female Athlete Triad Cumulative Risk Assessment is a clinical tool that categorizes athletes into low, moderate, and high risk for development of BSI based on low EA status/history of disordered eating or eating disorder, body mass index (BMI), age at menarche, history of oligo- or amenorrhea, low BMD, and history of prior BSI. When applied to a cohort of female collegiate athletes, those in the moderate- and high-risk groups were found to have relative risks for BSI of 3.4 and 10.4 when compared to low-risk athletes, respectively.[24] This clinical tool provides a method for risk stratification based on several factors reflective of metabolic state.

SEX-SPECIFIC RISK FACTORS IN MALE ATHLETES

It is now well recognized that, similar to female athletes, disruptions to the HPG axis cause deleterious effects on bone metabolism in male athletes. Low EA in male athletes may result in hypogonadotropic hypogonadism with suppressed sex hormones, including testosterone and estradiol, contributing to low BMD and increased risk for BSI.[18] The mechanisms for effects of low EA on sex hormone alterations and resulting impaired skeletal health in male athletes are less well understood than in female athletes. One report identified low estradiol as a more important contributor to impaired bone health than low androgens in male athletes as bioavailable estradiol levels were found to more closely correlate with BMD.[25]

Similar to female athletes, a modified version of the Female Athlete Triad Cumulative Risk Assessment was able to identify risk for BSI in male athletes. When applied to a population of collegiate male runners, excluding the menstrual variables, triad risk factors were found to be associated with BSI. Each risk factor point for low EA, BMI, BMD, and prior history of BSI was associated with a 27% increased risk for development of BSI.[26]

TABLE 3.2

TRABECULAR-RICH SITES OF BONE STRESS INJURY

Sacrum

Pelvis
   Pubic ramus
   Ischium
   Ilium

Femoral neck
Calcaneus

RISK BASED ON BONE MORPHOLOGY

When discussing metabolic risk factors for BSI, it is important to consider the site and composition of bone involvement. Trabecular bone has greater surface area and turnover and is thought to be more sensitive to changes in sex hormones compared to cortical bone; thus, more trabecular-rich sites appear to be at increased risk for BSI related to metabolic derangement rather than primarily mechanical factors (Table 3.2).[24,27,28] Changes in trabecular bone morphology from plate like to rod like with associated decreased connectivity are characteristic of postmenopausal osteoporosis.[29] Similarly, when comparing trabecular skeletal microarchitecture in amenorrheic versus eumenorrheic athletes via high-resolution computed tomography, athletes with menstrual dysfunction have been shown to have reduced plate-like trabecular bone volume fraction and connectivity compared to eumenorrheic athletes.[30] These changes are more pronounced in non–weight-bearing locations,[20] suggesting a partially protective effect of exercise itself regardless of menstrual status. Additionally, decreased energy to failure has been demonstrated in rod-like as compared to plate-like trabecular bone,[31] indicating increased susceptibility to microdamage potentially leading to stress injury. Reflective of this concept, amenorrheic athletes with a history of recurrent stress fractures have been found to have more abnormal trabecular bone morphology than amenorrheic athletes without recurrent BSIs.[30] Male athletes with BSI in the pelvis, sacrum, femoral neck, and calcaneus—all sites with increased trabecular composition—have been reported to have 4.6 times the risk for low BMD compared to those with cortical-rich sites of BSI.[27] Furthermore, BSI at trabecular-rich sites and low BMD, which often occur concurrently, have been found to be independent predictors of prolonged time to healing and return to sport.[32]

CONCLUSION

Adequate EA is essential for healthy bone metabolism in all athletes, and low EA serves as a key biological risk factor for BSI. In able-bodied athletes, triad risk factors of low EA, BMI, BMD, and a history of BSI are all observed cumulative risk factors in both sexes. Delayed menarche and secondary oligomenorrhea/amenorrhea are discernible risk factors specific to female athletes, while measures of hypogonadism in male athletes have not been clearly defined. Limited research has been performed to understand biological risk factors in adaptive sport athletes; available evidence suggests that this population is at high risk for low BMD but does not demonstrate traditional markers of low EA as risk factors for BSI. The involvement of trabecular-rich sites of BSI may

identify athletes with greater propensity for biological risk factors for injury. Risk stratification using clinical tools such as the Female Athlete Triad Cumulative Risk Assessment should be considered in all athletes, and development of screening tools more
specific for male and adaptive athletes is necessary. Further understanding related to
neurohormonal effects of low EA, as well as continued education regarding the importance of adequate EA, is necessary to improve prevention and treatment of BSIs in all
athletes.

KEY REFERENCES

Only key references appear in the print edition. The full reference list appears in the digital
product found on http://connect.springerpub.com/content/book/978-0-8261-4424-9/part/sec01/
chapter/ch03

6. Mountjoy M, Sundgot-Borgen J, Burke L, et al. International Olympic Committee (IOC) Con-
    sensus Statement on relative energy deficiency in sport (RED-S): 2018 Update. *Int J Sport Nutr
    Exerc Metab*. 2018 Jul 1;28(4):316–331. PubMed PMID: 29771168.

7. Blauwet CA, Borgstrom HE, Tenforde AS. Bone health in adaptive sports athletes. *Sports Med
    Arthrosc Rev*. 2019 Jun;27(2):60–66. PubMed PMID: 31046010.

13. Elliott-Sale KJ, Tenforde AS, Parziale AL, et al. Endocrine effects of relative energy deficiency
    in sport. *Int J Sport Nutr Exerc Metab*. 2018 Jul 1;28(4):335–349. PubMed PMID: 30008240.

23. Gordon CM, Ackerman KE, Berga SL, et al. Functional hypothalamic amenorrhea: an endo-
    crine society clinical practice guideline. *J Clin Endocrinol Metab*. 2017 May 1;102(5):1413–1439.
    PubMed PMID: 28368518.

24. Tenforde AS, Carlson JL, Chang A, et al. Association of the female athlete triad risk assess-
    ment stratification to the development of bone stress injuries in collegiate athletes. *Am J Sports
    Med*. 2017 Feb;45(2):302–310. PubMed PMID: 28038316.

26. Kraus E, Tenforde AS, Nattiv A, et al. Bone stress injuries in male distance runners: higher
    modified female athlete triad cumulative risk assessment scores predict increased rates of
    injury. *Br J Sports Med*. 2019 Feb;53(4):237–242. PubMed PMID: 30580252.

27. Tenforde AS, Parziale AL, Popp KL, et al. Low bone mineral density in male athletes is asso-
    ciated with bone stress injuries at anatomic sites with greater trabecular composition. *Am J
    Sports Med*. 2018 Jan;46(1):30–36. PubMed PMID: 28985103.

CHAPTER 4

Biomechanical Risk Factors

Richard W. Willy

INTRODUCTION

While the etiology of BSIs is complex and multifactorial, BSIs are thought to be a result of a loss of homeostasis between the rate of bone remodeling and the rate of bone microdamage due to repetitive, submaximal mechanical loading.[1,3,4] For the athlete, the etiology of a stress fracture can be more simply understood as the failure of skeletal remodeling to keep pace with the progression or volume of repetitive loading activities.[5]

This chapter aims to explore the biomechanical risk factors associated with BSIs in athletes by discussing the general influences of bone loading associated with BSI. Clinical measures to evaluate the biomechanics associated with BSI are explored. Since lower limb BSIs are more common, this chapter is largely dedicated to the biomechanics associated with lower extremity BSI.

BIOMECHANICS OF BONE LOADING

A basic understanding of bone loading is helpful to understand movement patterns that increase the risk of BSIs. Mechanical loading results in bone strain, that is, change in resting length, resulting in bone microdamage and signaling targeted bone remodeling.[3,6] In the case of the submaximal loads associated with BSIss, bone strain is relatively small but is applied in a highly repetitive manner such as during foot strike while running.[6]

Microdamage resulting from bone strain is dependent on a combination of cumulative bone loading cycles (i.e., number of foot strikes), strain magnitude (i.e., peak bone loads), and strain rate (i.e., rate of bone loading).[3] Activities that increase peak bone loads and/or the rate of bone loading will effectively reduce the number of bone loading cycles necessary to accumulate bone microdamage.[7] For instance, introducing fast downhill running to a run training program will theoretically reduce the number of bone loading cycles a runner can tolerate prior to bone fatigue. Even small increases in peak bone load result in an exponential decrease in the number of bone loading cycles to failure.[8] Conversely, a 10% reduction in peak bone load results in a 100% increase in the number of bone loading cycles to failure.[8,9] A rapid increase in the number of bone loading cycles, while keeping peak bone strain and strain rate static, typical of intense training periods, also increases the risk of bone stress fracture.[3,7,10]

Bone microdamage accumulates if rest is insufficient[7] or the athlete's physiology[11] is unable to adequately support bone remodeling. In the presence of continued loading, highly localized loss of bone mass and bone strength occurs due to the time lag between bone resorption in response to loading and subsequent bone formation.[6,7,12] This accumulation of microdamage results in a temporary decrease in localized load tolerance.[3] If load application continues unabated to this site of microdamage, the continuum resulting in BSI is initiated.[1,3,13]

Recognizing the lag between load application and new bone formation may assist the athlete, coach, and clinician in the prevention and rehabilitation of BSI. A cyclic training program that reduces training loads every 2 to 3 weeks would theoretically support bone adaptation and decrease the risk of BSI.[14] Indeed, BSIs tend to occur in the first 2 to 6 weeks as training loads are increased,[15–17] with the theoretical risk of BSI leveling off after the first 40 days of a new training program.[18] Rehabilitation programs for athletes recovering from a BSI should incorporate slow progressions in volume of loading cycles. For example, steps or jump landings during the initial weeks and provision for a temporary reduction in loading cycles periodically, every third week, may support bone adaptation.[19]

Bone loads are the net result of external forces (i.e., ground reaction forces) combined with internal forces (i.e., muscle forces).[20,21] Not surprisingly, the majority of BSIs occur in the lower extremities due to the important influence of ground reaction forces during endurance running or other repetitive landing activities, such as jumping.[2,3] Still, non–weight-bearing bones, such as ribs, are not immune to BSIs due to the large influence muscle forces have on internal bone loads.[2,20,22] In fact, the contributions of internal muscle forces to bone loads exceed the contributions of ground reaction forces during running and jumping. For instance, peak tibial bone loads (6–14 body weights) during running are the combination of ground reaction forces and the muscle forces that counter the ground reaction forces, namely, the soleus.[20,21,23,24] (Figure 4.1). Peak soleus muscle forces during running often exceed 6 to 7 body weights in force,[25,26] whereas peak vertical ground reaction forces are generally 2.5 to 3 times body weight.[27] As such, clinicians should consider both external ground reaction forces and the internal muscular influences acting on the bone when managing the athlete recovering from a BSI.

During functional activities, different types of forces act on bone. In vitro, bone is strongest under axial compression and weakest under tension and shear forces,[28,29] but these forces rarely occur in isolation in vivo (Figure 4.2). Instead, complex combinations of compression, tension, bending, torsion, and shear forces are experienced in vivo.[5] Bending forces, in particular, are often implicated in BSIs.[20,23] When a bone experiences a bending force, the convex side of the bone experiences tensile forces, whereas the concave side experiences compression forces.[5] Compared with other regions of the tibia, the posterior tibia experiences the greatest absolute bone stress during running and these stresses are predominately compressive due to soleus muscle forces.[20,26] In contrast, the anterior tibia experiences the greatest tensile stresses during running, with relatively lower amounts of compressive stresses.

At the extreme of BSI, a stress fracture may occur and the location contributes to its classification, with high-risk stress fractures and low-risk stress fractures occurring on the tensile and compression sides of the bending axis of the bone, respectively.[3,30] Staying with the example of the tibia during running, posterior tibial stress fractures are more common,[30–32] likely due to the high absolute bone stress in this region during running and jumping.[20,26] Yet a posterior tibial stress fracture is considered a low-risk stress fracture due to the low tensile stresses experienced in this region of the bone.[33] Conversely, the less common anterior tibial cortex stress fracture will experience relatively high tensile loads,[20] resulting in its classification as a high-risk stress fracture[30,33] Rehabilitation strategies for the athlete recovering from an anterior tibial cortex stress fracture

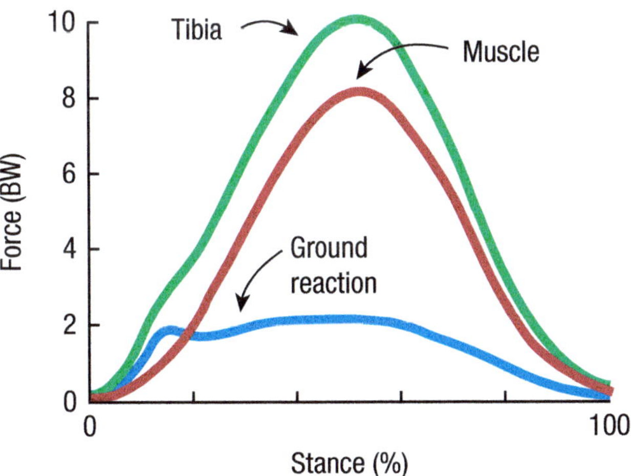

FIGURE 4.1 Tibia bone compressive forces during running are the net result of external forces (ground reaction forces) and internal forces (muscle). This figure demonstrates the importance of considering muscle forces in the study of bone loads.

Source: Reproduced with permission from Matijevich ES, Branscombe LM, Scott LR, Zelik KE. Ground reaction force metrics are not strongly correlated with tibial bone load when running across speeds and slopes: Implications for science, sport and wearable tech. *PLoS One.* 2019;14(1):e0210000.

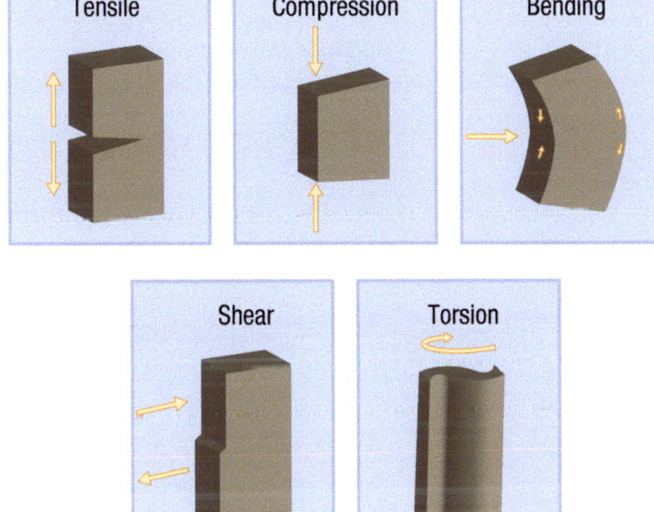

FIGURE 4.2 Various biomechanical loads experienced by bone. Bending loads are most commonly associated with bone stress injuries.

Source: Reproduced with permission from Mandell JC, Khurana B, Smith SE. Stress fractures of the foot and ankle, Part 1: Biomechanics of bone and principles of imaging and treatment. *Skeletal Radiol.* 2017;46(8):1021–1029.

are complex due to the challenge in managing tensile bone loads.[1,3,33] In summary, consideration of applied bone loads during an athlete's sporting activity of choice is crucial to understanding the risk factors for certain stress fractures and their rehabilitation.

THE ROLE OF BONE STRUCTURE IN THE RISK OF BONE STRESS INJURY

Bone structure has important influences on the risk of experiencing a BSI. Male and female runners who go on to experience a BSI or who have had a previous BSI tend to have compromised bone properties, including thinner bone cortices, and smaller bone structure and lower bone mineral density.[32,34–43] Consistent with these data, military cadets with a higher cross-sectional moment of inertia along the anterior–posterior axis of the tibia were reported to be at lower risk of sustaining a tibial stress fracture during basic training.[32] Changes in bone cortex diameter and bone size affect bending and torsional strengths to the fourth power, indicating that even small differences in cortex diameter have an exponential effect on resistance to bending and torsional bone loads[12] Narrow intermalleolar width, which can be easily measured with a caliper, is predictive of the occurrence of tibial stress injuries in soldiers[44] and in athletes,[42] suggesting that intermalleolar width may be an effective clinical surrogate for lower leg bone size. Overall, these data speak to the importance of assessing bone structure when determining the risk of BSIs in athletes.

Combining bone structure and movement pattern data provides important insights into the understanding of BSIs. For instance, if two runners experience identical training loads, the runner with lower bone strength will have a greater likelihood of developing a BSI. Popp et al.[45] found that competitive female runners with a previous history of stress fracture of any lower limb site had 11% to 17% lower tibial bone strength relative to their peak vertical ground reaction force during running compared with that of healthy uninjured runners. Intriguingly, these data indicated that runners with a history of *any* lower limb stress fracture do not have the same tibial bone strength relative to running load compared to runners without a history of stress fracture.[45]

Specific bony alignments may also increase the risk of BSI. While varus alignment (genu, tibial, subtalar, and forefoot varus) was observed by Matheson et al.[46] in athletes with lower leg stress fractures, only forefoot varus has been established as a risk factor for BSI. Specifically, forefoot varus is predictive of metatarsal stress fractures in the military[47] and has been observed in soccer players with a past history of fifth metatarsal stress fracture[48,49] and in athletes with recurrent stress fractures.[50] Leg length discrepancies may also contribute to the risk of BSI.[50,51]

MUSCULAR RISK FACTORS FOR BONE STRESS INJURY

Considering that muscle and the underlying bone are closely linked by anatomy and applied mechanical loads to generate human movements,[12,52–54] it is not surprising that muscle parameters are related to metrics of bone strength. Tibial bone strength closely relates to lower limb muscle size[36] and muscle performance.[37,52] The close relationship between muscle size and metrics of bone strength is also present in the upper limb in elite youth tennis players.[55]

Reduced muscle strength[56] and reduced muscle size[37,51,57] are risk factors for lower limb BSI. Smaller calf girth, associated with small muscle cross-sectional area, is a risk factor for stress fractures.[51] Bennell et al.[51] found that a 1-cm decrease in calf girth resulted in a fourfold increase in risk of BSI in female track and field athletes. Besides relating to the underlying bone strength, muscle plays an important role in diffusing bone compressive forces across the bone cortex during functional activities, such as jump landings.[12,22,58] Thus, enhanced muscle performance will reduce localized bone stresses. In contrast, short-term impairments in muscle function have a detrimental effect on bone loads. Specifically, muscle fatigue results in increased in vivo bone strain during walking[59] and elevated tibial shock,[60–62] vertical loading rates,[63] and tibial stress[23] during running. As such, excessive exposure to fatiguing workouts may elevate the risk of BSI.

Taken together, several recommendations specific to muscle and bone strength can be made. First, assessing the clinical metrics of muscle may provide an indication of the strength of the underlying bone. Simply measuring calf girth, particularly at 66% of lower leg length,[36] is a convenient clinical metric that may assist with identifying athletes at risk for BSI, particularly in female athletes. Second, improving muscle strength and endurance may be an important strategy to optimize underlying bone strength and bone loads during activities. For instance, young male runners who strength train at least once per week have higher bone mineral density than those who only run.[64] Athletes who regularly participate in resistance training have been shown to exhibit greater bone mineral content,[65] with just 12 weeks of heavy resistance training resulting in increased bone mineral density in young adult females.[66] In female Marine recruits, participation in less than 7 months of resistance training was associated with a fourfold greater risk of experiencing a stress fracture during basic training compared with female recruits who regularly performed resistance training.[67] The need to provide resistance training for the plantarflexors may depend on running mechanics and if loads are carried. Compared with a rearfoot strike pattern, a forefoot strike pattern exerts even greater plantarflexor forces during running.[68,69] Thus, runners who exhibit a non-rearfoot strike pattern may benefit the most from plantarflexor strengthening to enhance the conditioning of the plantarflexors and the underlying bone. Similarly, heavy loads carried by military cadets result in disproportionately large increases in plantarflexor demands.[70] Overall, these data suggest that optimal muscular strength via consistent resistance training is a likely important protective factor against the development of BSI. Despite these promising findings, it is not known if the addition of resistance training to a runner's overall training program lowers the risk of BSI.

MOVEMENT PATTERNS RELATING TO SPECIFIC RISK FOR BONE

The overwhelming majority of research on the biomechanics associated with BSI has been done in endurance runners due to (a) their propensity for BSI and (b) the repetitive nature of running, which lends itself to reproducible laboratory studies. Since the tibia is the most common site for BSI in running,[71] much of the literature focuses on this injury. The remainder of this chapter explores the specific movement patterns that are associated with BSI. When possible, the literature is reviewed relating to other athletic populations who are at high risk for certain BSI, such as gymnasts and soccer players.

The Etiology of Lower Limb Bone Stress Injury in Runners: The Role of Ground Reaction Forces

Ground reaction forces, readily measured in gait laboratories, represent the external load applied to an athlete's body. Compared with healthy runners, runners with a history of tibial BSI exhibit high rates of impact, that is loading rate of the vertical ground

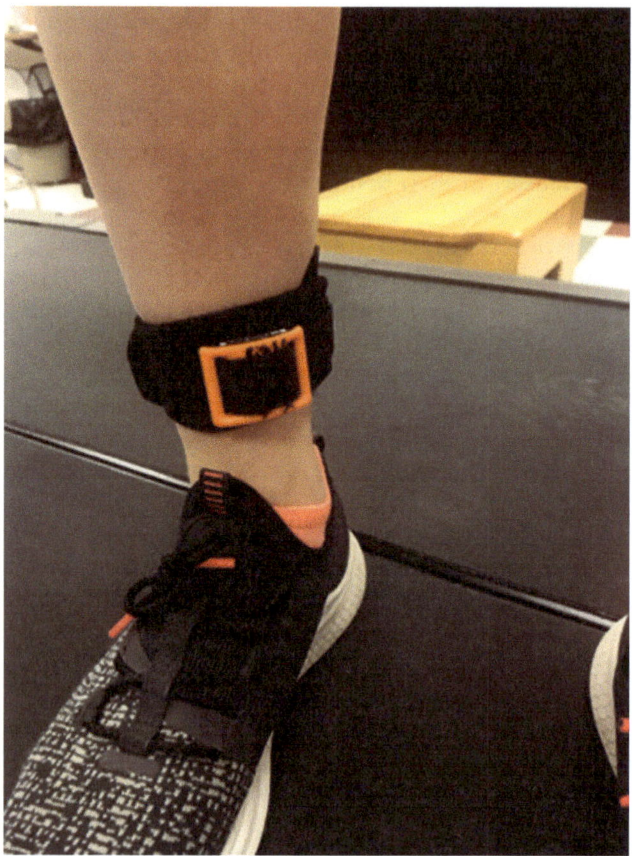

FIGURE 4.3 An accelerometer-equipped inertial measurement unit used to measure tibial shock during running.

reaction force.[72–75] Runners who exhibit a rearfoot strike pattern tend to exhibit a higher loading rate than non-rearfoot strikers.[76] Accelerometers, when mounted on the distal anterior tibia (Figure 4.3), measure tibial shock. Tibial shock is an attractive metric because it evaluates the shock wave propagating up the lower leg during the impact phase of running or landing from a jump. Tibial shock can also easily be measured during routine training sessions with commercially available wearable devices.[77] Tibial shock is higher in runners with a past history of tibial stress fracture.[75] Tibial shock increases while running downhill,[78] suggesting that downhill running should be carefully dosed in at-risk runners.

Quantification of loading rate requires a force plate, which is not likely feasible in most clinical settings. However, recent advances in wearable devices, such as accelerometers, now enable instrumented gait analysis to be completed in most clinical settings or outdoors in a runner's normal training environment.[77] Wearable accelerometers are portable and capable of data logging for extended periods of time.[77] Tibial shock is also highly correlated with the loading rate of the vertical ground reaction force during running[79–81] and is also higher in runners with a past history of tibial stress fracture.[75] Accelerometers are inexpensive and require only minimal software and technical expertise to use in the clinic. Furthermore, providing real-time feedback to lower tibial shock with an accelerometer also results in lower vertical loading rates,[82,83] suggesting that it is an effective means to reduce risk of tibial stress fracture in runners with high baseline impact loads. A low-tech assessment of impact forces requires merely listening to the sound intensity of a runner's footfalls[84] and can be easily quantified using a decibel meter application on a mobile phone.[85]

Nonvertical ground reaction forces during running are also associated with tibial BSI. Male runners with a history of tibial BSI run with a more medially directed ground reaction force, resulting in an increase in the medial bending (varus) moment acting on the tibia.[86] Milner et al. found that a greater twisting torque between the foot and the ground, known as the free moment, is observed in runners with a past history of tibial stress fracture compared with healthy runners. A higher free moment would result in greater torsional loads acting on the lower limb.[87] The free moment during running increases with fatigue,[62] suggesting that runners recovering from tibial stress fractures should avoid fatiguing runs. High amounts of rearfoot pronation also increase the free moment.[88]

Both the medially directed ground reaction force and the free moment require a force plate to measure, making it difficult to directly measure these risk factors clinically. However, assessing step width during running can provide insight into both medial loads and the free moment. A narrow step width increases varus loads acting on the knee and lower leg[89] and the free moment,[90] whereas running with a wide step width effectively reduces them. A narrow step width also results in greater hip adduction and rearfoot pronation of the stance limb.[91] A high level of hip adduction during running likely imparts a medial bending torque on the tibia, and excessive hip adduction has been noted in female runners with a history of tibial stress fracture.[74] Not surprisingly, running with a narrow step width increases tibial stress, whereas running with a wider step effectively reduces tibial stress.[92] Step width during running is easily assessed during a standard clinical gait evaluation with a high-speed camera (Figure 4.4). Running with a long step length, that is, overstriding, results in a narrow step width.[93] Step length can easily be reduced by cueing an increase in running cadence.[94,95]

Recent advances in musculoskeletal modeling suggest that the relationship between ground reaction forces and lower leg bone forces may not be as clear as once thought. As mentioned previously in this chapter, peak tibial bone force during running (6–14 body weights) is primarily influenced by peak vertical ground reaction forces (2.5–3.0 body weights of force) and peak soleus muscle forces (6–7 body weights in force).[25,26] Thus, considering only the vertical ground reaction force provides an incomplete picture of tibial bone forces during running. Compared with level running, uphill running is characterized by lower loading rate and peak vertical ground reaction forces and lower tibial shock,[78] which may lead one to incorrectly conclude that tibial bone forces will be lower during uphill running. However, plantarflexor muscle forces increase during uphill running,[21,78] resulting in potentially higher tibial bone forces than in level running. Unfortunately, precise estimation of tibial bone forces requires advanced musculoskeletal modeling techniques, which are not accessible to most clinicians. Determining better clinical estimates of internal bone loads during running is an area of study that is currently experiencing rapid development, particularly with recent advances in wearable technologies and machine learning.[9] Until better estimates are available, clinicians should be mindful of the influences of plantarflexor muscle forces when designing rehabilitation programs for runners recovering from lower leg BSI.

The Etiology of Lower Limb Bone Stress Injury: The Role of Plantar Loads

In contrast to more proximal anatomical regions, the foot is unique in that external loads are applied directly to the plantar surface. Thus, careful consideration of how the foot is interacting with the ground is critical to assessing risk and rehabilitation of BSI of the foot. Metatarsal BSI are common in runners, basketball players, soccer players, dancers,

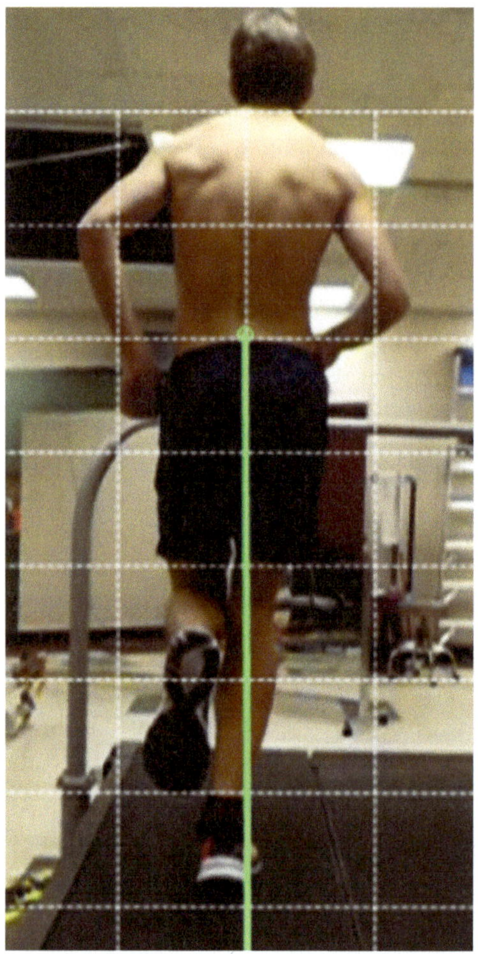

FIGURE 4.4 A runner with a past history of a right tibial stress injury exhibiting a narrow step width pattern, operationally defined as the ankle joint center passing midline to the 5th lumbar vertebra. This running mechanic increases the free moment (torsional loads) acting on the lower leg.

and the military.[33,96] The 2nd and 3rd metatarsals represent 52% and 35% of metatarsal stress fractures, respectively.[33,97] During the pushoff phase of running, plantar force is greatest under the 2nd and 3rd metatarsal heads, imparting a bending moment along the diaphysis.[98,99] A Morton's foot structure (long 2nd metatarsal) offloads the 1st metatarsal and shifts more force under the 2nd metatarsal head, resulting in an even greater bending moment on the 2nd metatarsal.[96] Royal Marine recruits with a history of 3rd metatarsal stress fracture exhibited a lateral shift in the resultant horizontal force, resulting in increased loading of the 3rd metatarsal head.[100] Elite male soccer players with a history of 5th metatarsal stress fracture exhibited greater peak plantar force on the lateral forefoot compared with heathy matched controls when performing soccer-specific movements.[101] Soccer players with a past history of navicular stress fracture exhibited a more medially directed center of pressure under the foot.[102] Similarly, runners with a past history of a navicular stress fracture exhibit greater rearfoot eversion and reduced forefoot abduction during the stance phase, which together would increase medial foot pressures. Together, these data suggest that deviations in the center of pressure acting on the plantar surface of the foot result in greater bone loads in distinct regions of the foot.

The Effect of Temporospatial Influences on Risk for Bone Stress Injury

Temporospatial metrics, for example, run speed and stride length, may play an important role in the risk for lower limb BSI. For instance, runners[103,104] and basketball players[105] experience greater tibial shock as run speed increases. In a probabilistic model, decreasing running speed from 4.5 m/sec to 3.5 m/sec reduced the likelihood of experiencing a tibial BSI by 7%, with a further 10% reduction in risk when running speed was decreased to 2.5 m/sec.[18] These data suggest that close management of the volume of higher velocity running in a training program may reduce the risk of BSIs.

Stride length or cadence, that is, step frequency, during running may also affect the risk of certain BSI. Adopting a 5% to 15% longer stride length (while maintaining the same running speed), contributing to lower running cadence, results in an increased probability of sustaining a tibial stress fracture[10] and an increase in loading rates.[106] Prospectively, high school cross-country runners who fell in the lowest quartile of cadence, that is, longer step length, were more than five times more likely (odds ratio = 5.85; 95% CI, 1.1–32.1) to experience shin pain than runners in the top quartile for cadence.[107] In contrast, a 7.5% to 15% reduction in stride length, that is, an increase in running cadence, resulted in reduced vertical loading rates[69,95] and reduced the probability of experiencing a tibial stress fracture.[10] However, reduced stride length does not reduce metatarsal strains,[99] suggesting that altered stride lengths have differential effects on bone load. Clinicians are cautioned, however, not to assume that a runner's naturally low cadence is associated with higher vertical loading rates. In fact, habitual running cadence does not appear to be associated with vertical loading rates during running.[108,109] Thus, adopting a higher cadence may be an effective means to reduce risk of tibial stress fracture but equating a lower habitual cadence with higher vertical loading rates appears to be problematic. With respect to walking, female military recruits were identified to be at elevated risk of pelvic BSI, which is thought to relate to the longer stride necessitated to maintain step with taller male cadets.[110] Overall, stride length appears to be an important factor in BSI in runners and military populations.

The Influence of Shoes and Landing Surfaces on Risk for Bone Stress Injury

Running shoe type has not yet been shown to reduce overall injury rates,[111] but specific running shoe types may play an important role in the prevention and risk of certain stress fractures. Minimalist shoes are proposed as a means to reduce vertical loading rates during running.[112] However, the introduction of a minimalist running shoe results in an immediate increase in vertical loading rates in runners[113–115] and elevated loading rates continue for at least the short term, for example, 3 to 6 weeks, with the continued use of the minimalist shoe.[116,117] Still, a minimalist shoe may more easily facilitate a transition to a forefoot strike compared with a traditional shoe; a forefoot strike results in reduced loading rates.[3,118,119] Thus, it appears that a minimalist shoe does not appear to lower vertical loading rates in the absence of instructed transition to a forefoot strike. More cushioning is not necessarily better, however, as maximalist shoes also result in immediate increases in vertical loading rates during running[120,121]; the same effect is noted in basketball shoes.[105] Interestingly, running in a shoe with the greatest perceived comfort (not necessarily the most cushioned shoe) resulted in the lowest tibial shock,[122] and basketball shoes with moderate levels of cushioning also demonstrated the lowest levels of tibial shock.[105] These data suggest that an optimal level of shoe cushioning may be runner specific. Regardless of the aforementioned studies, epidemiological evidence is currently lacking implicating specific running shoes in the etiology of tibial BSI.

Due to the direct interaction between the foot and the ground, shoe choice appears to have a stronger effect on risk of BSIs affecting the foot. Running in a minimalist shoe increases localized plantar pressures, affecting the 2nd to 5th metatarsal regions.[117,123] Compared with standard shoes, minimalist shoes also increase metatarsal strain during running due to an increase in bending moments,[99] and runners have been observed to exhibit bone marrow edema in the metatarsals after a 10-week transition to minimalist shoes although some runners were without associated symptoms.[124] Compared to less cushioned or minimalist shoes, softer-soled basketball shoes distribute plantar pressures more evenly during basketball maneuvers[125] and maximalist shoes reduce forefoot plantar pressures.[126] Soccer players are at high risk for lateral metatarsal BSI due to excessive cleat pressure in this region of the foot.[127] Running, kicking, and cutting in soccer shoes result in elevated plantar pressures to the lateral forefoot.[101,128,129] Localized plantar pressures from soccer cleats can be lessened with the addition of a specialized insole.[130]

The Role of Biomechanics in Bone Stress Injury in Gymnasts

Much of the gymnastics literature relating biomechanics to BSI focuses on the high ground reaction forces (6.8–13.2 body weights[131]) during landings and the high volume of training associated with this sport.[132–134] Unfortunately, no studies to date have followed gymnasts to determine if high ground reaction forces are related to BSI in this population. Compared to nongymnasts, gymnasts land from an elevated height with 25% greater peak vertical ground reaction forces,[133] indicating a stiffer landing. The stiffer landing was postulated to be the result of a training and competition emphasis on sticking landings by minimizing knee flexion.[133] Interestingly, gymnasts who use a landing strategy of increased lower limb flexion exhibit reduced vertical ground reaction forces.[134] While encouraging a softer landing may seem intuitive to reduce bone loads, a softer landing necessitates higher muscle forces and would apply more force to the underlying bone, potentially increasing the risk of BSI.[132]

Gymnasts experience lumbar spine BSI at a greater rate than do other athletes. Of likely clinical importance, 30% of gymnasts in a laboratory study experienced their peak vertical ground reaction forces while in end-range lumbar extension during various gymnastic landing maneuvers.[131] However, it is unknown if this movement pattern results in greater risk for spinal stress fractures. Clearly, additional research is needed to determine biomechanical risk factors for BSI in gymnasts.

In fact, chronic exposure to high impact forces over a prolonged period may impart an osteogenic, that is, bone building, response in gymnasts, provided sufficient recovery time is provided. Despite similar prevalence of amenorrhea and oligomenorrhea, female gymnasts exhibit greater bone mass than female runners,[135] suggesting an adaptive response to habitual high-impact loading. Prospective data suggest that adolescent female gymnasts gain bone mineral content and density in the femoral neck, lumbar spine, and distal radius at a faster rate than do matched controls who were active in ball sports.[136] Former collegiate gymnasts continue to demonstrate greater bone mineral density into the fourth decade of life, despite ceasing gymnastics participation at the conclusion of their college athletic careers.[137] Still, gymnasts are at high risk for BSI, suggesting that the aforementioned adaptive response of bone in these athletes is not entirely sufficient to eliminate their risk of BSI.

CONCLUSION

Based on the literature, several key points can be made relating biomechanical risk factors for BSI. Among these, optimizing bone mass and muscle strength appears to be critical components in reducing the risk of BSI in athletes. Specific biomechanics appear to increase the risk of BSI, including elevated localized plantar pressures and high vertical loading rates for foot and tibial BSI, respectively. Careful progression of fast running, jumping, and running distance likely reduces the risk of BSI. Finally, the use of minimalist footwear is a risk factor for metatarsal BSI, whereas a direct link between footwear and more proximal BSIs is currently unknown. The majority of the biomechanical literature on risk factors for BSI are related to runners, which is a limitation of this chapter. Overall, there is a large need for more investigations into prospective biomechanical risk factors for other athletic populations, such as gymnasts and rowers.

KEY REFERENCES

Only key references appear in the print edition. The full reference list appears in the digital product found on http://connect.springerpub.com/content/book/978-0-8261-4424-9/part/sec01/chapter/ch04

3. Warden SJ, Davis IS, Fredericson M. Management and prevention of bone stress injuries in long-distance runners. *J Orthop Sports Phys Ther*. 2014;44(10):749–765.

5. Mandell JC, Khurana B, Smith SE. Stress fractures of the foot and ankle, part 1: biomechanics of bone and principles of imaging and treatment. *Skeletal Radiol*. 2017;46(8):1021–1029.

9. Edwards WB. Modeling overuse injuries in sport as a mechanical fatigue phenomenon. *Exercise Sport Sci Rev*. 2018;46(4):224–231.

12. Hart NH, Nimphius S, Rantalainen T, et al. Mechanical basis of bone strength: influence of bone material, bone structure and muscle action. *J Musculoskelet Neuronal Interact*. 2017;17(3):114.

21. Matijevich ES, Branscombe LM, Scott LR, et al. Ground reaction force metrics are not strongly correlated with tibial bone load when running across speeds and slopes: implications for science, sport and wearable tech. *PloS One*. 2019;14(1):e0210000.

33. Mandell JC, Khurana B, Smith SE. Stress fractures of the foot and ankle, part 2: site-specific etiology, imaging, and treatment, and differential diagnosis. *Skelet Radiol*. 2017;46(9):1165–1186.

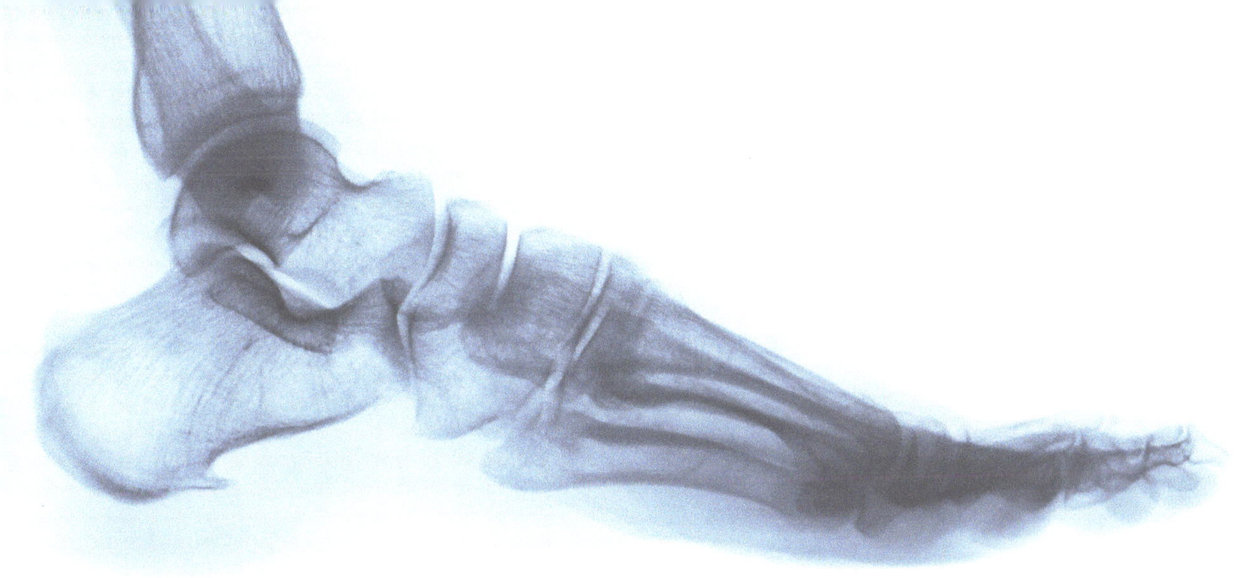

PART II

ANATOMICAL CONSIDERATIONS

CHAPTER 5

Upper Extremity Injuries

Kristine Karlson

INTRODUCTION

The ribs and upper extremities are not common locations for which clinicians have a high level of suspicion of bone stress injury (BSI) because, unlike the lower extremities, they are not traditionally weight-bearing bones. However, there are important biomechanical challenges to the upper extremity and ribs in some sports. Having a high level of suspicion for the possibility of a BSI when evaluating a patient with insidious onset of pain will aid the clinician in this evaluation. Asking the athlete to explain how the injured body part is used in their sport is useful if the clinician does not have prior knowledge of the specific sport. Commonly, it will be found, once the biomechanics are better understood, that somewhere there was a break in the kinetic chain of the sport or a specific overuse that was a cause of the injury. Muscle fatigue may lead to bad biomechanics and in some cases creates unique forces on the adjacent bones, which may be explained after understanding the sport and training program. An excellent review of probable mechanisms for many upper extremity BSIs based on sport biomechanics was written by Anderson.[1] In addition to the biomechanical challenges of sport, some upper extremity bones have anatomic narrow areas, which are vulnerable to stress. Attention to anatomy and muscle attachments to bone can also help clarify possible bone stress from muscular action or fatigue of the stress absorption of surrounding muscle.

Often, the upper extremity stress injury will generate pain only during sport, especially if the injury was due to weight bearing on the upper extremity. Commonly, a rib stress injury will be symptomatic with other things that provide stress to the rib, such as coughing. Rib or upper extremity stress injuries from throwing may or may not be symptomatic with other activities. This also differs from stress injury of the lower extremity, which will eventually cause pain with simple walking in most cases. Delay in diagnosis may be more likely with the injury in the upper extremity and rib due to this lack of clinical suspicion.

There are case reports in the literature of upper extremity BSIs in a wide variety of upper extremity locations, many of which are single cases and not always indicative of a pattern of injury common to that sport. However, some of these stress injuries are more common and fit into injury patterns that can be predicted based on the biomechanics of the sport. In their 1999 case review, Sinha et al.[2] proposed a categorization framework to make sense of the patterns of injury most commonly seen. This was revised by Miller et al.[3] in 2013:

- weight lifter, associated with stress injuries anywhere in the upper extremity
- rower, associated with rib stress injuries
- weight bearer (gymnastics, cheerleading, diving), associated with stress injuries distal to the elbow
- thrower (baseball, javelin), associated with stress injuries in the shoulder region
- swinger, renamed axial rotator (golf, tennis), associated with rib stress injuries

This categorization is not meant to be exclusive. Tennis players have been reported to have BSIs in the ulna and metacarpals for example,[4] and throwers have BSIs at and distal to the elbow. Still, this framework is useful in categorizing upper extremity stress injuries for further discussion and for considering the biomechanical risk factors in various sports.

RIB BONE STRESS INJURIES: ROWING AND GOLF

Evaluation

BSIs of the rib in rowing were uncommonly reported before the mid-1990s and then only in small case reports of elite rowers and golfers or as a consequence of coughing. Unfortunately, they are now a relatively common occurrence in rowers of all ages, from high school to master's. The increase in incidence has been a consequence of increased training program intensity at all levels and also probably due to more loads from more efficient equipment.

The mechanism of rib BSIs in rowing has not been fully explained. A comprehensive review of theories on mechanisms and rib biomechanics was published by McDonnell et al. in 2011.[5] The anatomy of the lower ribs is such that there is a fairly significant bend in the lateral rib, and that is the location of most BSIs, which occur in the anterior to lateral aspect typically of ribs 4 to 9. Attached to the rib in this region are the serratus anterior and the abdominal muscles. The rib is therefore an important kinetic chain link between the core and the upper extremity. In addition, there are bending forces exerted on the rib from the deep breathing required for strenuous exercise. High loads per stroke in longer distance off season training may be a risk factor as well, though these fractures are certainly also seen in the competitive season. It is possible that shoulder instability contributes to rib BSIs due to a loss of continuity in the kinetic chain. In golf, serratus anterior fatigue has been postulated as a contributor, and rib BSIs are more commonly seen on the leading side in the posterolateral ribs 4 to 6.[6]

Rib BSIs begin with insidious onset of pain, as with most BSIs. Rowers will report generalized chest pain not only with rowing but also with coughing, sneezing, rolling over in bed, and laughing. At this point, many clinicians assume the pain is intercostal or costochondral. As the BSI evolves, the pain location becomes more specific and may evolve to be point tender over a single rib.

Diagnosis of a rib BSI depends on high clinical suspicion early in the evolution of the pain, as time off early in the course may shorten the recovery time. Clinicians are therefore encouraged to presume that any rower with chest wall pain has a rib BSI unless proven otherwise. There is no association with side rowed versus sculling, position in the boat, or even experience level. Rib stress injuries are seen from high school to elite to master's rowers. Diagnosis is best confirmed with bone scan or MRI, depending on availability and cost, but ultrasound may be useful for diagnosis in experienced hands.

Treatment

Recovery from a rib BSI, whether in a rower or in a golfer, usually involves pain-free relative rest, as is typical for BSIs elsewhere. Cross training may be more difficult than with lower extremity stress injuries due to the need for rib motion in breathing and even swinging of the arms in running. A slow return to sport results, and rowers in particular may benefit from attention to correcting other weaknesses in their core and rotator cuff.[7]

THROWING-RELATED BONE STRESS INJURIES: BASEBALL, SOFTBALL, JAVELIN

Evaluation

There are numerous case reports in the literature of first rib BSIs in throwing athletes, to the point that this is considered a relatively common problem in baseball pitchers. Interestingly, these are not all in the throwing arm,[8] and they can also occur from swinging a bat. The first rib has unique anatomy, in that muscular action on the rib comes from the scalenes, which insert from above, and the serratus anterior and intercostals, which exert force from below. The first rib also has an anatomic area of weakness in the subclavian artery groove, and that is the area of most first rib bone stress failures. Though this is not unique to throwing athletes,[3] it is commonly thought of as being associated with throwing. Diagnosis of this BSI requires a high degree of clinical suspicion as the pain is relatively vague in the shoulder region, is dull, and may radiate to the sternum, though usually seen in the mid-clavicular region. Plain films may or may not find these injuries (as is common for stress injuries), and further imaging with MRI may be needed. If not seen via MRI, CT may be useful. This could be also found on bone scan, but due to higher radiation doses, bone scans are not currently commonly recommended for BSIs.

Treatment

These stress injuries typically respond to relative rest and progressive return to activity. Surgical intervention in this area is uncommonly pursued, but some cases go on to non-union, thoracic outlet syndrome, and first rib resection.[8]

HUMERUS

Evaluation

A BSI of the humerus from throwing is among the few BSIs that are typically diagnosed unfortunately only after the BSI has gone on to a completed fracture. These typically are spiral fractures of the mid-shaft and occur in bones without cysts or other clear structurally weak areas. Muscle fatigue has been implicated in these injuries, particularly the biceps and triceps, which may not be able to dissipate force normally as they fatigue. In adolescents, this is felt to be due to immature bone and high activity. Interestingly, this injury is also seen in healthy middle-aged pitchers, with the speculation that years of layoff from pitching and a relative lack of conditioning are important contributors to bone fatigue.[9] Athletes describe feeling or hearing a crack or pop following a specific incident of overuse, describe a crack or pop following an insidious onset of pain, or may have had progressive worsening of pain, as would be typical of BSIs elsewhere.[3]

Treatment

Because many of these are spiral fractures and may be displaced, surgical fixation is commonly the treatment of choice.

ELBOW

There are four commonly described areas of stress injury at the elbow, and each has a biomechanical cause, as discussed by Anderson[1] and Jones.[9] Medial epicondylar apophysitis in the adolescent throwing athlete is discussed in the following. BSIs of the olecranon tip are described in javelin throwers and are believed to be due to snapping the elbow into terminal extension while throwing. Repeated contraction of the triceps is implicated in BSIs of the mid-olecranon, and the proximal posteromedial olecranon is stressed in a valgus overload mechanism, which may be associated with weakness or injury to the ulnar collateral ligament, resulting in increased bone stress.

ULNA

The ulna is vulnerable in the windmill pitch of softball.[1] This is thought to be a torsional stress from forcible pronation at the release, where pitchers may also hit the ulna against the thigh. The ulna is also vulnerable to bending forces in weight lifting and the volleyball set. BSIs in the ulna are seen in other sports with repeated pronation and supination, such as the rotatory stress seen in the nondominant ulna in a two-handed backhand in lawn tennis.[9]

WEIGHT-BEARING BONE STRESS INJURIES: GYMNASTICS

Of all upper extremity BSIs, the possibility of stress injury in the arms and hands of gymnasts is most intuitively obvious, because these athletes are weight bearing, usually repetitively, on bones that are not necessarily designed for weight bearing in normal use. These injuries are reviewed by Wolf et al.[10] Most concerning among these injuries is a BSI of the scaphoid. The injury mechanism, in addition to loading, appears to be the combination of extension, radial deviation, and rotation common to many gymnastics maneuvers. This is a bone with poor healing ability, similar to traumatic fracture of the scaphoid, and stress injuries to the scaphoid require prolonged casting or screw fixation. Also relatively common is a physeal injury to the distal radius, which is discussed in the following.

Another region of stress injury in the wrist of gymnasts is known as ulnar abutment or impaction. This is seen in athletes with positive ulnar variance (ulna proportionally longer than average when compared to radius). This results in the ulna hitting against the lunate, seen on MRI as injury increased signal in the ulnar corner of the lunate.

PHYSEAL STRESS INJURIES: THROWING AND GYMNASTICS

Though not traditionally included in a discussion of BSI because they lack the metabolic risk factors seen in other stress injuries, overuse injuries to the physis probably should be considered BSIs. Prominent among these are the relatively common injuries known as Little League shoulder and Little League elbow. Little League shoulder is a BSI to the proximal humeral physis. In looking at the mechanics of this area, Anderson[1] emphasized the torsional stress placed on the humerus in late cocking and early acceleration of throwing. Adding to that biomechanical challenge is that throwing athletes may not obey pitch count limits if playing for several teams simultaneously. At the elbow, the BSI from throwing is at the medial apophysis, where the failure may be in the bone, instead of failure of the ulnar collateral ligament, as is seen in older throwing athletes. Rest is prescribed for both of these conditions, another similarity with other BSIs.

The distal radius is another physis that is at risk, this time in gymnastics, where the radius is loaded unlike most any other sport. Wolf et al.[10] also review this injury, where pain is localized to the distal radius in gymnasts without a history of specific trauma, and appears to be more common in athletes with ulnar negative variance. Injury to this physis can range from self-resolving pain to physeal growth arrest. Treatment therefore varies, and those with physeal arrest will likely require surgical intervention.

In general, most BSIs heal in 6 weeks, and stress injuries of the ribs and upper extremities are generally no different. There are some special cases in the upper extremity, such as the scaphoid, which has poor healing potential similar to the tarsal navicular in the foot. What is different is that upper extremity stress injuries may not cause pain with daily activities to the same extent as do the lower extremity stress injuries, and athletes may therefore be asymptomatic for all activities other than their sport and are more likely to assume that they are ready to return when in fact they are not. A gradual and stepwise return to the specific sport is therefore strongly recommended. Referral to a physical therapist familiar with the sport can be invaluable in guiding return to play. Rib stress injuries are somewhat different in that they cause pain with daily activities such as laughing, coughing, sneezing, rolling over in bed, and reaching, so athletes are likely to have a better sense that they have not yet recovered. Likewise, their return to sport needs to be gradual and stepwise in intensity.

CONCLUSION

BSIs of the ribs and upper extremities may not be as obvious as those in weight-bearing lower extremity bones. A high index of suspicion and attention to the biomechanics of sport and anatomy of the area as well as knowledge of reported BSI patterns in these anatomical sites should help guide clinicians in their assessment

KEY REFERENCES

Only key references appear in the print edition. The full reference list appears in the digital product found on http://connect.springerpub.com/content/book/978-0-8261-4424-9/part/sec02/chapter/ch05

1. Anderson MW. Imaging of upper extremity BSIs in the athlete. *Clin Sports Med.* 2006;25(3):489–504.

3. Miller TL, Harris JD, Kaeding CC. Stress fractures of the ribs and upper extremities: causation, evaluation, and management. *Sports Med.* 2013;43(8):665–664.

5. McDonnell LK, Hume PA, Nolte V. Rib BSIs among rowers: definition, epidemiology, mechanisms, risk factors and effectiveness of injury prevention strategies. *Sports Med.* 2011;41(11):883–901.

9. Jones GL. Upper extremity BSIs. *Clin Sports Med.* 2006;25:159–174.

10. Wolf MR, Avery D, Wolf JM. Upper extremity injuries in gymnasts. *Hand Clin.* 2017;33:187–197.

CHAPTER 6

Lower Extremity Injuries

Kevin M. Mullins and Michael Fredericson

INTRODUCTION

Lower extremity bone stress injuries may occur in weight-bearing bones, including the long bones of the femur, tibia, and fibula. Further, the patella is a key sesamoid bone of the lower extremity that can also be predisposed to overuse injury. Within each bone, the anatomical location may influence evaluation and management. Injuries to each bone are included here with details for evaluation and management based on specific anatomy.

Bone stress injuries of the femoral diaphysis and proximal femur can manifest as vague thigh pain. One of the most significant risk factors in developing injury is a recent alteration in a training program.[1-3] These changes may include any sudden increase in mileage, pace, volume, or cross-training activity, without adequate time for adaptation to the new workloads. Specifically, in long-distance runners, it has been documented that increased injury rate correlates most closely to increasing distance beyond 32 km/wk.[4] As with any stress reaction injury, it is also important to identify contributing risk factors. Sex-specific predispositions for low bone mineral density should be considered, including female athletes presenting with a stress injury in the setting of late onset menarche or irregular menses.[5] In this section, we review common types of stress reactions and fractures of the femur as well as important diagnostic workup and treatment strategies for the patella, tibia, and fibula.

FEMORAL SHAFT

Femoral shaft stress fractures make up a significant portion of all stress fractures in the body. Incidence has been reported to range between 20.6% and 22.5% among military recruits and varsity collegiate athletes, respectively.[6,7] Although the majority of femoral shaft fractures are considered to be diaphyseal lesions, distal femoral metaphysis stress fractures can also occur. In fact, these distal injuries in the past have commonly been labeled as a consequence of osteonecrosis of the knee; however, with greater understanding, we now know that many of these distal injuries are in fact truly subchondral insufficiency fractures.[8] Thus, it is important for the treating provider to approach all presenting patients with any possible concern for a femoral shaft fracture with careful due diligence and thoughtful diagnostic consideration.

Tubular in shape, the femur is a long bone with a thick cortex and an anterolateral bow in the proximal and middle third of the bone.[9] This anatomical structure is essential as it helps to accommodate the significant stresses placed on the bone during the running cycle, which is estimated to be on average three times the body weight mass.[10] As a result of the femoral shaft's bowed shape the lateral side of the shaft is under tension, while the medial side of the bone is under compression. Oh et al.[11] have shown via in vitro biomechanical studies that the greatest strain is placed on the posteromedial cortex of the proximal femur, making it especially susceptible to repetitive submaximal stresses. In a retrospective case series involving 25 track-and-field varsity and recreational runners over 10 years diagnosed with femoral shaft BSI, all but two injuries involved the medial femoral cortex on the compressive side, those being the anterior and posterior cortices of the proximal femoral diaphysis.[12]

Diagnosis

Femoral shaft stress injuries in athletes generally present as vague, poorly localized, insidious onset of discomfort in the anterior thigh. Early stages of pain can be misdiagnosed as a muscle strain or tear, when the pain is only aggravated while engaging in activity. Without intervention, the disease process may naturally progress to more significant bony insult, at which time the athlete may experience additional pain during ambulation or even at rest. Should an athlete dismiss these symptoms and continue to participate in heavy weight-bearing activity, there is a theoretical risk of further damage by advancing the fracture to the extent of displacement.[13,14]

Swelling, limited range of motion, and pain are not typically appreciated on physical exam.[15] Rather, the clinician should utilize the "fulcrum test" to help localize the anatomical site of impairment.[16] During this test, the athlete is seated with the lower leg hanging off of the examination table. Next, the clinician's arm is used essentially as a fulcrum beneath the thigh and is moved from distal to proximal thigh as the opposing hand then applies light pressure to the dorsum of the knee. A positive test includes one in which the light pressure on the knee results in a sharper and more focal pain discomfort. The clinician may also consider the "hop" test, during which the patient performs a series of single-legged hops on the affected limb. Pain in the region of interest would be indicative of a positive test.[17]

Radiography is recommended for initial screening purposes, although the radiographs may be normal early in the disease process; however, as noted earlier, the sensitivity is very low.[18] Longitudinal femur stress fractures may be diagnosed on radiography with a visible fracture line on the anterior–posterior view of the hip.[19] More recently, there has also been growing evidence in the literature to support the use of ultrasound with deep array transducers as an alternative and equally accurate diagnostic tool for femur stress fractures when compared to traditional radiography.[16] A hypoechoic, hypervascular rim around the cortex of painful bone would represent the earliest sonographic findings of a stress fracture, indicative of periosteal reaction. Soft tissue edema may also be seen, and in later stages of the disease process, cortical irregularity and subsequent callus formation might also be visible.[20]

CT might also have a role in early stage injuries, as it has been found to be the best option for detecting osteopenia, which is the earliest sign of fatigue damage for cortical bone.[21] Nuclear scintigraphy (i.e., bone scan) is not recommended as the imaging modality of choice due to low specificity, high dosage of ionizing radiation, and additional limitations.[18] MRI provides more detailed anatomical information than bone scan, including periosteal edema, bone marrow edema, and fracture line (Figure 6.1).[12] MRI remains the imaging method of choice for stress injuries of the femoral shaft as there is no ionizing radiation (compared to CT and nuclear scintigraphy). Findings typically include periosteal

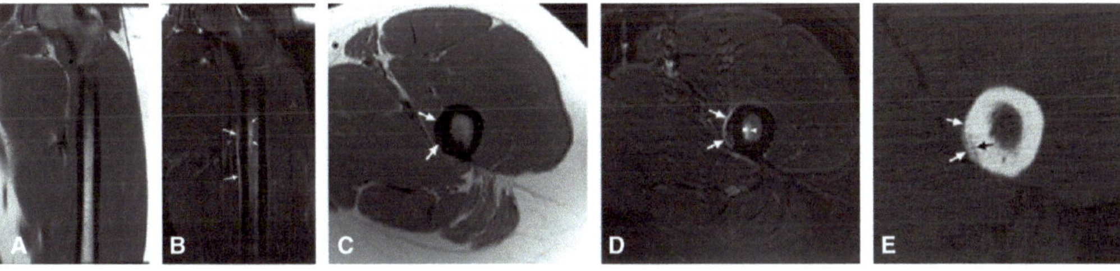

FIGURE 6.1 Femoral diaphyseal stress fracture in a 21-year-old female basketball player. Patient had insidious onset of pain during the season. (A) Coronal T1-weighted image shows an essentially normal appearance of the proximal femoral shaft. (B) Coronal T2-weighted image with fat suppression shows periosteal reaction (*large arrows*) as well as endosteal edema (*small arrows*). (C) Axial T1-weighted image shows thickening of the medial femoral cortex. (D) Corresponding T2-weighted image with fat suppression shows periosteal reaction with a thin curvilinear area of intracortical signal as well as endosteal edema (*arrowhead*). (E) CT image (1.25 mm of section thickness, bone reconstruction kernel) obtained on the same day as MRI shows periosteal reaction (*white arrows*) and intracortical lucency (*black arrow*) consistent with limited intracortical fracture.

Source: Reproduced with permission from Fredericson M, Jennings F, Beaulieu C, et al. Stress fractures in athletes. *Top Magn Reson Imaging*. 2006;17(5):309–325.

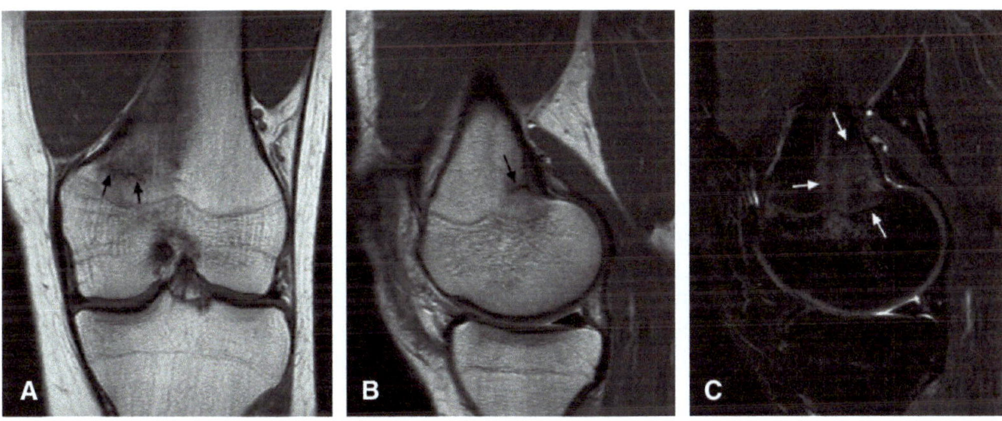

FIGURE 6.2 Stress fracture of distal femoral metaphysis in a 19-year-old male recreational athlete. (A) Coronal T1-weighted image shows low signal line (*arrows*) in the medial femoral diaphysis. (B) Sagittal proton density Y- weighted image shows fracture line (*arrow*). (C) Sagittal fat-suppressed T2-weighted image shows geographic marrow edema (*arrows*) surrounding area of fracture.

Source: Reproduced with permission from Fredericson M, Jennings F, Beaulieu C, et al. Stress fractures in athletes. *Top Magn Reson Imaging*. 2006;17(5):309–325.

and bone marrow edema of the medial aspect of the femur between the proximal and middle thirds of the femoral diaphysis. Depending on the severity of the injury, there may also be a fracture line visible at this approximate junction.[22]

Distal femur stress fractures are relatively uncommon in comparison to diaphyseal and femoral neck lesions (Figure 6.2). However, when distal femoral metaphysis injuries do occur, they can sometimes be misinterpreted as spontaneous osteonecrosis of the knee (SONK) due to the adjacent anatomical location. It has been proposed that the manifestation of a linear component in association with a subchondral marrow abnormality on imaging can better clarify appropriate categorization of these lesions into either those of subchrondral insufficiency fractures or those of osteoarthritis.[23,24]

Treatment

In the absence of full cortical break or displacement on imaging, recommended initial treatment is conservative. An assistive device such as crutches may be considered if the patient is experiencing pain with day-to-day ambulation. Once the patient is able to ambulate without any discomfort, then a prescription for cross-training program would be reasonable. Subsequently, when the patient is pain free with all normal weight-bearing activities, one may recommend gradual return to athletics. In addition, the fulcrum test, as described in detail earlier in this chapter, can be utilized as an indicator of bone healing for the femoral stress fracture.[7] The typical duration for return is approximately 8 to 12 weeks after the initial injury.

One specific algorithm that can serve as guidance for the treatment of femoral stress fractures has been described by Ivkovic et al.[26] In this scenario, recovery time is to be divided into four distinct phases, each covering a 3-week duration, for a total of 12 weeks. In order to progress into the next phase, the patient must complete a series of tests within that given phase. Once all phases have been completed, theoretically one can return to sport without limitation.

Nonunion or delayed union of femoral diaphyseal stress fracture is unlikely following a course of conservative therapy. In the rare instances of such complication, however, referral for surgical evaluation of possible intramedullary rod placement would be warranted.[12]

PATELLA

Stress fractures in the patella are uncommon.[28,29] When they do occur, they can be classified as either transverse or vertical, depending on the orientation of the fracture line. Initial symptoms typically include vague, anterior knee pain without any specific traumatic injury. Radiography is the initial imaging of choice, but careful attention should be directed not to misdiagnose a patella fracture as a bipartite patella.[30,31] Longitudinal stress fractures typically are found in the lateral patella facet but are especially difficult to detect when nondisplaced.[32–34] MRI is a more accurate diagnostic tool and may be used in similar fashion to other stress fracture workup algorithms. Specifically, the axial T2-weighted fat-suppressed sequence is the best to demonstrate bone marrow edema, while the axial T1-weighted sequence can show the potential fracture line, localized to the lateral aspect of the patella.[34] Should nonoperative treatment fail and displacement occur, then surgical excision of the lateral fragment may be considered.[35] Similarly, transverse fractures are prone to displacement, and immobilization is recommended for initial nonoperative treatment when these do occur.[36]

TIBIA

Tibial stress injuries account for the majority of stress fractures in the body. For athletes presenting with exertional leg pain in the sports medicine clinic, up to 75% of cases have been found to be secondary to medial tibial stress syndrome and tibial stress fractures.[37] Risk factors for developing tibial stress injuries are similar to those in other weight-bearing regions of the body, with an increased injury rate as distance increases beyond approximately 32 km/wk.[4] In this section, we discuss the diagnostic and treatment considerations for the medial tibial cortex, anterior tibial cortex, and medial tibial plateau injuries.

The tibia is the second largest bone in the body and provides the majority of weight bearing through the leg as opposed to its lower extremity counterpart the fibula.[38] The tibial shaft is triangular in cross-section and is made up of three borders and three surfaces.[39] The anterior border divides the medial and lateral surface of the tibia, while the medial border divides the medial and posterior surfaces. Dividing the lateral and posterior surfaces is the interosseous border.[38] The most common site for tibial stress fractures is the posteromedial border of the tibia on the compressive side of the bone.

Increased subtalar pronation due to reduced ankle dorsiflexion in the setting of tight gastrocsoleus musculature can predispose athletes to excessive subtalar joint pronation and the development of tibial stress injuries. Additional biomechanical risk factors include a standing foot angle less than 140° with weight bearing, hindfoot, and forefoot varus, as well as greater hindfoot movement during running.[1,40,41] It has also been reported that the velocity of pronation, in addition to the degree of pronation, serves as an important risk factor for development of medial tibial stress syndrome or tibial stress fracture.[40]

Lastly, it is important to note that there is greater impact to the tibia with a heel-strike versus forefoot-strike patterned running gait. Specifically, with a heel-strike pattern, the ankle is dorsiflexed, tibia angulated, and knee extended. In contrast, during a forefoot strike, the ankle is generally plantarflexed, knee flexed, and the tibia is vertical (see Chapter 17 for more details on gait retraining for tibia bone stress injuries).[42]

Diagnosis

Patients with a tibial stress injury often present with pain along the medial border of the tibia. Many times, it can be difficult to differentiate between medial tibial stress syndrome (i.e., grade 1 bone stress injury) and a more significant tibial stress fracture.[41,42] The key to differentiating these two diagnoses lies with the timing and duration of pain symptoms. Specifically, it is important to delineate whether or not the pain persists after running and during daily ambulation, which may be indicative of a more extensive injury as well as more diffuse symptoms along the periosteum versus more focal, deep bone pain. Additional differential diagnosis includes that of exertional compartment syndrome and popliteal artery entrapment syndrome. In the former, the athlete often reports exertional aching or cramping in the leg, with associated tightness or weakness. These symptoms are commonly bilateral, are localized over the muscle, and may have numbness or tingling, reflecting nerve involvement in the respective compartment.[43–48] In contrast, popliteal artery entrapment presents with intermittent claudication symptoms, including calf discomfort, cramping, coolness, and numbness of the foot.[43]

On physical exam, in early stage grade 1 injuries, there is often a diffuse area of tenderness over the posterior medial edge of the tibia. Pain may be aggravated by active muscle strength activation, specifically in those muscles that have origin over the posterior medial tibial border, including the posterior tibialis, flexor digitorum longus, and soleus, of which the latter is best tested with repetitive toe raises.[21] However, it is important for the examiner to test for both localized tenderness over the tibia and direct and indirect percussion over the bone, which has been shown to correlate with greater severity of marrow involvement and cortical abnormalities on imaging.[77] In addition, pain or discomfort in the proximal portion of the tibia is unusual for medial tibial stress syndrome but can be found in up to 43% of tibial stress fracture injuries.[49,50]

Similar to the femoral stress fracture workup, screening radiographs may be considered as an initial imaging modality, although often findings are normal in the presence of early disease. Alternatively, ultrasound is another viable tool, with the first reported use of musculoskeletal ultrasound to diagnose a bone stress injury described in 1992 by Howard et al.[51] The five ultrasound hallmarks of bone stress injury include hyperechogenicity of the surrounding soft tissue, increased periosteal color Doppler flow, thickening of the periosteum, posterior shadowing, and cortical disruption. More recently, it has been suggested that fracture and soft-tissue interface by real-time strain elastography might also be a useful tool for obtaining information regarding tissue stiffness and elasticity, providing valuable information on bone injury and healing.[52] Much like femur fractures, CT may have a role in early stage injuries, as it has been found to be the best option for detecting osteopenia, which is the earliest sign of fatigue damage for cortical bone.[21]

MRI is the imaging method of choice for diagnosing tibial stress injuries. The aforementioned recent systematic review found the sensitivity for detecting lower extremity stress fractures to be up to 99% and specificity up to 97%.[18] When comparing bone scan and MRI to diagnose tibial stress injuries, it has been determined that periostitis is likely the initial finding on the spectrum of injury severity. The Fredericson classification system is recommended to grade the severity of stress injury based on marrow involvement, as well as to help guide anticipatory recovery timeline. In this classification system, a grade 1 injury represents periosteal edema. Progressive marrow involvement visible on T2 is a grade 2 injury, while grade 3 injury is when the marrow is seen on both the T2 and the T1 sequences.[77] Eventually, cortical stress fracture is the final grade, grade 4, which can further be delineated as either a grade 4a or a grade 4b, depending on if there are multiple discrete areas of intracortical signal changes or linear areas of intracortical signal change correlating with a frank stress fracture.[53]

Treatment

The management for compressive side tibial stress injuries is almost always nonoperative, with a focus on temporary cessation of running in order to allow for adequate bone remodeling and repair.[21] The estimated delay in returning to impact activity can best be determined based on MRI and utilizing the previously discussed Fredericson criteria. Grade 1 stress injuries typically require 2 to 3 weeks, grade 2 to 4a approximately 6 to 9 weeks, and grade 4b 9 to 12 weeks or longer.[53] If there is severe pain with daily activities, then a pneumatic tibial brace is recommended to immobilize distal and mid-tibial injuries.[54] Additional consideration should also be made for injury prevention, such as the incorporation of a foot orthosis to help control pronation and dissipate increased stress to the tibia and supporting musculature.[21,55] Alternative consideration in management strategies may be warranted in anterior tibial cortex or medial tibial plateau fractures, which is detailed in separate sections.

ANTERIOR TIBIAL CORTEX

Mid-tibia stress fractures of the anterior cortex are atypical and necessitate a separate discussion and unique treatment approach. Unlike the previously reviewed posteromedial tibia stress fractures, injuries to the anterior cortex most commonly occur in jumping or leaping athletes.[56,57] They have high risk for progression into nonunion due to their anatomical location on the tension side of bone, a region with lessened vascularity. On imaging, radiographs demonstrate a radiolucent cortical defect surrounded by sclerosis, a finding termed the "dreaded black line."[21] Bone scans may show a linear uptake compatible with periostitis or can be negative if the lesion is metabolically inactive.[21] Treatment for this injury typically entails a period of non–weight-bearing immobilization for 6 to 8 weeks, although some athletes may elect to have intramedullary rod placement earlier to allow for quicker healing and return to play. There has also been significant success in the development of shockwave as an added modality for bone healing, which can be used during the time of protected weight bearing.[58] See Chapter 19 for more information and further reading on this. However, should conservative management fail after 3 to 6 months of management, then referral for possible surgical excision and bone grafting or placement of an intramedullary rod is indicated.[59–61]

MEDIAL TIBIAL PLATEAU

The medial tibial plateau also represents another rare yet important potential site of stress fracture.[62,63] On physical exam, tenderness is typically found just inferior to the medial joint line, along the anteromedial aspect of the proximal tibia. Due to anatomical orientation, it can be misinterpreted as a pes anserine bursitis or tendinitis by the untrained examiner or attributed to medial tibiofemoral osteoarthritis or joint disease. Radiographic imaging will often show a linear transverse region of sclerosis of 2 or 3 mm thickness in the medial tibial plateau. Alternatively, if x-rays are negative during the early disease process, then MRI may be used to demonstrate bone marrow edema of the medial tibial plateau as well as periosteal edema.[22] Treatment includes utilization of long-leg brace for immobilization.

LONGITUDINAL TIBIA

While the majority of tibia stress fractures occur in a transverse plane, perpendicular to the cortical shaft, there are rare occasions when the fracture may actually present longitudinally.[64–66] Of the longitudinal tibial stress injuries described in the literature, most have been classified as insufficiency stress fractures, as opposed to fatigue stress fractures.[67–69] Depending on the demographic and clinical history of the patient, differential diagnosis for this type of injury should also include neoplasms and osteomyelitis.[70] While plain films may be normal in many cases, advanced imaging as in CT can confirm radiographic findings and can more easily detect a fracture line when compared to MRI.[71] MRI, however, will still typically show cortical thickening adjacent to the fracture line as well as bone marrow edema association. Conservative management with protected weight bearing is recommended.

FIBULA

Stress fractures in the fibula are the fourth most common location for stress fractures, accounting for 15.5% of all stress injuries.[72] These fractures typically occur more distally within the fibula bone, just superior to the tibiofibular ligament attachment.[64,73] Predisposing anatomical risk factors for developing a fibula stress fracture include the cavus-type foot.[21] On physical exam, due to the superficial location of the fibula, the examining provider can easily palpate the bone for tenderness within the region. Similar to other lower extremity stress fractures, radiographs should be used for initial screening, followed by MRI if indicated. If initial radiographs are negative in early disease, MRI may still show evidence of bone marrow edema or a fracture line. Differential diagnosis should always include exertional compartment syndrome, popliteal entrapment, or peroneal nerve entrapment injury or peroneal tendinopathy. In general, these fractures can be managed nonoperatively with an initial period of protected weight bearing followed by a gradual return to running once symptoms have resolved.

MEDIAL MALLEOLUS

Medial ankle pain secondary to a medial malleolus stress fracture is rare, but when it does occur, the diagnosis warrants close attention given the high-risk nature of the injury. Found in running and jumping athletes most often, with an average age of 24.5 years in one report, initial presentation is typically that of vague gradual increasing pain and swelling over the medial aspect of the ankle.[74] As such, medial malleolus fractures typically originate as a vertical stress line starting at the junction of the tibial plafond and medial malleolus with extension both medially and proximally from this site. Radiographs are typically negative, while MRI shows focal bone marrow edema similar to other lower extremity bone stress injuries discussed previously. In some instances, a well-defined vertical fracture line can be appreciated.[22,75] In the case that imaging does show signs of a medial malleolar fracture, then referral for open reduction and internal fixation may be considered for athletes with aspirations of returning to sport early.[76] Otherwise, nonoperative management is the treatment of choice, in conjunction with a pneumatic ankle brace. A recent systematic review found that the average time missed for patients undergoing operative treatment was 2.4 weeks, with a 13.7-week average healing time, while those who elected for nonoperative management missed 7.6 weeks of activity with 14.3 weeks on average of healing time.[74] The theoretical benefit of earlier return to play should always be compared to the risk for any patient undergoing operative surgery, and as such, a careful, thoughtful discussion should take place before committing to any surgical intervention.

CONCLUSION

Lower extremity bone stress injuries of the femur, tibia, and fibula are common among endurance athletes and require judicious workup in the setting of heightened clinical suspicion. It is important to recognize when initial radiographs may be falsely negative, warranting the need for further advanced imaging to aid in the development of an appropriate management strategy and treatment plan. While the vast majority of lower extremity stress fractures can be dealt with in a nonoperative manner, one must be able to successfully distinguish in which scenarios a prompt surgical referral is required. Developing a comprehensive understanding of the topics and concepts discussed in this chapter plays an important role in the process of becoming a fully competent and capable sports medicine provider.

KEY REFERENCES

Only key references appear in the print edition. The full reference list appears in the digital product found on http://connect.springerpub.com/content/book/978-0-8261-4424-9/part/sec02/chapter/ch06

5. Tenforde AS, Sayres LC, McCurdy ML, Sainani KL, Fredericson M. Identifiying sex-specific risk factors for stress fractures in adolescent runners. *Med Sci Sports Exerc* 2013;45:1843–1851.

12. Fredericson M, Jiang KU, Bergman G, et al. Femoral diaphyseal stress fractures: results of a systematic bone scan and magnetic resonance imaging evaluation in 25 runners. *Physc Ther Sport*. 2004;5:188–193.

21. Fredericson M, Jennings F, Beaulieu C, Matheson G. Stress fractures in athletes. *Top Magn Reson Imaging*. 2006;17:5:309–325.

22. Bergman AG, Fredericson M. MR imaging of stress fractures, muscle injuries, and other overuse injuries in runners. *Magn Reson Imaging Clin N Am*. 1999;7:151–174.

75. Fredericson M, Bergman AG, Hoffman KL, Dillingham MS. Tibial stress reaction in runners: correlation of clinical symptoms and scintigraphy with a new magnetic resonance imaging grading system. *Am J Sports Med* 1995;23:472–481.

CHAPTER 7

Pelvis and Hip Injuries

Kate Temme and Rahul Kapur

INTRODUCTION

Bone stress injuries (BSIs) occur rarely in the general population but represent up to 20% of all sports medicine clinical diagnoses.[1–3] BSIs are overuse injuries that develop when insufficient repair of bony microtrauma occurs in the setting of repetitive submaximal skeletal load. BSIs occur along a continuum from mild stress reaction to cortical stress fracture.[4–6] Certain athletic populations have a higher incidence of BSIs, including long-distance runners, gymnasts, and track and field athletes.[7,8] Female athletes are at a greater risk for BSI than their male counterparts in comparable sports.[8,9]

The vast majority of BSIs reported are those below the knee.[1,10,11] Among NCAA collegiate athletes, stress fractures of the tibia and metatarsals represent over half of all reported BSIs.[8] However, pelvic, femoral neck, and upper extremity BSIs are likely underreported and require a high degree of suspicion for accurate diagnosis and management.[10]

Historically, trabecular stress fractures of the sacrum and pelvis had been considered low-risk stress fractures. More recently, several studies have noted that these trabecular-rich stress fracture sites are associated with prolonged healing and return to sport, which lends importance to early identification and management of these injuries to minimize length of disability.[4] Trabecular-rich sites of BSIs of the femoral neck, sacrum, and pelvis are weighted more heavily than cortical sites in the Female Athlete Triad Coalition cumulative risk factor assessment[12] and are more often associated with disordered eating and menstrual dysfunction than stress fractures at predominantly cortical sites (tibia, fibula, metatarsals).[4] Low bone mineral density is associated with a higher risk of trabecular BSI in both male and female athletes.[4,13] This highlights the importance of the female athlete triad[12,14,15] and relative energy deficiency in sport (RED-S)[16–18] evaluation and management in this subset of BSIs.

FEMORAL NECK BONE STRESS INJURIES

Evaluation

Femoral neck bone stress injuries (FNBSIs) were first reported in the military in 1905 and in athletes in 1965.[19] They are most commonly reported in endurance athletes, especially runners and military recruits.[20,21] The femoral neck experiences significant tensile and compressive forces. Loads to the femoral neck are high during impact activities and may exceed 4 to 8 times body weight when running.[20] While rare, FNBSIs are considered high-risk injuries due to the possibility of fracture progression, displacement, nonunion, and avascular necrosis most often occurring in tension-sided (lateral) injuries. Given the high risks of morbidity, careful evaluation and early detection of FNBSIs are critical to allow for appropriate management, recovery, and successful return to sport.

Athletes with FNBSIs may present with vague or deep groin pain that worsens with weight-bearing activity. Pain may radiate to the anterior thigh or buttock, and patients may demonstrate a C-sign. Initially, pain presents with prolonged exercise but with progression may also occur with activities of daily living and at rest. Unlike the distal lower extremity, palpation of the hip is limited by structural depth. Hip range of motion deficits, pain at extreme ranges of motion, and axial loading may be present but are nonspecific findings on examination. A single-leg hop test is often positive but is also nonspecific.[22] Log roll or active straight leg raise may reproduce groin pain. A positive forced flexion, adduction, and internal rotation test suggestive of femoroacetabular impingement, and acetabular labral pathology and have been associated with FNBSI.[23,24] Increased forces on the femoral neck may result from repetitive end-range hip motions in the setting of acetabular over-coverage and predispose athletes to FNBSI. A positive fulcrum test may suggest a femoral shaft stress fracture. Given physical exam limitations, imaging is indicated whenever clinical suspicion exists for this high-risk BSI.

Plain radiographs are often the initial BSI imaging modality, due to availability and cost considerations, but demonstrate low sensitivity.[25,26] Only 10% of early BSI are identified on x-ray,[26] and complete stress fractures are often radiographically occult. Bone scintigraphy is highly sensitive for acute fractures but is limited by specificity and radiation exposure. CT is most helpful when confirmation of a fracture line would alter management. MRI demonstrates superior sensitivity and specificity, without ionizing radiation exposure, and provides diagnostic evaluation of surrounding soft tissue injuries (Figure 7.1).[27] Several MRI grading systems exist for BSI,[4-6] and higher-grade BSIs have been associated with prolonged recovery.[4,28]

A comprehensive risk factor assessment including training and biomechanical errors, triad and RED-S components, calcium and vitamin D status, and family- and medication-related bone health history should be performed and addressed when appropriate.

Differential diagnosis is vast and includes hip osteoarthritis, femoroacetabular impingement and acetabular labral tears, hip flexor tendinopathy, core muscle injury/athletic pubalgia, osteitis pubis, osteomyelitis, inguinal hernia, and various vascular, neoplastic, or gynecologic etiologies.

Treatment

Tension-sided (lateral, superior) FNBSIs often require urgent surgical referral and fixation due to the risk of fracture progression, nonunion, and avascular necrosis. Rarely, complete rest with serial imaging may be successful as long as cortical fracture widening does not occur.[29] Compression-sided (medial, inferior) FNBSIs are much more common than tension-sided BSI. They are usually managed with non–weight bearing on crutches with weight-bearing progression initiated after initial healing and pain resolution. Depending on injury severity, compression-sided FNBSI may require 4 to 6 weeks of non–weight bearing followed by 4 to 6 weeks of weight-bearing progression.[30] Rehabilitation is initially focused on rest and pain relief. During the initial rehabilitation phase, athletes may use nonimpact cross-training activities such as swimming, deep water running, or cycling to maintain cardiovascular fitness and prevent performance deficits upon return to sport. Antigravity treadmill training (ATT) may be utilized when

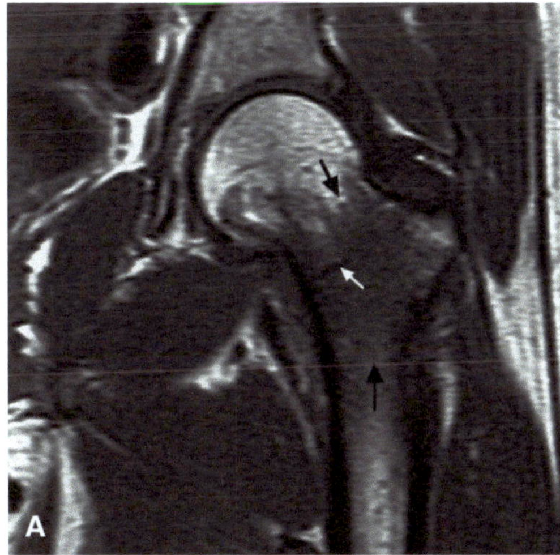
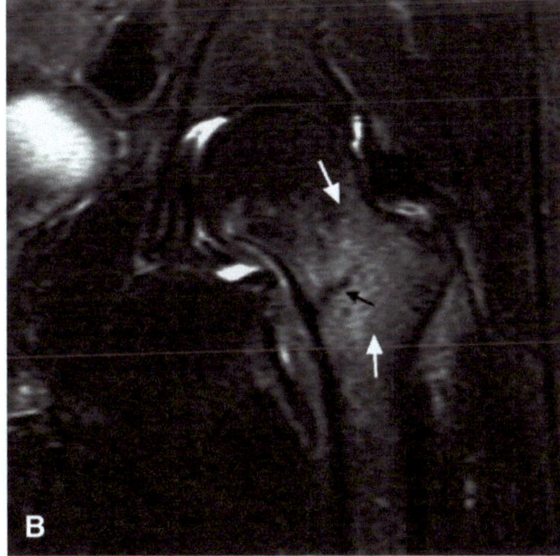

FIGURE 7.1 Midfemoral neck stress fracture in a 20-year-old female collegiate basketball player. (A) Coronal T1-weighted MRI (TR = 600, TE = 15) of the left hip shows extensive marrow edema (*black arrows*) and a low-signal fracture line (*white arrow*) along the medial compressive aspect of the femoral neck. (B) Coronal T2-weighted MRI with fat suppression (TR = 4500, TE = 72) shows marrow edema (*white arrows*), partial fracture (*black arrow*), and periosteal edema.

TR, repetition time; TE, time to echo.

Source: Reproduced with permission from Fredericson M, Jennings F, Beaulieu C, et al. Stress fractures in athletes. *Top Magn Reson Imaging*. 2006;17(5):309–325.

available to prepare runners for an eventual return to ground running through a progressive bodyweight protocol. After athletes reach 85% to 90% bodyweight with ATT, they should be transitioned to a gradually progressive ground running program. Return to running is considered when full weight-bearing and cross-training remain asymptomatic and healing is noted on imaging.

Analgesics should be used with caution, as they may mask pain and allow for a more rapid activity progression than is safe for recovery. Additionally, prolonged use of nonsteroidal antiinflammatory drugs may impede bony healing.[31,32]

LESSER TROCHANTER BONE STRESS INJURIES

Evaluation

Lesser trochanteric BSIs are rarely reported in the literature. One study of femoral BSI in 71 runners found that 20% had abnormal uptake in the lesser trochanter on bone scintigraphy.[22] In a retrospective study of nine runners with stress injury at the lesser trochanter, all were found to have iliopsoas tendinopathy, periostitis near the lesser trochanter, and marrow edema of varying degrees from the lesser trochanter to the femoral neck (Figure 7.2).[33] Fracture lines were noted in the femoral neck in three of the runners on initial imaging. In one noncompliant runner, progression from localized lesser trochanter marrow edema and iliopsoas abnormalities to a complete femoral neck stress fracture was demonstrated on follow-up imaging.[33] Consideration of BSI should occur in runners with marrow edema at the lesser trochanter, due to the risk of FNBSI, as treatment for BSI would vary greatly from iliopsoas insertional tendinopathy or enthesopathy.

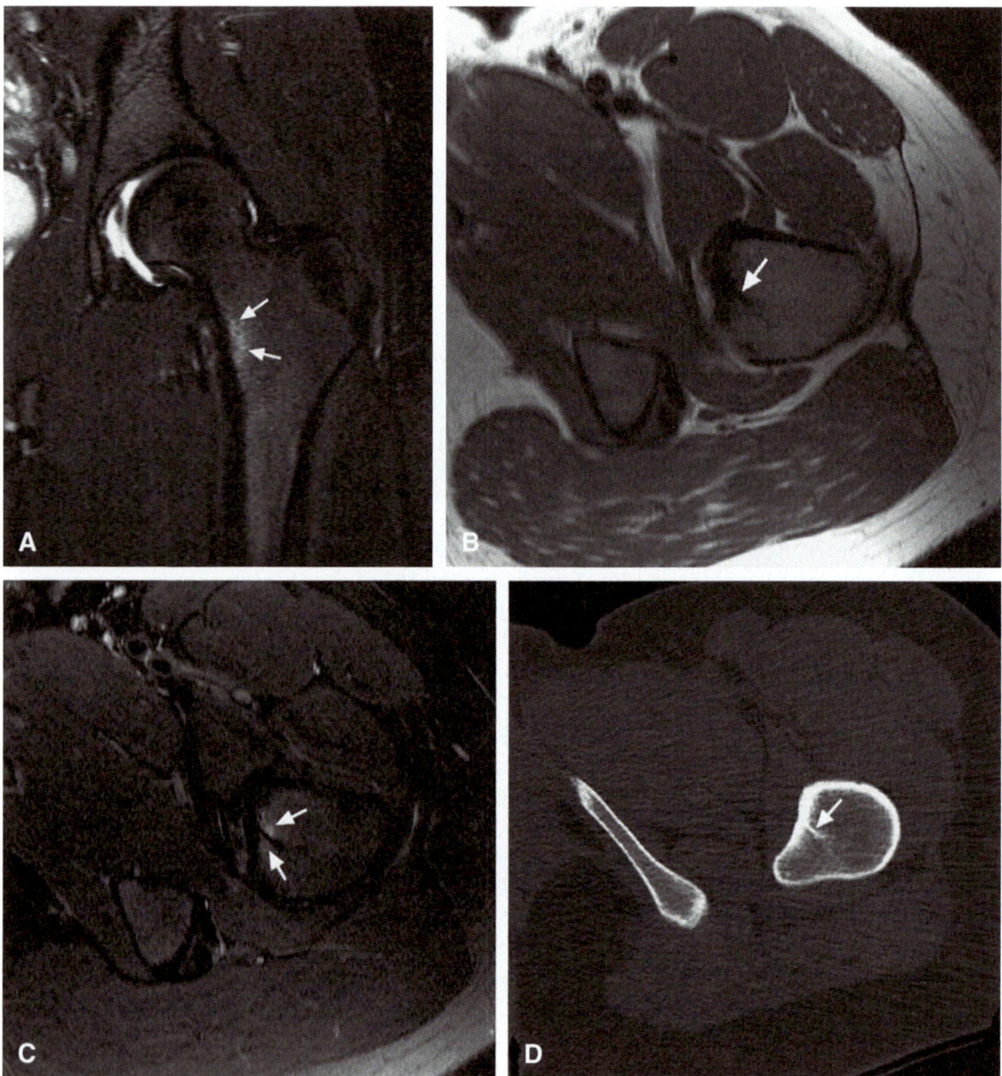

FIGURE 7.2 Stress reaction at the level of the lesser trochanter in a 20-year-old female soccer player. (A) Coronal T2-weighted scan with fat suppression (TR = 4650, TE = 54) shows marrow edema along the endosteal surface of the inferomedial femoral neck. (B) Axial T1-weighted image (TR = 600, TE = 14) shows a normal low signal line (*arrow*) known as the calcar femorale, which should not be confused with a fracture line. (C) Axial T2-weighted image with fat suppression (TR = 4266, TE = 64) shows that the marrow edema (*arrows*) is near the calcar femorale. (D) Axial CT image in a different patient, showing that the calcar (*arrow*) is a normal dense condensation of bone and not a fracture line.

TR, repetition time; TE, time to echo.

Source: Reproduced with permission from Fredericson M, Jennings F, Beaulieu C, et al. Stress fractures in athletes. *Top Magn Reson Imaging*. 2006;17(5):309–325.

Mechanism of injury may include chronic traction injury secondary to repetitive iliopsoas activation in runners, which places undo stress on the adjacent femoral neck. Alternatively, muscle fatigue during distance running may decrease bony shielding[33] and increase fracture risk.

Treatment

Evaluation and management of lesser trochanter BSIs follow the same algorithm as FNBSIs and should include a period of non–weight bearing to prevent progression to a FNBSI.

SACRAL BONE STRESS INJURIES

Evaluation

Sacral BSIs are rare compared to those of the femoral neck and lower extremities. Sacral stress fractures are classified as insufficiency or fatigue fractures. Sacral insufficiency fractures were first reported in 1984[34] and 1985[35] and are far more prevalent than fatigue stress fractures.[36] Sacral fatigue fractures were first reported in military recruits in 1989.[37] Subsequently, multiple case reports have been published in both male and female athletes and military recruits as well as in children and adolescents[38] and postpartum women.[39]

Endurance running is the most common sport associated with sacral BSI,[36,40,41] and they occur more commonly in female runners.[9,42,43] Case reports of other sports include basketball, volleyball, soccer, tennis, field hockey, and gymnastics.[40,41] Risk factors include training overload, rapid change in training regimen, impaired shock absorption, muscle fatigue, and leg-length discrepancies.[36,44] As with all stress fractures, and especially trabecular BSIs, the presence of the female athlete triad and RED-S risk factors increases risk for BSI.[44–46]

Sacral BSI should be suspected in all athletes with insidious onset of unilateral low back or buttock pain, as this symptom is present in up to 95% of cases.[40] Pain is aggravated by weight-bearing activities and in rare cases can mimic a lumbar radiculopathy.[47] Physical exam may reveal tenderness, which can be focal or diffuse along the sacrum, adjacent paraspinal muscles, or buttock. Sacroiliac (SI) joint maneuvers such as Flexion, Abduction and External Rotation (FABER) test, Gaenslen test, thigh thrust, distraction, compression, or sacral thrust test may be positive.[48] Single leg hop may localize pain to the affected sacrum, and special attention should be paid to evaluating for leg-length discrepancy.[41,48,49] Differential diagnosis includes SI joint dysfunction, sacroiliitis, spondylolysis, gluteal muscle injury, lumbar sprain, facet arthropathy, or radiculopathy.[49,50]

The study of choice for diagnosis of sacral BSI is MRI, due to superior sensitivity and specificity.[47] There is no specific classification for sacral BSI. Instead, the Denis classification, which was developed for traumatic sacral fractures, is most commonly utilized.[51] This classification separates fractures into three zones based on location relative to the sacral foramina, with zone 1 being lateral, zone 2 at the level of the sacral foramina, and zone 3 involving the body and central canal. The majority of sacral stress fractures occur in zone 1 and affect the superior aspect of the sacral ala and run parallel to the SI joint (Figure 7.3).[44] Fractures of zones 2 and 3 are more likely to present with neurologic symptoms. Early sacral BSI may not be evident on MRI or bone scan. If clinical suspicion exists, empiric treatment with repeat imaging several weeks later is recommended for diagnostic confirmation.[52]

Treatment

Prolonged return to play among collegiate track and field athletes with trabecular BSIs[4] supports a proposed medium-/moderate-risk classification for BSIs of the sacrum.[48] Most sacral BSI showed evidence of high-grade bone stress injury on MRI, which was also an independent risk factor for delayed return to sport.[4]

Management plans incorporate three main phases, which may vary in duration based on fracture location risk classification and stress injury grading on imaging as well as on underlying biological and biomechanical risk factors for healing such as nutrition and

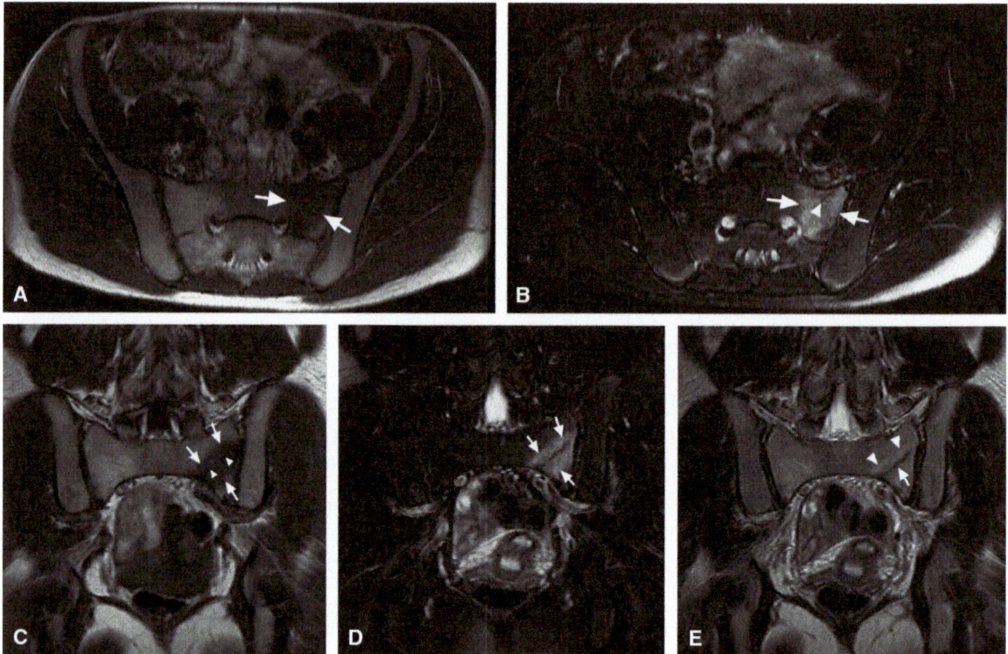

FIGURE 7.3 Sacral stress fracture in a 22-year-old female distance runner. (A) Axial T1-weighted image (TR = 520, TE = 14) shows hypointense edema signal in the left sacral ala (*arrows*). (B) Axial T2-weighted image with fat suppression (TR = 5460, TE = 75) shows a subtle low signal line (*arrowhead*) centered in the area of marrow edema (*arrows*). (C) Coronal T1-weighted image (TR = 500, TE = 14) again shows the marrow edema in the left sacrum (*arrows*), with a low signal line allowing the diagnosis of fracture. (D) Coronal T2-weighted image with fat suppression (TR = 4666, TE = 105) better demonstrates the fracture line centered in the edema (*arrows*). (E) Coronal T2-weighted scan inadvertently performed without fat suppression (TR = 4166, TE = 105) demonstrates the fracture line (*arrow*), but the extensive area of edema revealed with fat suppression (B and D) is barely detectable because of the bright marrow fat signal (*arrowheads*). Because of such diminished sensitivity for marrow changes, suppression of fat is considered mandatory for detection of stress injuries

RT, repetition time; TE, time to echo.

Source: Reproduced with permission from Fredericson M, Jennings F, Beaulieu C, et al. Stress fractures in athletes. *Top Magn Reson Imaging.* 2006;17(5):309–325.

bone health.[53] Phase 1 involves modified weight bearing until pain-free ambulation is achieved. Phase 2 involves early mobilization and nonimpact loading activities focused on correction of pelvic obliquity, strength imbalances, and core weakness.[50] Phase 3 involves sport-specific training and return to activity.[54] Most of the literature supports return to full activity in 3 to 4 months.[36,42,48,49,53]

OTHER PELVIC BONE STRESS INJURIES

Evaluation

Pubic rami BSIs have been reported in runners, Australian football players,[55] and military recruits.[56,57] They occur most often at the inferior pubic ramus near the pubic symphysis.[53,55] BSIs of the pubic symphysis are likely due to shearing forces created by repetitive contraction of the muscle groups attached to the bony pelvis, including the adductors, hamstrings, and rectus abdominis. They occur more commonly in women, possibly due to increased trabecular bone composition in the pelvis, which is sensitive to estrogen deficiency.[53] In female military recruits, inferior pubic rami BSIs were felt to be associated with overstriding, in which women were forced to keep in step with men despite shorter limb lengths. When these recruits were allowed to maintain a natural stride length, the incidence of pubic rami BSIs sharply declined.[56,57] Additionally, pubic rami BSIs may also occur in association with hip surgery.

Pain is usually of insidious onset in the inguinal, perineal, or adductor region and becomes worse with activity. Examination often reveals point tenderness at the pubic ramus and increased pain with loading such as the hop test. Differential diagnosis includes osteitis pubis, adductor or rectus injury, intrinsic hip pathology, or referred pain from the genitourinary and gastrointestinal systems. Plain radiographs may reveal increased sclerosis with or without a fracture line. MRI is the definitive test if initial radiographs are negative.

Treatment

Management is similar to that of sacral BSIs with a focus on pain-free ambulation, rehabilitation focused on adductor stretching, hip and core strengthening, and progression to sport-specific activities. Return to play is also similar to that for sacral BSIs as pubic rami BSIs are also considered moderate risk.[48] Most require 6 weeks of protected activity before sport-specific progression is begun, with return to sport in approximately 12 weeks.[48,53]

BSIs of the acetabulum are rare but have been reported in military endurance athletes, dancers, and cyclocross athletes.[58–60] Acetabular rim stress fractures have been associated with both femoroacetabular impingement and developmental dysplasia of the hip.[61,62]

Finally, ischial BSIs are exceedingly rare, with only a few case reports in the sports literature.[63,64] They usually present as insufficiency fractures or in association with hip surgery, such as acetabular osteotomies. Surgical fixation of a nonunion fracture has been reported in a collegiate football player.[64]

CONCLUSION

Trabecular BSIs of the femoral neck, sacrum, and pelvis have been associated with prolonged healing in comparison to the more prevalent cortical BSIs of the lower extremity. These BSIs often present with higher-grade injury on MRI at diagnosis, which is also predictive of a longer healing time frame.[4] These injuries require a high index of suspicion for early diagnosis and appropriate management to limit resultant morbidity and time away from sport. Multistep rehabilitation protocols that incorporate gradual increases in bone strain while addressing biomechanical and training errors will be most effective for injury recovery. Given that trabecular BSIs are more often associated with triad and RED-S risk factors than cortical BSIs, prevention through screening and multidisciplinary management of these underlying intrinsic risk factors are especially critical for injury prevention and treatment.[12,17]

KEY REFERENCE

Only key references appear in the print edition. The full reference list appears in the digital product found on http://connect.springerpub.com/content/book/978-0-8261-4424-9/part/sec02/chapter/ch07

13. Tenforde AS, Parziale AL, Popp KL, Ackerman KE. Low bone mineral density in male athletes is associated with bone stress injuries at anatomic sites with greater trabecular composition. *Am J Sports Med*. 2018;46(1):30–36. Epub 2017/10/06. doi:10.1177/0363546517730584. PubMed PMID: 28985103.

23. Goldin M, Anderson CN, Fredericson M, et al. Femoral neck stress fractures and imaging features of femoroacetabular impingement. *PM R*. 2015;7(6):584–592. Epub 2015/01/13. doi:10.1016/j.pmrj.2014.12.008. PubMed PMID: 25591871.

28. Ramey LN, McInnis KC, Palmer WE. Femoral neck stress fracture: can MRI grade help predict return-to-running time? *Am J Sports Med*. 2016;44(8):2122–2129. Epub 2016/06/03. doi:10.1177/0363546516648319. PubMed PMID: 27261475.

30. Liem BC, Truswell HJ, Harrast MA. Rehabilitation and return to running after lower limb stress fractures. *Curr Sports Med Rep*. 2013;12(3):200–207. doi:10.1249/JSR.0b013e3182913cbe. PubMed PMID: 23669091.

33. Nguyen JT, Peterson JS, Biswal S, et al. Stress-related injuries around the lesser trochanter in long-distance runners. *AJR Am J Roentgenol*. 2008;190(6):1616–1620. doi:10.2214/AJR.07.2513. PubMed PMID: 18492915.

36. Eller DJ, Katz DS, Bergman AG, et al. Sacral stress fractures in long-distance runners. *Clin J Sport Med*. 1997;7(3):222–225. PubMed PMID: 9262893.

42. Johnson AW, Weiss CB, Stento K, Wheeler DL. Stress fractures of the sacrum: an atypical cause of low back pain in the female athlete. *Am J Sports Med*. 2001;29(4):498–508. doi:10.1177/03635465010290042001. PubMed PMID: 11476393.

60. Williams TR, Puckett ML, Denison G, et al. Acetabular stress fractures in military endurance athletes and recruits: incidence and MRI and scintigraphic findings. *Skeletal Radiol*. 2002;31(5):277–281. Epub 2002/04/04. doi:10.1007/s00256-002-0485-0. PubMed PMID: 11981604.

CHAPTER 8

Spine Injuries

Erin Moix Grieb, Aleksei Dingel, James Policy,
and Kevin G. Shea

INTRODUCTION

Low back pain is a common complaint in pediatric and adolescent patients. Spondylolysis and spondylolisthesis are the most common causes of back pain in this population. Spondylolysis is an abnormality of the pars interarticularis of the neural arch. It can be unilateral or bilateral, with the L5 vertebrae the most commonly affected followed by L4,[1] although it can occur at other parts of the spine. It is thought of as a continuum of disease, including stress reaction, stress fracture, true spondylolysis, and spondylolisthesis.[2] Bone stress injury (BSI) is the continuum of disease from stress reaction to stress fracture. Stress reaction is "interosseous edema with surrounding sclerosis without cortical or trabecular disruption."[3] Stress fracture is a "disruption of trabecular or cortical bone of the pars without a bony gap or lysis."[3] Spondylolytic defect is a "complete disruption of the pars interarticularis with a gap and surrounding sclerosis at the edges of the defect."[3] Spondylolisthesis is "translation of one vertebral segment relative to the next caudal segment."[3]

Spondylolysis is an overuse BSI of the spine. Sheer stress of the lumbar spine is particularly high at the pars interarticularis,[4] contributing to risk of injury at this location in the vertebrae. The inferior articular process stresses the adjacent pars interarticularis of adjacent vertebrae during lumbar spine extension. Repetitive impacts can produce a stress reaction or stress fracture of the pars interarticularis. Bone marrow edema, noted on MRI, without visible fracture line is considered an early response to stress.[5,6] Injury to the bone may present initially as an early BSI and may progress into true fracture (spondylolysis) and potentially spondylolisthesis if not managed properly.[7]

Spondylolysis may be congenital or acquired. Family history, sex, and race may all play a role and may predispose an individual to spondylolysis.[8,9] Repetitive stress and overuse may be the primary culprit. A genetic predisposition to weak points in the pars has also been suggested,[9] as spondylolysis occurs in 15% to 70% of first-degree relatives.[9,10] It occurs in males two to three times more frequently than females; however, spondylolisthesis occurs in females two to three times more than males.[11] There are racial differences with prevalence in the white population two to three times more compared to that in the black population,[8] and the Inuit population has a rate of up to 25%.[12]

EPIDEMIOLOGY

The incidence of spondylolysis is 4.4% at the age of 6 years,[8] 4.4% to 4.7% in the general pediatric and adolescent populations, and 6% in the adult population.[13] The incidence in adolescent athletes is higher than in nonathletes, with reported incidence of symptomatic defects in young athletes varying between 15%[2,14] and 47%.[15] There is an increased incidence in those who participate in certain higher-risk sports that involve repetitive axial loading and rotation, particularly with hyperextension of lumbar spine. Gymnastics, weight lifting, ballet, wrestling, diving, rowing, volleyball, and football are sports that have some of the highest rates of spondylolysis among athletes.[4,16,17]

HISTORY AND EXAMINATION

Spondylolysis may be asymptomatic in many athletes. Athletes with symptomatic lesions generally present with low back pain that is made worse with sports-related activities. Insidious onset of pain is more common than symptoms following acute injury. Pain can be dull or achy to sharp; it typically worsens with activity, particularly lumbar hyperextension. The onset of pain often coincides with the onset of puberty and the adolescent growth spurt. The mean age of onset is between 15 and 16 years.[18] Pain may also be reported in the buttocks or posterior thigh.[2] Patients may also present with shoulder and/or localized neck pain.[19]

IMAGING

There is no universally accepted consensus for the imaging protocol to evaluate spondylolysis. Imaging used includes plain film radiographs, MRI, CT, bone scintigraphy (bone scan), and single-photon emission CT (SPECT) or SPECT-CT.[20]

Plain films, two views that include the anteroposterior and lateral views of the lumbosacral spine, are the initial study of choice due to low cost, low radiation, and efficacy (example of spondylolysis seen on AP view in Figure 8.1). With refractory courses or atypical presentations, advanced imaging should be considered.[21]

The gold standard to diagnose BSI of the pars interarticularis is MRI due to high sensitivity and no ionizing radiation. Prior to true spondylolysis, lower-grade BSI may be seen with bony edema,[22] which cannot be seen on plain films or CT. Pars abnormalities can be detected without the use of special sequences, such as with sagittal T2 and short tau inversion recovery (STIR) images (Figures 8.2 and 8.3); however, these may not be routine at all imaging centers and so may be useful in additional instructions when ordering. When possible, a 3 Tesla MRI should be obtained; the higher signal-to-noise ratio results in improved image quality and clinical efficiency.[23]

MRI findings in acute-to-subacute injuries include edema on T2 and STIR images at the pars interarticularis and/or pedicle. These are treated nonsurgically as outlined previously. MRI findings in chronic injuries include lytic lesion at pars interarticularis and are initially treated nonsurgically; if treatment fails, a CT may be obtained as a preoperative study.

CT and SPECT are sensitive diagnostic tools; however, high sensitivity comes with ionizing radiation use, often during periods of growth spurts. CT may be helpful in advanced cases to detect if a lytic defect has occurred (Figure 8.4).[21] To decrease the exposure to ionizing radiation, a limited CT should be obtained; thin cuts with 3D reconstruction should be requested for better visualization and potential surgical planning.

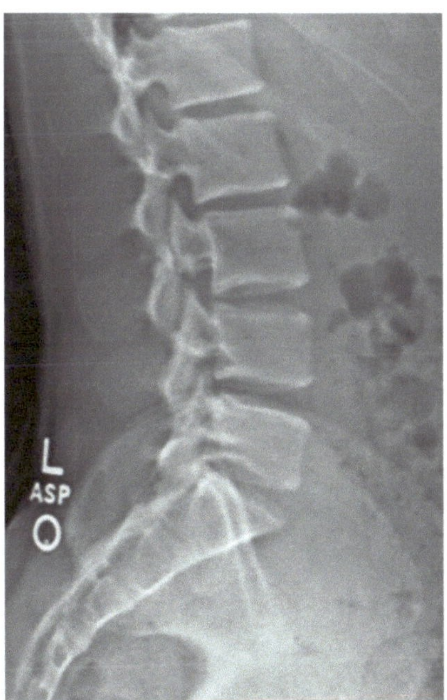

FIGURE 8.1 L3 pars defect without spondylolysthesis.

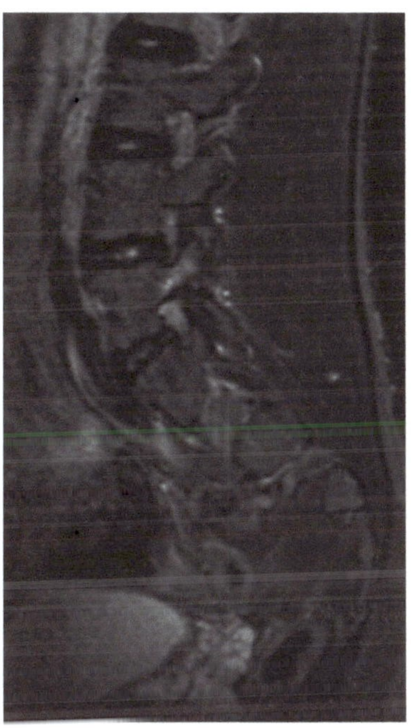

FIGURE 8.2 MRI sagital STIR sequence with bilateral L5 pars edema without lytic defect.

STIR, short tau inversion recovery.

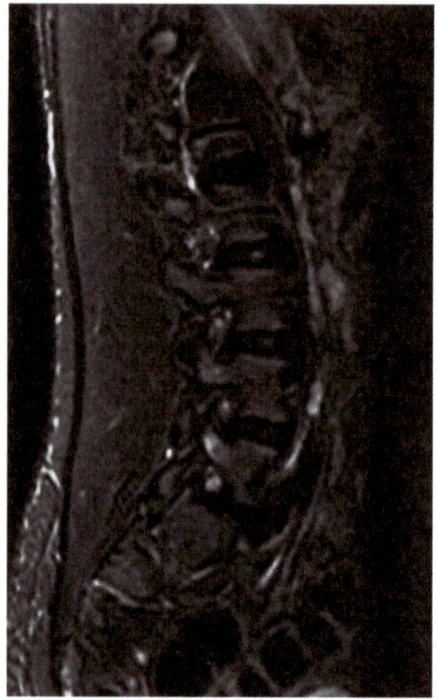

FIGURE 8.3 MRI sagital STIR sequence demonstrating L5 pars edema without lytic defect, less pronounced than in Figure 8.2.

STIR, short tau inversion recovery.

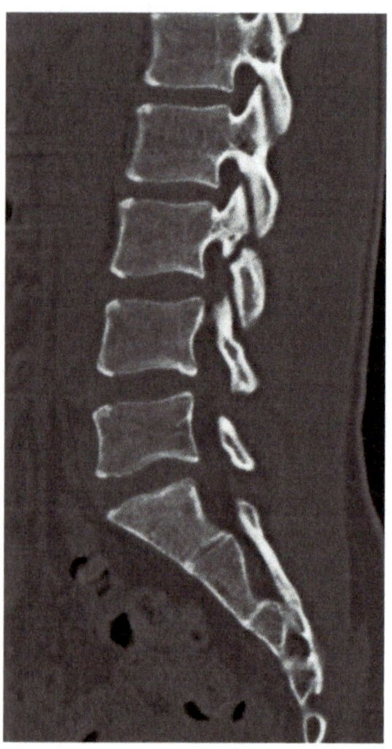

FIGURE 8.4 CT demonstrating L3 lytic lesion of the pars without spondylolysthesis.

TREATMENT/MANAGEMENT

Initial therapy of symptomatic spondylolysis should focus on conservative management to reduce pain and allow bony union, including rest, activity modification, and physical therapy, with or without adjunctive orthosis brace. Surgery is rarely indicated but may be considered after prolonged conservative treatment. Asymptomatic spondylolysis that is discovered incidentally does not typically require intervention.

Nonsurgical Treatment

Rest

There should be a period of rest from physical activities and sport until the patient is asymptomatic with hyperextension. Best outcomes may be achieved with 3 months' restriction from sports.[24] Pain management may also be a component of conservative management.

Activity Modification

For those with BSI, activity modification in which the patient refrains from all dynamic mobility and impact activities is recommended.

Physical Therapy

Intervention typically includes flexibility exercises, body mechanics, and strengthening of core and upper and lower extremities accomplished through physical therapy (PT). Tightness of hamstrings and hip flexors can lead to compensatory lumbar extension, so these deficiencies need to be addressed. The final portion of PT focuses on return to sport activity with sport-specific conditioning and achievement of proper mechanics prior to returning to sport. With return after lumbar spine BSI, athletes should avoid exercises that

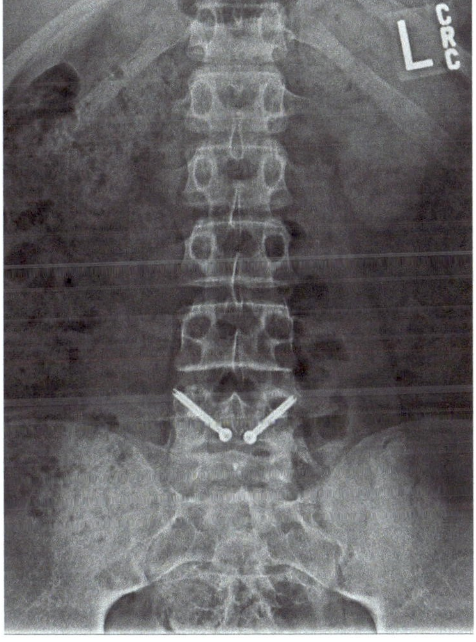

FIGURE 8.5 AP view, showing bilateral L5 Buck's screws.

AP, anteroposterior.

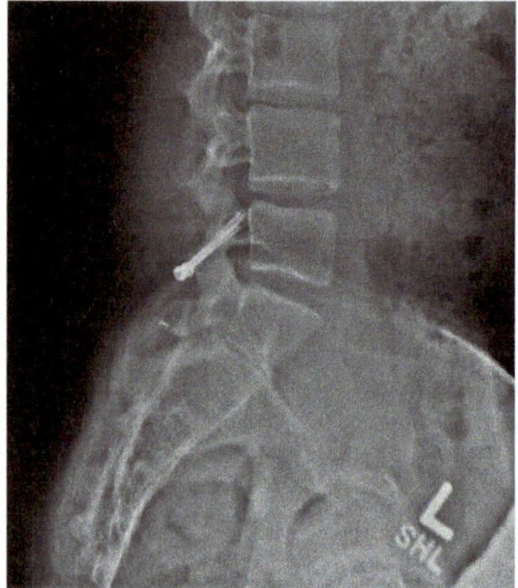

FIGURE 8.6 Lateral view showing bilateral L5 Buck's screws.

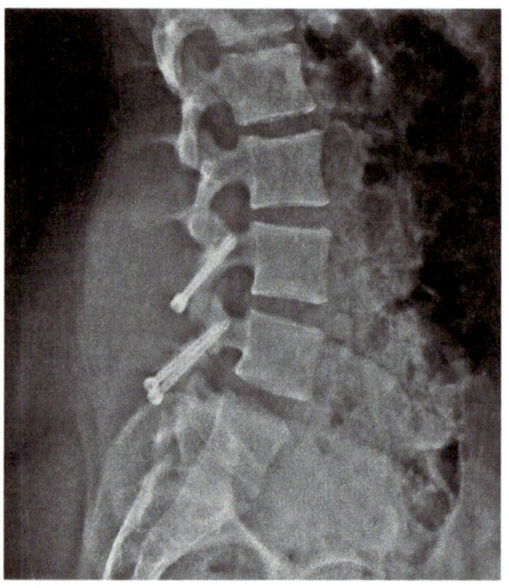

FIGURE 8.7 Lateral view showing bilateral L4 and L5 Buck's screws.

encourage lumbar extension (deadlifts, Olympic squats) and avoid excessive rotation through thoracic spine as this can contribute to recurrent injury. Time of initiation varies, though early initiation (<10 weeks) has been shown to make full return to sport sooner.[25]

Brace

Thoracolumbosacral and lumbosacral[26] orthoses are available in rigid and flexible variations. Antilordotic orthotic treatment can be used, but its effectiveness has been debated. Klein et al.[26] found that bracing did not affect clinical outcome in nonoperative patients. Sairyo et al.[27] found that those with early stage defects had a 90% heal rate at 3 months. Recommendations for full-time rigid orthosis include use for 4 to 12 weeks (20 hours/day) until asymptomatic.[28–29]

Authors are divided on brace use. In patients with edema on MRI at pars interarticularis and/or pedicle, James Policy (JP) recommends rigid brace wear for 23 hours/day × 6 weeks (modified Boston Brace protocol), followed by a course of PT. Erin Moix Grieb (EMG) recommends activity modification followed by PT once pain free; if PT fails, brace

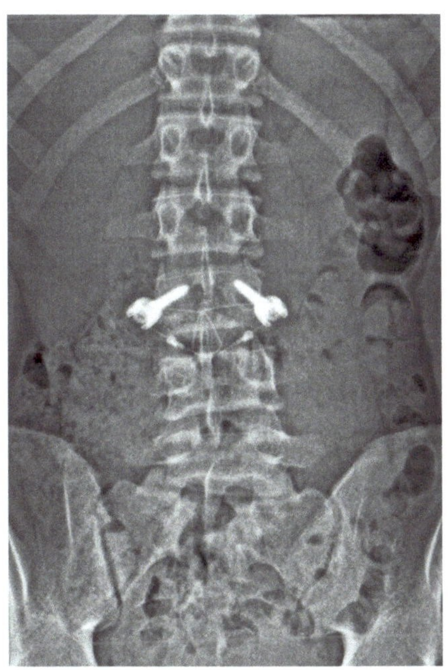

FIGURE 8.8 AP view showing bilateral L3 pedicle screw/tension band fixation technique.

AP, anteroposterior.

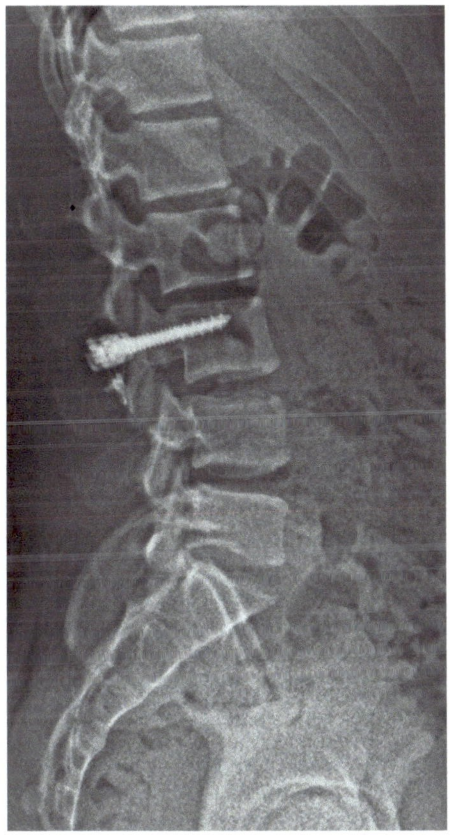

FIGURE 8.9 Lateral view showing bilateral pedicle screw/tension band technique.

use is then considered. Of note, JP rarely requires treatment of patients with less than 3 months of back pain, while EMG treatment for patients with acute onset of back pain.

Ultrasound

Recent research suggests that low-intensity pulsed ultrasound, when combined with standard conservative management techniques, is an effective treatment for promotion of healing early state spondylolysis; treatment duration was shortened with earlier return to sport.[30] While this is not currently a standard technique used in the management of early state spondylolysis, recent research is promising.

Surgical Treatment

Surgical management is typically reserved for cases of spondylolisthesis or disabling symptoms despite conservative care.[31,32] Preserving segmental spinal motion typically results in best outcomes and is achieved with direct pars interarticularis repair.[32] Multiple operative techniques are used: Buck repair, Scott repair, Morscher repair, and pedicle screw-based repair (examples seen in Figures 8.5–8.9). A comparison study by Mohammed et al. demonstrated that the pedicle screw-based direct pars repair had the highest fusion rate and the lowest complication rate.[32]

Adolescents diagnosed and treated conservatively early prior to true spondylolysis (negative radiographs, positive MRI) achieve "good" or "excellent" outcomes at the rate of 93% at an average of 13 months[33] and 91% at 9 years.[34] Return to sport is achieved in 92.2% and 90.3% of adolescent athletes treated nonoperatively and operatively, respectively.[35]

CONCLUSION

Pediatric and adolescent athletes are specializing at earlier ages and are at increased risk for overuse injuries, including spondylolysis. Appropriate diagnosis is achieved through detailed history and physical examination, with initial confirmatory studies of AP and lateral radiographs, MRI, and/or rarely a CT scan. Most patients heal with conservative management consisting of rest, activity modification, possible antilordotic orthosis, and subsequent PT. When conservative management fails, surgical repair may be needed but is rarely indicated.

KEY REFERENCES

Only key references appear in the print edition. The full reference list appears in the digital product found on http://connect.springerpub.com/content/book/978-0-8261-4424-9/part/sec02/chapter/ch08

1. Blanda J, Bethem D, Moats W, Lew M. Defects of pars interarticularis in athletes: a protocol for nonoperative treatment. *J Spinal Disord*. 1993;6(5):406–411.

17. Congeni J, McCulloch J, Swanson K. Lumbar spondylolysis. A study of natural progression in athletes. *Am J Sports Med*. 1997;25(2):248–253.

26. Klein G, Mehlman CT, McCarty M. Nonoperative treatment of spondylolysis and grade I spondylolisthesis in children and young adults: a meta-analysis of observational studies. *J Pediatr Orthop*. 2009;29(2):146–156.

28. Steiner ME, Micheli LJ. Treatment of symptomatic spondylolysis and spondylolisthesis with the modified Boston brace. *Spine (Phila Pa 1976)*. 1985;10(10):937–943.

32. Mohammed N, Patra DP, Narayan V, et al. A comparison of the techniques of direct pars interarticularis repairs for spondylolysis and low-grade spondylolisthesis: a meta-analysis. *Neurosurg Focus*. 2018;44(1):E10.

CHAPTER 9

Foot and Ankle Low-Risk Injuries

Stephanie R. Douglas, Karen L. Troy, and Adam S. Tenforde

INTRODUCTION

The metatarsals are a common site of bone injuries in the athletic population, with an incidence second only to injuries of the tibia.[1] Bone stress injuries (BSIs) result when repetitive stress to the bones of the forefoot or midfoot, such as with running, jumping, dancing, and other repetitive weight-bearing activities, exceeds the bone's capacity for remodeling.[2–4]

Metatarsal stress injuries make up 38% of all stress fractures of the lower extremity, with 90% of all metatarsal stress fractures occurring in the 2nd, 3rd, and 4th metatarsals.[5,6] First metatarsal stress fractures are rare due to the larger diameter of the bone. Stress injuries of the metatarsal shaft are generally considered low risk due to their tendency to heal with conservative treatment without complications.[3] Cuboid injuries are less common but may be seen in ballet dancers, runners, and gymnasts or in association with injury to the plantar fascia.[7] Injuries to the cuneiform are rare and have been reported in track and field sprinters, who experience high stress through the medial cuneiform during the propulsive phase of the gait cycle.[4]

This chapter describes the risk factors associated with metatarsal shaft, cuboid, and cuneiform injuries as well as their clinical evaluation and management. Injuries to the navicular, sesamoid, and base of the 5th metatarsal are considered high-risk injuries and require more aggressive management and are discussed in Chapter 10.

A number of biological risk factors are thought to contribute to a predisposition to BSIs, primarily by serving as causes or indicators of diminished bone strength (Table 9.1). Prior fracture is perhaps the most robust predictor of future bone injury, with one study showing a sixfold increased risk for developing a fracture seen among girls with a history of fracture.[8,9] Genetics are known to influence fracture risk, and associations have been identified at loci both with and without a known role in bone biology.[10] Low bone mineral density (BMD) is an independent risk factor for BSIs in females and increased healing time from a BSI in males.[9,18] Medications that affect BMD, interfere with cell turnover or inhibit absorption of nutrients involved in bone integrity can increase susceptibility to fracture and include contraceptives, steroids, antacids, anticonvulsants, and antidepressants.[9,11,12] Nutritional deficiencies, particularly of calcium and vitamin D, resulting from disordered eating, restrictive diets, or malabsorption syndromes, can likewise contribute to poor bone health and elevated fracture risk.[9,11,13–17] Female athletes

RISK FACTORS FOR DEVELOPING MIDFOOT AND METATARSAL BONE STRESS INJURIES

BIOLOGICAL	BIOMECHANICAL
Prior fracture[8,9]	Anatomic factors
Genetics[10]	Leg-length discrepancy[20–23]
Medications (contraceptives, steroids, antacids, anticonvulsants, antidepressants)[9,11,12]	Smaller calf girth[23]
Nutritional deficiencies (calcium, vitamin D)[9,11,13–17]	Dorsal or plantar-flexed metatarsals[20]
Disordered eating	Excessively tight gastrocnemius muscles[20]
Restrictive diets	Thin tibial cortex/lower tibial cross-sectional area[24]
Malabsorption syndromes	Longer metatarsal length[3,37]
Female sex[38–40]	Pes planus[26]
Amenorrhea[39,41]	Plantar fasciotomy[28]
Low BMD[9,18]	Foot weakness/fatigue[27–29]
	Dynamic loading patterns
	Low dynamic arch index, low foot abduction, or delayed forefoot loading[30]
	High average and instantaneous vertical loading rate[31]
	Non-rearfoot strike pattern[32,33]
	Extrinsic factors
	Chronic overload or abrupt increase in training volume or intensity[8,34]
	Changes in training surface or footwear[34–36]

BMD, bone mineral density.

are at greater risk for BSIs than males, with sex-specific differences arising from the interrelationship of energy availability, menstrual function, and BMD.

Anatomic factors that increase forces through the metatarsals and bones of the midfoot confer elevated risk of bone injury. Leg-length discrepancy, smaller calf girth, dorsal or plantarflexed metatarsals, and excessively tight gastrocnemius muscles are all associated with increased BSI risk in an athletic population.[19–23] A thinner tibial cortex and lower tibial cross-sectional area have been noted in females with lower limb stress fracture.[24] Longer metatarsal length increases the lever arm of the ground reaction force during running, causing a larger bending moment. This increased bending moment is transmitted through the associated ray of the foot and may contribute to fractures of the metatarsal base, as seen with injury to the 2nd metatarsal.[3,4] Of note, one study of the contributions of BMD and geometry to 2nd metatarsal strength demonstrated that failure load was most strongly influenced by mid-shaft cortical volumetric BMD and metatarsal base height, with larger values being associated with stronger bone.[25]

A greater incidence of 2nd and 3rd metatarsal stress fractures is seen with pes planus, which may be associated with foot weakness.[26] Foot weakness may more generally increase BSI risk as well, as the foot intrinsic muscles attenuate skeletal loading and may decrease metatarsal bending. A study of college soccer players found weaker toe flexion in the 5th metatarsal BSI group compared to the noninjury group, and a cadaveric model demonstrated increased strain on the 2nd metatarsal in a simulation of plantarflexor fatigue.[27,28] Similarly, increased maximal force, peak pressure, and impulse were observed under the 2nd and 3rd metatarsal head and the medial forefoot at the end of a fatiguing run.[29] In a cadaveric study using a gait simulator, 2nd metatarsal strain increased by 100% with plantar fasciotomy, suggesting that this and other structures supporting the arch play an important role in preventing overload of the metatarsals.[28]

Dynamic loading patterns associated with 2nd metatarsal injury include lower dynamic arch index and lower foot abduction, while delayed forefoot loading during running is a risk factor for 3rd metatarsal injury.[30] In a meta-analysis of the relationship between ground reaction force and tibial and metatarsal stress fractures, higher average and instantaneous vertical loading rates were observed in the stress fracture group compared to the noninjured group.[31] A non-rearfoot strike pattern results in transmission of higher loads to the forefoot and may increase rates of metatarsal injury.[32,33] Notably, studies investigating the influence of load rates on metatarsus and midfoot BSIs have not been published.

Extrinsic factors related to training progression and training context can contribute to bone injury risk. Abrupt increases in training volume or intensity, or chronic overload, may result in the accumulation of microdamage that exceeds the ability of bone to remodel. Running volumes in excess of 32 km (20 miles) per week correlate with BSI risk.[8,34] Changes in training surface or footwear can lead to altered biomechanical forces and stress fracture development.[34] In particular, transitioning from standard to minimalist footwear has been shown to increase strain on all metatarsals by 28.7% and increase the probability of bone failure according to a mathematical model.[35] Additionally, case reports suggest that an abrupt transition to minimalist footwear may contribute to the development of metatarsal stress fractures in some individuals.[36] Hypothetically, poorly fitting shoes may elevate injury risk as well, due to abnormal shear forces and altered foot strike mechanics.

METATARSAL SHAFT

Evaluation

Fractures of the metatarsal shafts are considered low-risk injuries with a good prognosis for healing. With BSIs of metatarsal shafts 2 to 5, an early finding on MRI is periosteal reaction with possible cortical lucency (Figures 9.1 and 9.2).[42] This is in contrast to 1st metatarsal injuries, which often show sclerosis with no periosteal reaction.[42] More advanced injuries demonstrate periosteal edema, bone marrow edema, and fracture line and may be associated with surrounding soft tissue edema.[42]

Presenting symptoms of a BSI of the foot are often insidious and include localized pain at the site of injury exacerbated by impact or weight bearing, sometimes with edema or skin discoloration in the case of advanced injuries.[3,42,43] When there is suspicion for a BSI, clinicians should take a thorough history with assessment of the risk factors outlined above. In athletes, a training history should be obtained, including baseline training volume and intensity, type of footwear, frequency of competition, and any recent changes from the normal pattern of activity.[8,34-36] A dietary history should be recorded, including estimated daily servings of calcium and vitamin D and any foods typically avoided.[9,11,13] Female athletes should be screened for triad risk factors such as disordered eating behaviors, menstrual dysfunction, history of fractures, and history of low BMD.[8,9,39,41] Patients should be asked about any family history of low BMD or orthopedic issues. Medications should be noted, with particular attention paid to hormonal

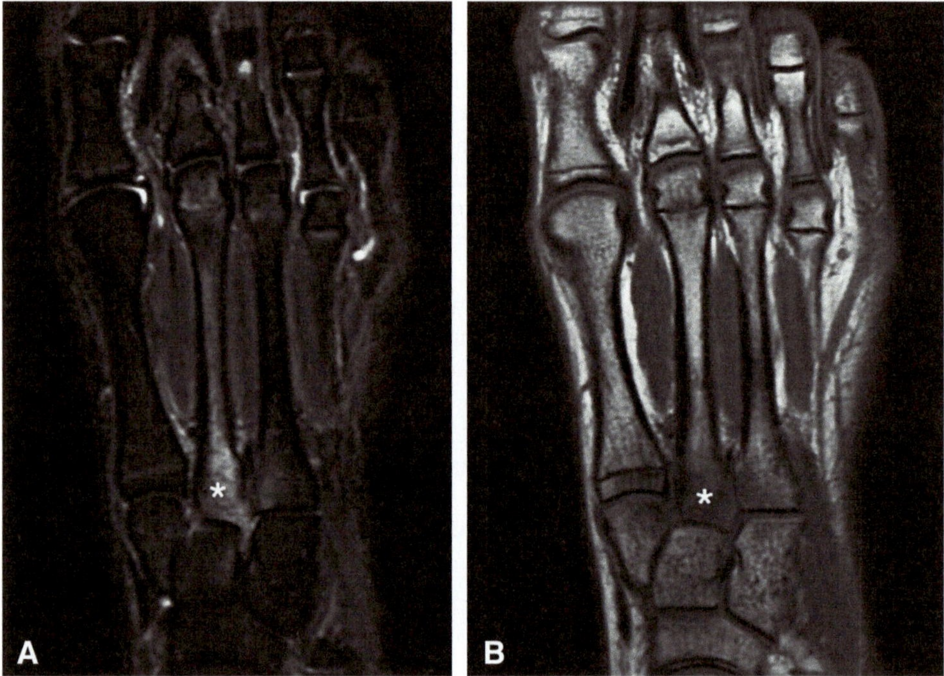

FIGURE 9.1 (A) MRI with long axis STIR showing marrow edema of the left 2nd metatarsal (*indicated by asterisk*) consistent with grade 3 bone stress injuries. (B) Corresponding loss of T1 signal indicating grade 3 injury.

STIR, short tau inversion recovery.

medications (contraceptives, estrogen, and progesterone), steroids, antacids, anticonvulsants, and antidepressants.[9,11,12]

In the setting of BSIs, physical examination often reveals focal bony tenderness to palpation as well as pain with percussion. Swelling or bruising may be evident.[3,43] The single-leg hop test is sensitive to bone injuries of the foot and is positive if it reproduces the index pain, although caution is needed in using this test if a more advanced injury is suspected to avoid further injury.[3] Following a history and physical examination, x-ray is often the first step in diagnosis but it has a poor sensitivity for early BSIs and injury to certain anatomic locations (cuboid, cuneiform).[2,42,44] MRI is the preferred modality for evaluating suspected bone injury, as it allows for assessment of injury severity (particularly important in athletes) and avoids exposure to ionizing radiation.[2] MRI demonstrates periosteal or bone marrow edema with lower-grade BSIs as well as a low-signal intensity fracture line, defined as grade 4 BSIs or stress fracture.[45] Ultrasound is a low-cost alternative to MRI, with good sensitivity and specificity for diagnosis of early metatarsal stress fractures.[46]

Management varies by location but primarily consists of activity restriction and immobilization with a gradual return to sport following a period of healing. Considerations for specific sites of injury are outlined in the following. If needed, pain can be managed with ice and acetaminophen. Nonsteroidal antiinflammatory drugs are controversial due to concerns that they may have a detrimental effect on bone healing.[47,48]

In conjunction with treating the injury, clinicians should seek to reduce modifiable risk factors to prevent future injury. Physical therapy plays an important role in correcting biomechanical risk factors as well as addressing the stiffness and mobility deficits

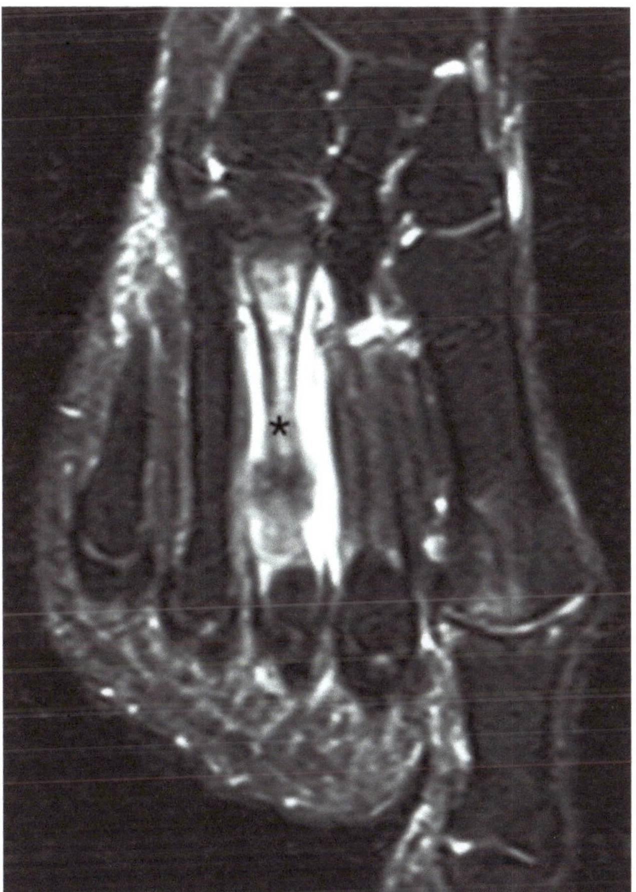

FIGURE 9.2 MRI with T2 images showing significant bone marrow and periosteal edema with fracture line consistent with grade 4 injury of the 3rd metatarsal.

resulting from immobilization and activity restriction. Educating the patient on appropriate training techniques, training progressions, and recovery, as well as proper footwear, may be helpful.[8,34-36] Nutritional optimization is important due to its critical role in maintaining bone health, and patients should be counseled to obtain adequate calcium and vitamin D in addition to meeting their energy requirements.[49,50]

Treatment

The mainstay of treatment of metatarsal shaft BSIs is activity restriction and avoidance of activities that cause pain. For many injuries, a firm-sole shoe with metatarsal pad may allow for pain-free ambulation; however, immobilization with a walking boot may be required for some if walking is painful.[51] Repeat radiographs may be considered at 4 to 6 weeks if a fracture line was present on initial imaging or by clinical judgment.[3] Gradual return to sport may begin when the site of injury is nonpainful and radiographs provide evidence of healing. Most injuries of the metatarsal shaft show sufficient healing by 6 to 8 weeks to tolerate progressive loading.[3] Experimental evidence suggests that shockwave therapy may speed healing by increasing blood flow and stimulating cell growth and proliferation.[52-54] The majority of metatarsal shaft injuries heal with nonoperative treatment, but early operative intervention may be considered if there is dorsiflexion of the fracture. Late operative intervention is indicated for symptomatic nonunion.[6]

BASE OF 2ND METATARSAL

Evaluation

Injuries to the base of the 2nd metatarsal are distinct from injuries to metatarsal shafts 2 to 5 and demonstrate a high rate of nonunion, especially if the fracture involves the metatarsal–cuneiform joint.[42,56] Fractures of the 2nd metatarsal base are most commonly seen in ballet dancers and occur as a result of repetitive extreme plantar flexion, but they may also be seen in runners. A long 2nd metatarsal (Morton toe) and a naturally pronated foot are risk factors for this injury due to increased force transmission through the 2nd ray of the foot.[3,4] Additionally, poor ankle plantarflexion may lead to early heel lift off during running, which increases metatarsal forces and causes excessive plantar flexion at the Lisfranc joint.[55] Both of these factors have been associated with elevated risk of injury.[4,43]

Treatment

Treatment consists of rest and weight-bearing immobilization for a minimum of 4weeks along with use of crutches for non–weight-bearing status, with possible adjunctive shockwave therapy.[52,56–58] In some cases of persistent pain or site of injury at 2nd metatarsal, bone healing may be confirmed with radiographs and a pain-free clinical examination prior to weaning from a walking boot. Risk of reinjury can be reduced by use of custom foot orthosis with metatarsal pad beneath the 2nd metatarsal.[3]

CUBOID AND CUNEIFORM

Stress injuries of the cuboid and cuneiform are rare, though this may be partially due to under-diagnosis as they are often radiographically occult.[4,42] MRI is the preferred modality for evaluating suspected injury and shows bone marrow edema, along with a low-signal intensity line if fracture is present. Other causes of cuboid bone marrow edema include altered foot mechanics and reactive edema from peroneal tendon injury.[42] Plantar fascia rupture or plantar fasciotomy can lead to destabilization of the lateral column of the foot and increased force on the peroneus longus tendon, which runs along the undersurface of the cuboid.[42,59] Likewise, risk of cuneiform injury is elevated in the setting of plantar fascia pathology.[60] Stress fractures of the cuboid and cuneiform rarely displace and are usually responsive to conservative treatment. Successful treatment has been reported using immobilization in a walking boot followed by gradual reintroduction to sport as early as 6 weeks.[61]

CONCLUSION

BSIs of the foot and particularly the metatarsals are common among athletes. Risk factors are both biological and biomechanical and include behavioral, anatomic, and external contributors. MRI is the preferred modality for diagnosis when x-ray is negative, and imaging may demonstrate periosteal and bone marrow edema with possible fracture line depending on the severity of the injury. With the exception of injuries to the 5th metatarsal and 2nd metatarsal base, injuries of the metatarsals, cuboid, and cuneiforms are often responsive to conservative treatment consisting of activity modification and a possible period of immobilization followed by a gradual return to sport upon clinical and radiographic evidence of healing.

KEY REFERENCES

Only key references appear in the print edition. The full reference list appears in the digital product found on http://connect.springerpub.com/content/book/978-0-8261-4424-9/part/sec02/chapter/ch09

3. Tenforde AS, Kraus E, Fredericson M. Bone stress injuries in runners. *Phys Med Rehabil Clin N Am.* 2016;27:139–149. doi:10.1016/j.pmr.2015.08.008

8. Tenforde AS, Sayres LC, McCurdy ML, et al. Identifying sex-specific risk factors for stress fractures in adolescent runners. *Med Sci Sports Exerc.* 2013;45:1843–1851. doi:10.1249/MSS.0b013e3182963d75

42. Mandell JC, Khurana B, Smith SE. Stress fractures of the foot and ankle, part 2: site-specific etiology, imaging, and treatment, and differential diagnosis. *Skeletal Radiol.* 2017;46:1165–1186. doi:10.1007/s00256-017-2632-7

45. Fredericson M, Gabrielle Bergman A, Hoffman KL, Dillingham MS. Tibial stress reaction in runners: correlation of clinical symptoms and scintigraphy with a new magnetic resonance imaging grading system. *Am J Sports Med.* 1995;23:472–481. doi:10.1177/036354659502300418

50. Mountjoy M, Sundgot-Borgen JK, Burke LM, et al. IOC consensus statement on relative energy deficiency in sport (RED-S): 2018 update. *Br J Sports Med.* 2018;52:687–697. doi:10.1136/bjsports-2018-099193

CHAPTER 10

Foot and Ankle High-Risk Injuries

David E. Oji

INTRODUCTION

Bone stress injuries (BSIs) in the foot and ankle can be divided into higher risk- and lower-risk anatomical locations for injury (Figures 10.1 and 10.2). This is based on differences in biomechanics, anatomical factors such as blood supply, and the specific considerations for populations treated such as athletes. The focus on this chapter is to review BSIs in high-risk locations, separated by anatomy, with details on evaluation and management.

TARSAL NAVICULAR BONE STRESS INJURY

Evaluation

Tarsal navicular BSIs are high-risk injuries that account for 14% to 25% of all stress fractures, with the highest incidence of these injuries occurring in sports that involve explosive movements, rapid cutting, and jumping.[1-4] These sports include basketball, football, track and field sports, rugby, and basketball.[5-7] These injuries are important to identify as nonunion risk is much higher compared to other BSIs in the body.

The navicular is a concave bone that articulates with the talus, cuneiform, and cuboid. The posterior tibialis tendon inserts on the medial aspect of the bone. The talus and navicular, along with the cuboid and calcaneus, make up the transverse tarsal joints.

Biomechanically, the navicular and the rest of the transverse tarsal joints play an important role in allowing the hindfoot to pivot with the forefoot during the gait cycle. When the heel is inverted due to the pull of the posterior tibialis tendon, the transverse tarsal joint becomes rigid, preparing the foot for push off. It is during this push-off phase when the compressive forces to the navicular are generated through the 1st and 2nd metatarsocuneiform joints.[1] In conjunction with the pull of the posterior tibialis tendon medially, this creates a zone of maximal tensile load at the central third of the navicular body.

Furthermore, the central third is a watershed area of relatively poor blood supply, where the medial aspect is supplied by the posterior tibialis artery and laterally by the dorsalis pedis artery. As a result, this relatively avascular central third is prone to BSIs.

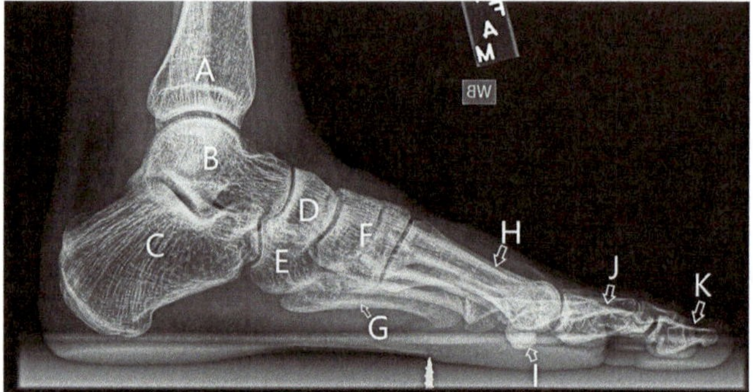

FIGURE 10.1 Bony anatomy of the foot and ankle on a lateral x-ray: (A) tibia, (B) talus, (C) calcaneus, (D) navicular, (E) cuboid, (F) cuneiform, (G) 5th metatarsal, (H) 1st metatarsal, (I) sesamoid, (J) proximal phalanx, and (K) distal phalanx.

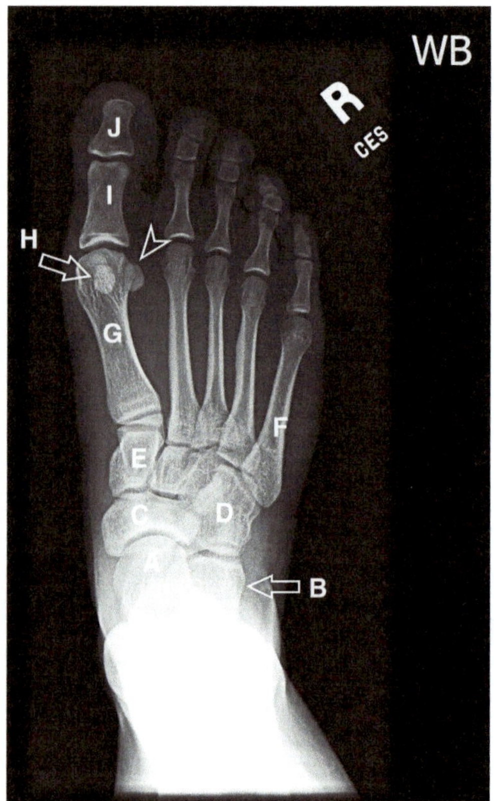

FIGURE 10.2 Bony anatomy of the foot and ankle on an AP x-ray: (A) talus, (B) calcaneus, (C) navicular, (D) cuboid, (E) cuneiform, (F) 5th metatarsal, (G) 1st metatarsal, (H) tibial sesamoid, (I) proximal phalanx, (J) distal phalanx, and (*arrowhead*) fibular sesamoid.

AP, anteroposterior.

Risks for navicular BSI can be divided into biological and biomechanical factors. Biological factors include medications (i.e., steroids), consequences of low energy availability, and insufficient vitamin D. Biomechanical factors are improper training regimen, changes in exercise intensity, and low bone mineral density.[8] Navicular BSI–specific risks include the hypovascularity seen in the central third of the bone, long 2nd ray or shortened 1st ray, metatarsus adductus, reduced ankle dorsiflexion, cavus foot, talar beaking, and stiffness in the subtalar joint.[9]

Clinically, patients present with vague pain around the dorsal proximal midfoot or the area overlying the navicular bone. The discomfort can be dorsal and even on the plantar aspect of the foot. Symptoms are generally worsened by activities especially when pushing off or landing. Many athletes have point-specific pain overlying the navicular on palpation, described as the "N" spot.[10] Swelling is uncommon. Hopping may reproduce the index pain.[1] Plain radiographs are typically normal, with sensitivity of detecting a fracture at only 33%.[2,3]

Advanced imaging is recommended when suspecting BSI of the navicular. MRI is the best modality to identify bone edema and stress reaction. Furthermore, it can help rule out other soft tissue or bony injuries to the area. If there is a high suspicion of a stress fracture on MRI as opposed to a stress reaction even if a fracture line is not visible on the MRI, a CT scan is recommended (Figure 10.3).[11] MRI alone may miss a potential fracture with a sensitivity of 71.4%.[12] Furthermore, CT scan can be used during treatment to evaluate fracture healing and ensure that union of the fracture has been obtained prior to returning to play.

A classification based on CT scan has been described.[13] Type I involves fracture through only the dorsal cortex. Type II involves fracture through the navicular body, with type III involving the second cortex. Severity of the fracture pattern such as a complete fracture, displacement, presence of avascular necrosis, subchondral sclerosis, and cystic changes may be associated with increased risk of nonunion and delay in fracture healing.[13,14]

Treatment

Navicular BSI have been shown to have a high union rate with the appropriate treatment that involves non–weight bearing for a minimum of 6 weeks. Whether the patient is treated with a short leg cast or operative fixation, non–weight bearing is critical for fracture union. Treatment involving protected weight bearing or partial weight bearing has a high rate of delayed union or nonunion. A meta-analysis done by Torg et al. in 2010 reported that only 47% of patients treated with weight bearing and rest had a successful outcome, with return to play at 5.7 months compared to 96% when treated with 6 weeks of non–weight bearing in a cast. Return to play for the non–weight-bearing group was 3.7 months.[15] Khan et al. reported a similar high rate of union with conservative management, with an 86% union rate and return to play at 5.6 months. In patients treated with non–weight bearing for a duration less than 6 weeks, only 69% of patients were able to return to activities. Finally, in individuals who had no activity restrictions, only 20% were able to return to play.[2]

Complications from nonoperative treatment in general are low especially when treated with non–weight-bearing casts or tall walking boots for 6 weeks to maintain proper foot position in neutral dorsiflexion. Unfortunately, there are no studies that report specifically on fracture recurrence treated conservatively. In one study, the authors reported a recurrence rate of 11.2% in patients treated without surgery and 6 weeks of non–weight bearing.[12]

Other conservative treatment methods can augment standard treatment, such as bone stimulator, vitamin D supplementation, and teriparatide use. However, these

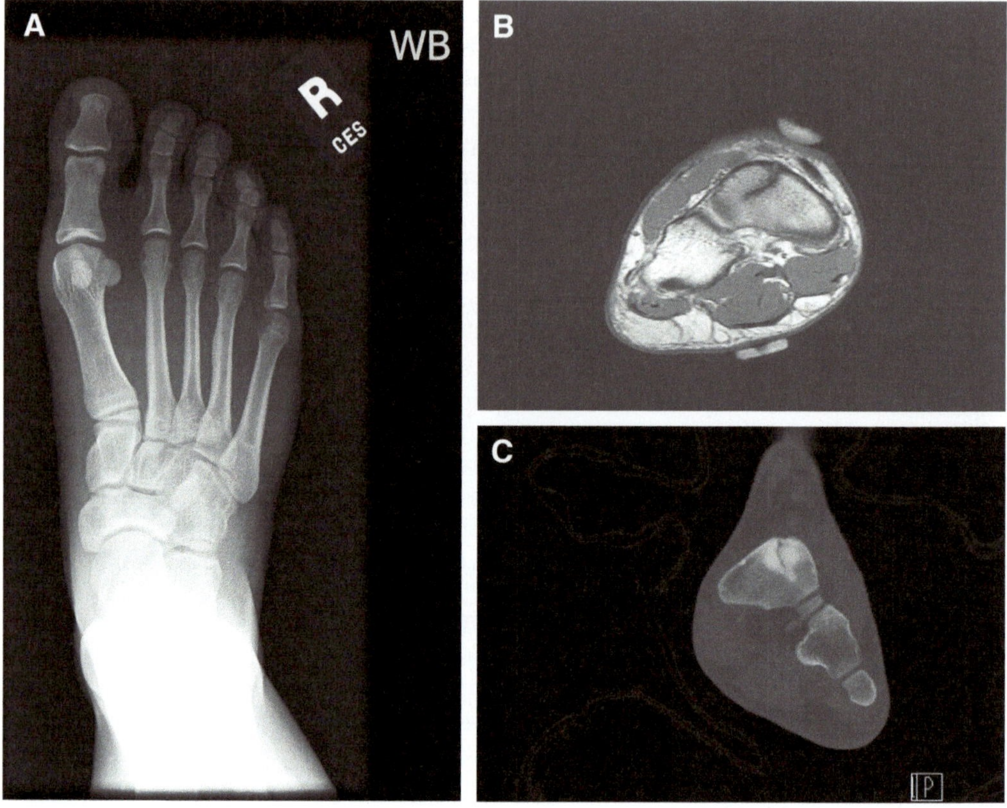

FIGURE 10.3 Eighteen-year-old gymnast with several weeks of dorsal proximal foot pain. (A) Initial x-rays were normal. MRI and subsequent CT were obtained. (B) Coronal T1-weighted MRI demonstrating a dorsal cortical defect of the navicular consistent with a stress fracture. (C) Coronal CT scan showing the type II navicular stress fracture with sclerotic bone.

modalities should not be used to supplant standard treatment methods as evidence for their efficacy is limited.

Absolute indications for surgical treatment include displaced fractures, presence of cystic formation, avascular necrosis, sclerotic bone, and fracture nonunion. Relative indications are delayed union, recurrence of the fracture, and complete fractures (type III) in elite athletes who cannot tolerate conservative management. For partial fractures or nondisplaced complete fractures, percutaneous screw fixation can be done without need for open reduction internal fixation. If there is fracture displacement or dorsal sclerotic bone, resection of the sclerotic bone and bone graft is recommended. Complications include hardware pain, nerve irritation, infection, nonunion, and recurrence of fracture. Saxena et al. reported that 7 of the 42 surgically treated patients required hardware removal (11.2%) and 1 patient (2%) developed complex regional pain syndrome that resolved with removal of hardware.[12] In individuals with more severe fracture patterns, such as displaced fractures and presence of cyst formation, time to healing may be delayed. In these individuals, surgery is recommended.[13,16] In displaced fractures, nonunion risk even with bone graft can be as high as 20%.[14]

Torg et al. in their meta-analysis reported that 82% of patients had a successful outcome when treated with surgery.[15] In a systematic review done by Mallee et al., the mean time to return to play was 16.4 weeks in the surgically treated patients versus 21.7

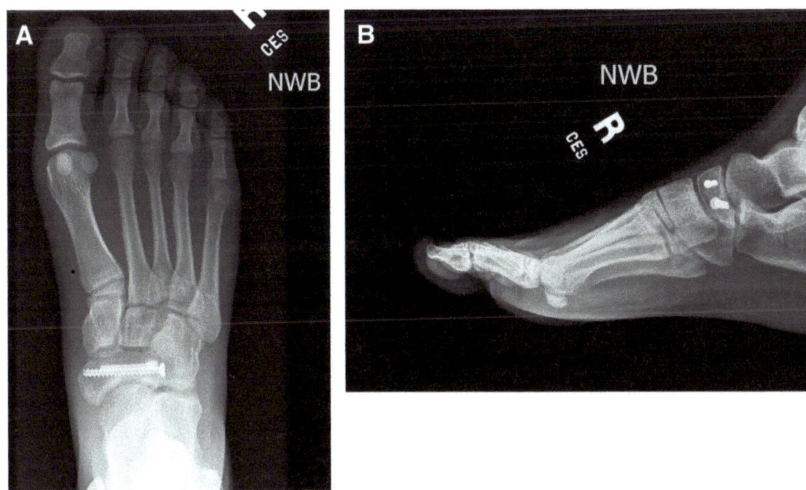

FIGURE 10.4 (A) Postsurgical plain radiographs demonstrating lateral to medial screw fixation. (B) Screws are placed on the dorsal and plantar halves of the navicular.

weeks in patients treated in non–weight-bearing casts for greater than 6 weeks.[17] Other studies reported no difference in return to play with non–weight-bearing treatment versus surgical fixation.[12,15,16] The rates of long-term posttraumatic arthritis after a stress fracture to the navicular regardless of treatment are unknown.

The author's preferred treatment for elite athletes is surgical fixation with a single partially threaded cannulated screw for type I fractures or two parallel screws for type II and type III fractures. Screws are placed lateral to medial to reduce injury to the posterior tibialis tendon and minimize hardware irritation. It is imperative that the screws be placed where the fracture is located and perpendicular to the fracture line (Figure 10.4). Iliac crest bone graft is used to augment fixation with any fracture displacement. If the navicular stress fracture has areas of avascular necrosis, subchondral sclerosis, or cystic formation, debridement of the abnormal bone and bone graft is done. Postoperative rehabilitation involves 6 weeks of non–weight bearing in a tall controlled ankle motion (CAM) boot with initiation of gentle active and passive motion including hindfoot mobilization at 2 weeks after surgery. Weight bearing as tolerated in a CAM boot is started after the 6th week. Closed chain exercise with physical therapy is allowed at 8 weeks. Repeat CT scan is done at 10 to 12 weeks to evaluate fracture healing (Figure 10.5). Once full union is obtained, patients are weaned out of the boot and advanced as tolerated back to their respective sport.

In summary, navicular BSIs are a high-risk injury that can have long-term consequences if they are not properly identified and treated. In an athlete with pain over the navicular in the setting of negative x-ray findings, MRI should be done to rule out navicular stress reaction or stress fracture. If there is high suspicion for a navicular stress fracture on MRI even if a fracture line is not visible, a CT scan is highly recommended. Both nonoperative and surgical treatments are effective in treating navicular BSIs. Regardless of treatment option, a minimum of 6 weeks of non–weight bearing in a cast or boot is needed to prevent delayed union or nonunion. Whether surgery can improve return-to-activity time is still unknown and debated. However, in more severe fracture types, surgical fixation may improve fracture union and reduce the time needed to return to play.

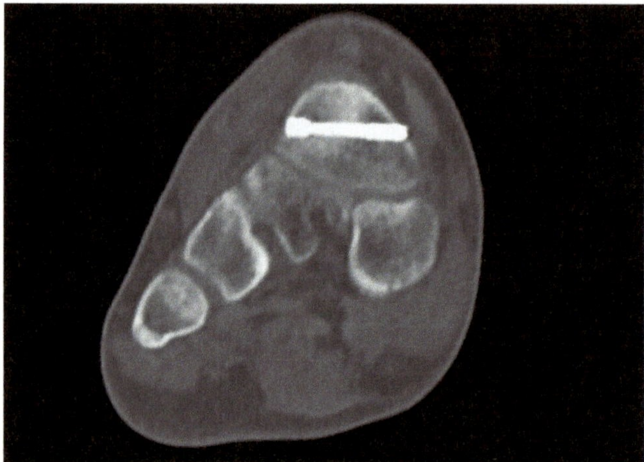

FIGURE 10.5 Repeat CT scan obtained at 10 weeks after surgery. The scan showed complete healing of the stress fracture, and the athlete was allowed to advance to full activities as tolerated.

CALCANEAL BONE STRESS INJURY

Evaluation

Unlike some of the stress fractures of the foot and ankle, which have a high rate of fracture nonunion without surgical intervention, most calcaneal stress injuries have a propensity to heal with conservative management. Calcaneal stress fractures are the second most common stress fracture in the foot and ankle among military recruits, with a higher incidence in female soldiers. The study found an incidence of all stress fractures in female recruits to be 1.09% with calcaneal fractures accounting for 39% of those injuries. Incidence in male recruits for all stress fractures was 0.91%, with calcaneal stress fractures making up 20%.[18] Outside of military personnel, they most commonly occur in long-distance runners.[19]

The calcaneus is the largest bone in the foot. It articulates with the talus superiorly and cuboid distally. There are three muscular insertions on the calcaneus. The gastrocnemius and soleus insert on the posterior calcaneal tuberosity through the Achilles tendon. The third is the plantaris muscle, which can insert directly or through the Achilles tendon to the posterior calcaneal tuberosity. The bone is composed predominately of trabecular bone with a thin cortical shell.[20] The trabecular structure of the calcaneus runs in an arc extending from the subtalar articular surface to the posterior cortex (Figure 10.6A).

The mechanism of calcaneal BSIs may be due to the eccentric pull of the Achilles tendon on its calcaneal insertion with repetitive heel strike. As a result, the majority of fractures occur on the posterior aspect of the calcaneus with the fracture line perpendicular to the trabecular lines distal to posterior calcaneal tuberosity (Figure 10.6A).[21] Fractures can also occur in the middle and anterior aspects of the calcaneus.[22]

The most common risk factor for developing these injuries is being a military recruit. Other factors associated with stress fractures, such as the female athlete triad, relative energy deficiency in sport, changes in duration or frequency of exercise, poor nutrition, and medication use such as steroids, are also common. Calcaneus has greater trabecular bone content, and low bone mineral density has been observed to be more common with this injury.[23] There is also a small subset of older patients with osteoporosis

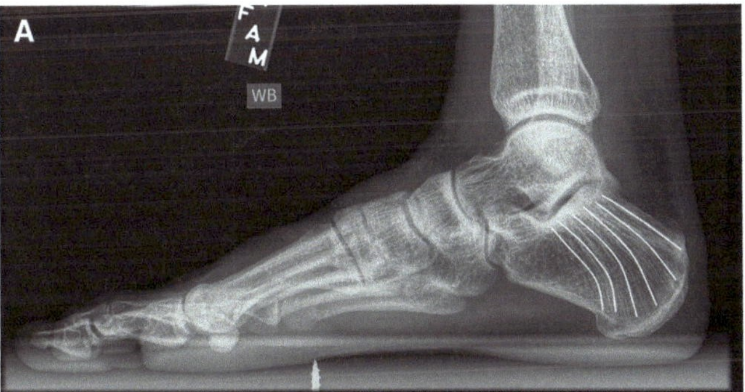
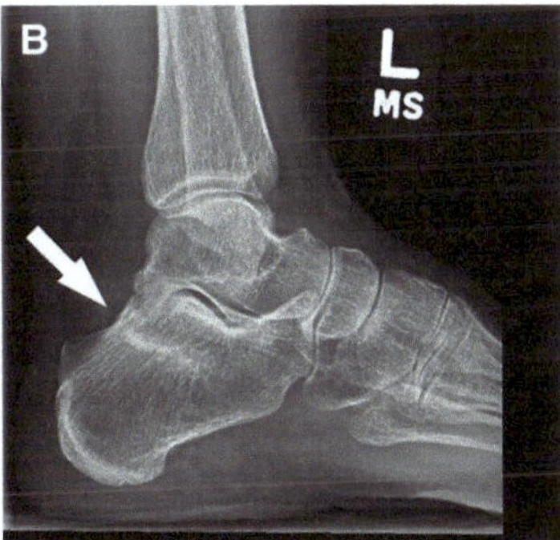

FIGURE 10.6 (A) Normal trabecular lines of the calcaneal body. Fractures occur perpendicular to these lines. (B) Central calcaneal stress fracture in a 45-year-old avid runner. Fracture extends anteriorly. Note that the fracture line is perpendicular to the calcaneal trabeculae.

developing calcaneal stress fracture in the postoperative period after a total hip arthroplasty or total knee arthroplasty.[24,25] On average, the fractures occurred 10 weeks after a total hip arthroplasty.[24] This could be due to changes in gait after surgery. Another etiology could be increased mechanical load from reduced pain after joint replacement or postoperative analgesics.[26] In addition, the elongated anterior process of the calcaneus and navicular–calcaneal coalitions has been associated with stress fractures of the anterior process of the calcaneus.[27]

Symptoms typically occur 1 to 3 weeks after changes in frequency, duration, or difficulty in exercise. Pain is localized along the posterior aspect of the tissues overlying the calcaneus. Patients can have pain along the medial and lateral wall of the calcaneus. Calcaneal squeeze test may provoke pain. Differential diagnosis includes plantar fasciitis, insertional Achilles tendonitis, retrocalcaneal bursitis, Baxter's neuritis, and calcaneal apophysitis in patients with open growth plates.[28] The location of where the patient is tender can help narrow down the differential diagnosis (Figure 10.7).

Identification of the fracture on plain radiographs may lag behind symptoms by up to 3 to 4 weeks. Typically, when seen, a sclerotic line will be identified on the lateral view of the foot in the posterior calcaneus (Figure 10.6B). If there is high suspicion for calcaneal BSIs, MRI is the modality due to its high sensitivity and specificity.

Treatment

Conservative treatment consisting of protected weight-bearing, cessation of the inciting activity, and gradual resumption of impact sports is the standard of care as these injuries have a high rate of healing without long-term consequences or loss in the activity level.[22,29–35] Outside of exercise modification, cast immobilization is rarely required.[36] A short period of boot immobilization with no weight-bearing restrictions can be done to rest the painful extremity.

Recurrence of the calcaneal BSI can occur with premature return to vigorous activity before resolution of the patient's symptoms or within 8 weeks from initiation of treatment.[37] To prevent this, a two-phase treatment regimen is recommended. In the initial phase, rest with protected weight bearing and activity restriction is provided until the patient is pain free with weight bearing. This phase may take up to 8 weeks. The second phase consists of gradual reintroduction of activities over a 6- to 12-week period. If pain returns, the activity level should be decreased.

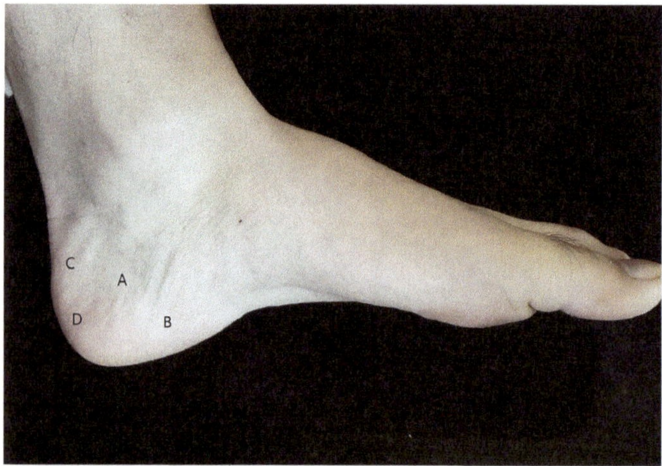

FIGURE 10.7 Typical location of pain when palpating the medial hindfoot. (A) Calcaneal stress fracture, (B) plantar fasciitis, (C) Achilles tendonitis/retrocalcaneal bursitis, and (D) Achilles tendonitis/apophysitis.

Additional nonoperative treatment measures for BSIs should be considered. These include vitamin D and calcium supplementation, identification and treatment of any nutritional deficits along with consideration for workup for underlying impaired bone density with dual-energy x-ray absorptiometry, and treatment of any endocrine or metabolic irregularities.

There is one case report of surgical treatment of bilateral displaced posterior calcaneal stress fractures in a 67-year-old female who sustained the injury from a 3-week hiking trek.[38] In addition, there are reports of anterior calcaneal stress fractures, especially in the setting of a calcaneal—navicular coalition that required surgical treatment including resection of the coalition and screw fixation of the stress fracture.[27,39,40] Outside of these reports, however, there are no other reported surgical treatment of calcaneal stress fractures.

The author's preferred treatment involves controlled ankle boot immobilization and cessation of the inciting activity level with no restriction on weight bearing until the patient is able to ambulate with no discomfort or pain. Once the pain is resolved, the patient is weaned out of the boot and initiation of nonimpact activities can be done. A slow gradual return to activities is done over the subsequent 6-week period. A return to run progression including antigravity treadmill may be considered starting 6 to 8 weeks from initiation of treatment. Return to vigorous activity level is resumed only after the patient is completely asymptomatic. An exercise regimen including intensity, duration, and frequency is adjusted to prevent recurrence. Physical therapy to optimize strength and mobility of the foot and ankle should be considered, especially if the injury required immobilization. Vitamin D, calcium, and maintenance of good caloric intake are continued even after fracture healing.

In conclusion, calcaneal BSI is a common injury that can be confused with other foot and ankle ailments such as plantar fasciitis. This injury needs to be considered in any patient with suspicion of a stress injury. MRI may be needed to identify the fracture if plain radiographs are negative. Conservative treatment is the mainstay of care. Care should be taken to gradually return the patient to impact activities as recurrence of the fracture can occur.

PROMIXAL 5TH METATARSAL JONES FRACTURE

Evaluation

Stress fractures of the 5th metatarsal account for only 2% of all metatarsal stress fractures.[41] Compared to a traumatic fracture of the 5th metatarsal, which occurs most commonly as a tuberosity avulsion fracture at the insertion of the peroneus brevis, 5th metatarsal BSIs occur generally at the metaphyseal and proximal diaphyseal portions of the bone. Although he described it first, in 1902, Sir Robert Jones himself suffered from the fracture due to dancing.[42] Proximal 5th metatarsal fractures are classified into zones 1, 2, and 3 depending on the location of the fracture. Zone 1 fractures are a tuberosity avulsion fracture. Zone 2 involves the metaphysis or the articulation between the 4th and 5th metatarsals extending to the metaphyseal/diaphyseal junction. Finally, zone 3 fractures occur at the proximal diaphysis (Figure 10.8).[43-45] A majority of stress fractures to the 5th metatarsal occur in the distal zone 2 and zone 3 areas of the bone or approximately 1.5 cm distal from the tuberosity.[46] These injuries are often associated with basketball and football. However, an athlete participating in any sport that involves

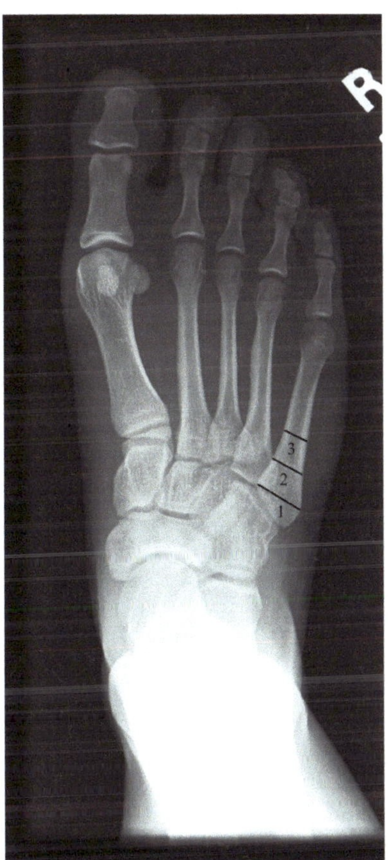

FIGURE 10.8 Locations of zone 1, zone 2, and zone 3 fractures of the base of the 5th metatarsal. Zone 1 fractures involve the proximal tubercle. Zone 2 fractures are located at the 4th and 5th metatarsal articulation and the metaphyseal/diaphyseal junction. Zone 3 fractures involve the proximal diaphysis or are distal to the metaphyseal/diaphyseal junction.

repetitive loading to the lower extremity, such as lacrosse, soccer, running, gymnastics, and dance, can result in a 5th metatarsal BSI.[47–51]

There are two main tendon attachments to the proximal 5th metatarsal. The peroneus brevis inserts on the proximal tuberosity, a site common for avulsion fractures from inversion ankle injuries. The peroneus tertius inserts on the proximal diaphysis on the dorsal surface.[52] The main blood supply to the 5th metatarsal comes from the metaphyseal arteries on both the proximal and distal aspects of the bone and the nutrient artery entering the bone at the middle third of the diaphysis. The nutrient vessels divide into the proximal and distal branches. The proximal branch is shorter compared to the distal branch and does not fully reach the metaphyseal and diaphyseal junction of the metatarsal.[18] This watershed area can decrease the healing potential in the bone accounting for the propensity to develop stress fractures in the proximal 5th metatarsal and the delay in fracture healing.

There are multiple risk factors for base 5th metatarsal BSI including biological factors such as insufficient metabolic intake, female athlete triad/relative energy deficiency in sport, medications (i.e., steroids and anticonvulsants), and vitamin D deficiency. Biomechanical factors include an increase in volume or intensity in training regimen. This results in continued repetitive submaximal load, leading to failure of bone integrity and a stress fracture.[8] Other factors more specifically associated with base 5th metatarsal stress fractures include cavus foot and varus hindfoot.[50,53,54] These foot deformities can lead to increased load to the lateral column during ambulation, thereby increasing the risk of BSI in the area. Although cavus foot and/or hindfoot varus can be a risk factor for 5th metatarsal BSIs, surgical treatment of the deformity is typically not needed. Shoe modifications consisting of orthotics with a lateral post and forefoot posting was enough to allow fracture healing and prevent recurrence.[53]

Patients typically present with localized pain over the lateral aspect of the 5th metatarsal. These symptoms can be present up to 18 months from presentation.[55] However, in some individuals, repetitive load stress reactions can manifest in a subclinical manner without the typical prodromal symptoms. An acute-on-chronic injury may occur, resulting in the localized typical pain overlying the base 5th metatarsal.

Initial radiographic assessment should begin with three view plain radiographs of the foot. Early radiographic findings can include cortical thickening at the lateral base of the 5th metatarsal.[51] This can progress to a radiolucent fracture line (Figure 10.9).

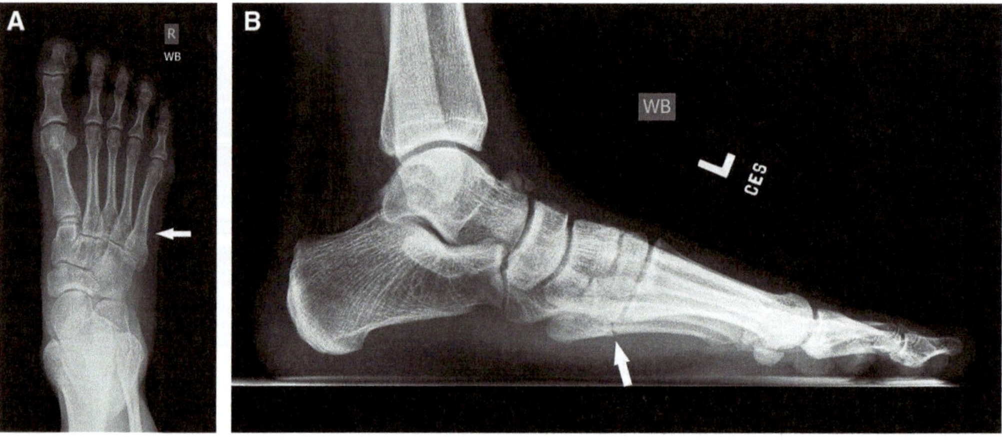

FIGURE 10.9 Fifth metatarsal stress fracture in a 20-year-old football athlete involving zone 2 and extending into zone 3. (A) AP view and (B) lateral view.

AP, anteroposterior.

However, negative x-ray findings may not rule out an early BSI. In a setting of stress reaction without periosteal reaction, a fracture may not show up on plain radiographs. As a result, if there is continued clinical suspicion for a Jones fracture, an MRI should be obtained. An MRI is a much more sensitive modality compared to x-rays and can show localized bone edema, periosteal reaction, and cortical fracture line in higher grade injuries.[36,56]

Treatment

Conservative treatment for BSIs of the base of the 5th metatarsal involves non–weight-bearing immobilization in a short leg cast or CAM boot for a minimum of 6 to 8 weeks or until radiographic evidence of fracture healing is identified. Clapper et al. reported 72% successful union in patients treated with non–weight-bearing immobilization with an average time to union of 21.2 weeks.[57]

Due to the risk of delayed union and nonunion in this area, athletes should not be allowed to weight bear during this period. Weight bearing even in a cast or boot can lead to delayed union and high risk of a nonunion. Zelko et al. reported only 2 of 15 patients treated in a weight-bearing cast healed fully without surgical intervention. In those two individuals in whom healing occurred without surgery, time to union was 7 and 20 months.[58]

Kavanaugh et al. reported a high rate of delayed union and nonunion in athletes treated conservatively. In their study, 12 of 18 patients had incomplete fracture healing at 6 months.[49] Konkel et al. reported delayed union in 4 of 13 patients with a Jones fracture or stress fracture of the base of the 5th metatarsal. Although in their series the delayed unions did heal, there was a considerable delay with average full union ranging from 3.5 months in Jones fractures to 4.8 months in stress fractures.[59]

Case series of treatment with extracorporeal shockwave treatment exist in the literature for primary treatment of nonunion or in rare instances in failure to achieve union following surgical management; high-level evidence studies are currently lacking for evaluation of success in healing this injury.[60,61]

Due to the delay in fracture healing, athletes may benefit from surgical treatment for earlier fracture healing and return to sport.[55,57,62–64] Surgical treatment typically consists of an intramedullary screw fixation (Figure 10.10). If an area of sclerotic bone is observed in a chronic nonunion, curettage of the site with bone graft is recommended. Clapper et al. reported 100% union in their series of patients who underwent surgery for failure of conservative management. Average time to healing was 12.1 weeks versus 21.2 weeks for 18 patients treated with non–weight-bearing cast alone.[57]

DeLee et al. were the first to report the use of percutaneous intramedullary screw fixation with a 4.5-mm solid screw for 5th metatarsal diaphyseal stress fractures. They reported an average healing time of 7.5 weeks and return to sport in 8.5 weeks on average with no postsurgical complications or refracture.[55] Similar earlier fracture healing and return to play has been seen in other studies by Porter et al.[62] and Pecina et al.[64] A systematic review of the literature between 1994 and 2010 demonstrated a return to sport at an average of 12 weeks for athletes treated with surgery versus 24 weeks for athletes treated conservatively.[65]

Surgical technique options include solid screw fixation versus cannulated screws and which size screw to place at the fracture site. There is no clear clinical advantage between a solid and a cannulated screw. Theoretically, the solid screw will be less likely to break. However, Pietropaoli et al. in their biomechanical study found no difference between the two screws from a biomechanical standpoint.[66]

Screw width should be a minimum of 4.5 mm or larger. Smaller screws have been shown to be correlated with delayed union and nonunion.[67] However, increasing the

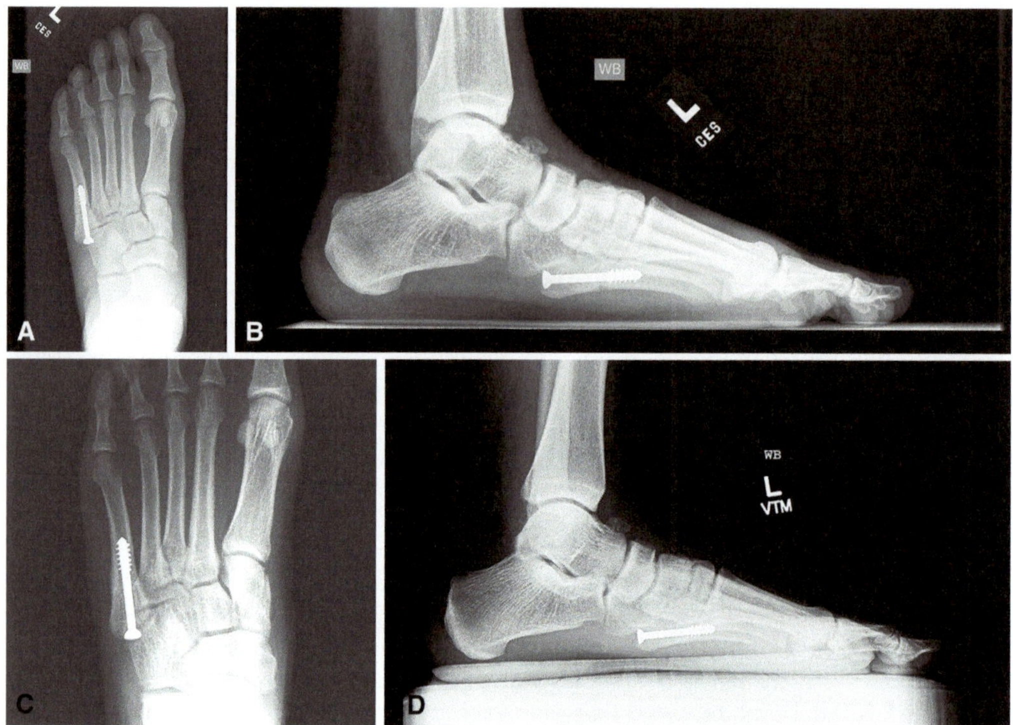

FIGURE 10.10 Postoperative radiographs of the previously mentioned 20-year-old football athlete. (A) AP x-rays at 2 weeks after surgery. (B) Lateral view at 2 weeks after surgery. Note the screw threads extending just past the fracture line and filling the medullary canal to provide stability by improving pullout strength. (C and D) Radiographs obtained at 12 weeks after surgery demonstrating complete healing of the fracture.

AP, anteroposterior.

screw size to 5.0 and 6.5 mm has not been shown to improve fracture healing or improve fracture stiffness after fixation.[68-70] One advantage of a larger screw compared to a 4.5-mm screw is the increased pull-out strength due to improved thread purchase.[70] In general, the widest screw that is needed to fill the medullary canal just distal to the fracture line should be placed (Figure 10.10). Although the 5th metatarsal can accommodate a 6.5-mm screw, this can result in stress shielding across the fracture and stress reactions distal to the screw fixation.

Another consideration for surgical fixation is screw length. Due to the lateral curvature and plantar bow, a long screw can result in perforation of the medial distal cortex and lead to fracture distraction or even a distal diaphyseal fracture.[71,72] Based on the study done by DeSandis et al., screw length should be 50 mm or less with typical lengths of 40 mm or less.[71] The distal screw threads of a partially threaded screw only need to pass the fracture site and should not extend to the distal diaphyseal cortex of the metatarsal (Figure 10.10).

Complications after surgical fixation include continued delayed union, refracture, hardware irritation, and sural nerve injury. The most common causes of delayed union or nonunion after surgical treatment are incomplete reaming of the sclerotic canal, undersized inlay bone graft, undersized screw, or early return to vigorous activity.[67,73] Refracture can also occur from use of an undersized screw or after screw removal. In these situations, placement of a larger screw after reaming the canal is recommended.

In addition, resection of the sclerotic bone and autologous bone graft may be beneficial.[74] Athletes can also develop pain from the screw head and finally sural nerve injury. Pain from the hardware can typically be managed with shoe modifications.

The author's preferred treatment for athletes with a stress fracture in zones 2 and 3 is a solid, partially threaded intramedullary screw to allow earlier weight bearing, continuation of nonimpact conditioning, and earlier return to play.[55,62–64] The widest screw that fills the intramedullary canal distal to the fracture on the anteroposterior fluoroscopy view is chosen to improve pull-out strength. Screw length is kept to the minimum needed to assure that all the threads are distal to the fracture line. If the fracture has a large area of sclerotic bone, the area is debrided and bone grafted using cancellous chips combined with iliac crest bone marrow aspirate.

Postoperatively, athletes are kept toe touch weight bearing for the first 1 to 2 weeks in a boot. They are then made weight bearing as tolerated in a boot for additional 4 weeks and progressed into a foot orthosis until radiographic fracture healing is observed. Athletes are not allowed to return to play until radiographic union of the fracture is observed. If the athletes have a cavus foot or varus hindfoot, they are placed into a custom orthotic with a lateral heel wedge and 1st metatarsal head well to reduce pressure to the lateral column.

To review, BSI localized to the base of the 5th metatarsal has a higher than typical risk of developing a delayed union or nonunion. Although there is evidence that these fractures can be treated with conservative management, elite athletes heal their fracture more reliably and with earlier return to play with surgical treatment. Fixation should consist of the widest screw that is needed to fill the distal intramedullary canal. Care should be taken to not place a screw that perforates the distal medial cortex. Athletes should return to play once fracture healing is observed radiographically. Activity level should be increased in a stepwise controlled manner as recurrence of the fracture can occur even with surgical fixation with early vigorous return to play.

SESAMOID BONE STRESS INJURY

Evaluation

Sesamoid is a bone that travels within a tendon typically situated near an angular structure in the body to improve mechanical strength of the tendon. An example of a large sesamoid bone is the patella of the knee. In the foot, the two main sesamoid bones are the tibial (medial) and fibular (lateral) hallucal sesamoid located plantar to the first metatarsal head. Stress fractures to these structures represent approximately 4% of foot and ankle injuries and less than 1% of all running disorders.[75]

Of the two sesamoids, the tibial sesamoid is larger and slightly elongated in morphology. The tibial sesamoid is subjected to greater weight-bearing forces compared to the fibular sesamoid and thus is more commonly injured.[46,76,77] Mechanically, the hallucal sesamoids have multiple functions, all of which help to improve the push-off ability of the hallux. First, they elevate the 1st metatarsal head to improve the strength of the flexor hallucis brevis as the tendon travels through the bone. Second, they function to protect the flexor hallucis longus as it travels between the two sesamoids. Finally, they modify and help dissipate the forces at the metatarsophalangeal joint.[46,78] This last function is critical as greater than 50% of the body weight is transferred through the 1st metatarsophalangeal joint during gait cycle.[79]

The main blood flow to the tibial and fibular sesamoid is from the medial plantar metatarsal artery and the plantar arch vessels.[80] The major vascular vessels enter the sesamoid at the proximal pole supplying up to two thirds of the blood flow to the bone with a small capsular vessel supplying the distal portion.[81,82] The distal third with its tenuous blood vascular supply along with the watershed area between the two vascular structures can lead to stress injuries in the sesamoid.

Ossification occurs between 9 and 11 years of age in multiple areas of the sesamoid.[11] The multiple ossification centers in a minority of individuals fail to fuse together during development. The incidence of tibial bipartite sesamoids ranges from 7.2% to 30.6%. The incidence of fibular bipartite sesamoid is from 0.6% to 2.5%.[83–85] The rates of having a bipartite sesamoid on the contralateral side are approximately 25%.[86] The incidence of bipartite sesamoids can have significant implications in athletes as the presence of bipartite sesamoid on imaging studies, particularly x-ray can be interpreted as a sesamoid fracture in individuals having plantar first metatarsal head pain. It can be difficult to distinguish between the two.

Although the specific incidence of sesamoid BSIs in individual sports is not well studied, these injuries are most commonly observed in individuals participating in activities that require repetitive forced dorsiflexion such as dance, American football, gymnastics, and running.[86–88] Rates of sesamoid stress fractures are more common in females than in males.[88] The mean age at the time of presentation ranged from 16.8 to 36.5 years.[87,89] Similar to other stress fractures, biological and mechanical risk factors can be present, such as inadequate caloric intake, vitamin D deficiency, and improper training regimen.

Pain related to sesamoid BSIs typically has an insidious course with no specific acute injury or trauma. As a result, there can be a delay in presentation. Pain is localized to the plantar first metatarsal head. Symptoms are exacerbated by weight bearing, participating in impact sports, and climbing stairs. In addition, pain is worse with activities that require forced dorsiflexion at the 1st metatarsal phalangeal joint.[87] Discomfort and pain are generally improved with rest. On examination, athletes may have an effusion at the 1st metatarsophalangeal joint or swelling over the sesamoid. Pain is exacerbated by forced dorsiflexion.

Radiographic analysis includes a weight-bearing three view of the foot. Additional views to visualize the sesamoids can be done. This includes a medial oblique to help visualize the tibial sesamoid better and an axial sesamoid view (Figure 10.11A). However, initial radiographs may be negative as a periosteal reaction or fracture line may not be present if the athlete is evaluated soon after symptoms occur.

A true acute fracture of the sesamoids will exhibit sharp irregular borders on either side of the fracture, possible comminution, and fracture gap. In contrast, a bipartite sesamoid will have smooth cortical edges and may have a bipartite sesamoid on the contralateral side. Stress fractures are rarely bilateral.[11] Finally, the size of the bipartite sesamoid when measured together is larger than the nonpartite sesamoid.[90]

MRI is sensitive and specific in evaluating for stress reaction consisting of sesamoiditis versus stress fracture as initial plain radiographs are routinely negative (Figure 10.11B).[46] In addition, MRI can help assess for osteonecrosis of the sesamoids and rule out adjacent tendinous and ligamentous injuries. A CT scan can also be obtained to identify a fracture line if there is high suspicion for a stress fracture on MRI or x-rays.

A bone scan can have a high rate of false positives. In one study of military recruits, it was shown that a mild to moderate increase in scintigraphic activity at the sesamoids was visualized in asymptomatic patients.[91]

Pain related to surface anatomy can be very helpful in narrowing the differential diagnosis. Sesamoid BSIs have pain localized directly over the bone at the plantar aspect of the first metatarsal head. Most commonly, it is pain over the tibial sesamoid. Pain at the dorsal, medial, or lateral aspect of the hallux can be due to other injuries such as collateral ligament tears, abductor hallucis tendonitis, and chondral injuries of the metatarsal head (Figure 10.12). Symptoms related to stress fractures of the sesamoids typically have an insidious course. An acute injury or trauma to the hallux with pain plantarly and inability to ambulate should direct you to consider turf toe until proven otherwise.

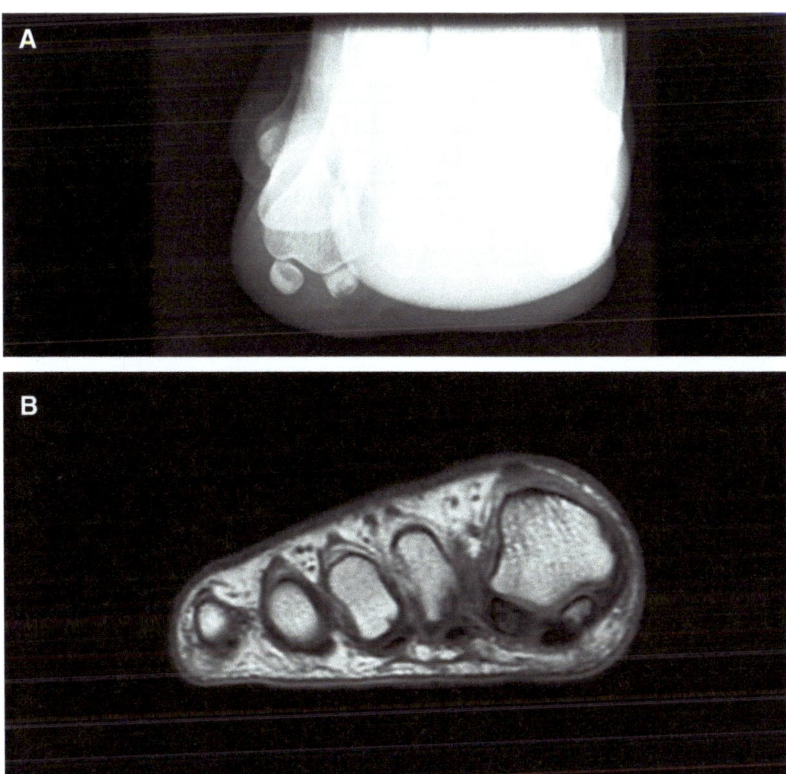

FIGURE 10.11 22-year-old runner with a 2-month history of increasing pain at the tibial and fibular sesamoids. (A) x-rays demonstrated a fibular sesamoid stress fracture best seen in the sesamoid view. (B) T1-weighted coronal MRI with findings consistent with those of a chronic stress fracture to the fibular sesamoid and patchy edema at the tibial sesamoid due to sesamoid stress reaction.

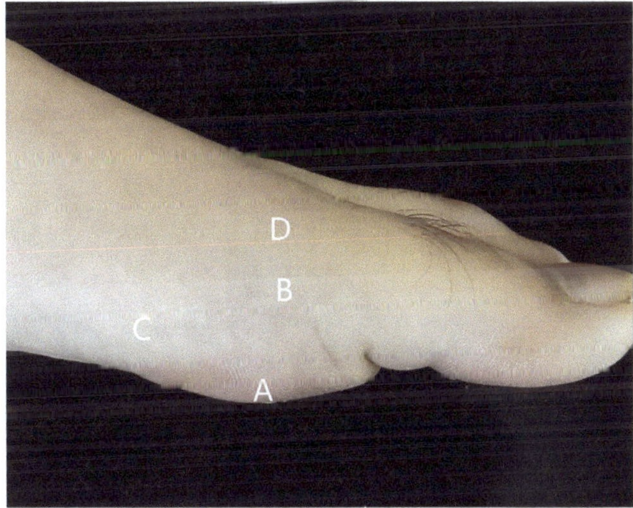

FIGURE 10.12 Typical location of pain in the forefoot due to the sesamoid injury/turf toe (A), medial collateral ligament injury (B), abductor hallucis injury (C), and 1st metatarsal chondral injury (D).

Treatment

Conservative treatment is the treatment of choice for sesamoid BSIs as a majority of athletes will improve without surgical intervention (Figure 10.13). Treatment involves anti-inflammatory medications, cessation of activities, treatment of any metabolic risk factors, and placement of the extremity into a short leg cast or boot and kept non–weight bearing for 6 to 8 weeks.[86] The athlete is then weaned into a custom-molded full-length orthosis with a proximal metatarsal pad and a relief well or viscoelastic polymer under the sesamoids. This can be combined with a carbon fiber forefoot plate or metal shank to restrict both forefoot motion and dorsiflexion.[11] Gradual resumption of activities can then be initiated. Other orthotic modifications include a Morton's extension once the fracture has healed to limit forced dorsiflexion through the 1st metatarsophalangeal joint. Cortisone injection is not recommended as this can be detrimental in fracture healing along with concerns of atrophy to the surrounding tissue. Low heel shoes should be utilized to reduce pressure to the metatarsal head.[11]

Treatment of sesamoid stress reaction is similar to that of a stress fracture with activity modification and treatment of any risk factors. However, if symptoms are mild, they may be allowed to weight bear as tolerated in a boot for several weeks and weaned into an over-the-counter orthosis with a metatarsal pad. The orthotic can be placed into the boot for further comfort. A steel or carbon fiber shank can also be utilized to limit great toe dorsiflexion in their shoes. A custom-molded orthosis can also be used with the same modifications for a stress fracture.

Return to play with conservative treatment can take up to 14 weeks or longer. A recent meta-analysis demonstrated a return time to sport of 13.9 weeks with return rate of athletes to preinjury level of 64%.[88]

The use of electromagnetic and low-intensity pulsed ultrasound bone stimulators can be considered. However, there are no reported studies that describe their efficacy in the treatment of sesamoid stress fractures.

Surgical indication is a failure of conservative management with symptoms occurring for greater than 6 months. Operative treatment can involve partial sesamoidectomy, complete sesamoidectomy, bone grafting without screw fixation, and percutaneous

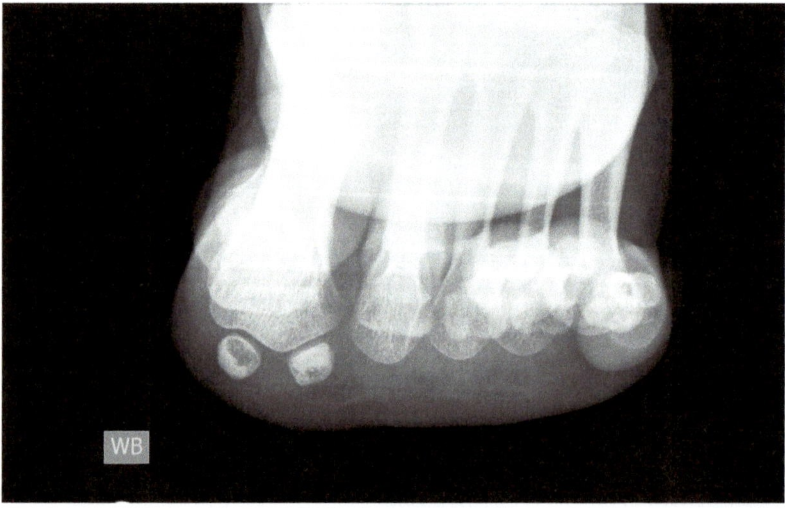

FIGURE 10.13 The previous 22-year-old runner with fibular sesamoid and tibial sesamoiditis after 3 months of conservative management. Repeat radiographs demonstrated a healed stress fracture to the fibular sesamoid.

screw fixation. A complete sesamoidectomy should be done with caution as there can be a loss of up to 10% of push-off strength with this procedure.[11] Furthermore, tibial sesamoidectomy can increase the hallux valgus angle and intermetatarsal angle. In contrast, a fibular sesamoidectomy can decrease the hallux valgus angle and intermetatarsal angle. Athletes with a baseline hallux valgus deformity should be cautioned before proceeding. However, in a study done by Kane et al., the change in the hallux valgus angle and intermetatarsal angle was on average less than 1.1° and 0.8°, respectively, and did not result in any loss of function or activity level.[92]

Biedert and Hintermann reported on a series of five athletes treated with proximal fracture fragment excision and repair of the flexor hallucis brevis. Four of the five patients returned to their sport without restrictions.[87]

To avoid loss of push-off strength with a sesamoid excision, Anderson and McBryde described using bone autograft without internal fixation. Fracture gap was less than 3 mm. Of the 24 patients who underwent surgery, 19 healed radiographically and 17 athletes returned to their preinjury athletic activity and level.[93]

Percutaneous screw fixation of a transverse sesamoid stress fracture has also been described with good results.[89,94,95] Blundell et al., in their series of nine patients, used screw fixation. All of the patients had fracture union by 6 months and were able to return to their preinjury activity levels and sport with no complications.[94]

Contraindications to both bone grafting and screw fixation include cartilage loss, hallux rigidus, and avascular necrosis of the sesamoid. Furthermore, sesamoidectomy should not be done if there is a congenital absence of the other sesamoid as this can significantly reduce push-off strength and result in a dorsiflexion deformity of the great toe.

A meta-analysis comparing conservative versus surgery treatment demonstrated that athletes returned to their sport significantly quicker with operative care by 2.9 weeks. Athletes with fractures treated with sesamoidectomy returned to play faster than those treated with internal fixation. In addition, athletes with fibular sesamoid BSIs regardless of treatment were found to return to play quicker than those with tibial stress fractures.[88]

The author's preferred treatment for stress fracture to the sesamoids is conservative, nonoperative treatment for minimum of 6 months. Athletes are placed into a boot and kept non–weight bearing for 6 weeks. They are then allowed gradual weight bearing in a boot and weaned into a custom-molded orthosis with a 1st metatarsal pad and relief well at the sesamoids. Gradual resumption of activities is allowed thereafter (Figures 10.11 and 10.13).

If the athlete has failed 6 months of conservative management with continued fracture line or is unable to return to their activity level, repeat MRI is done to rule out avascular necrosis of the sesamoids and to evaluate for arthritis at the sesamoid metatarsal complex. If the fracture line is present with a fracture gap of 2 mm or less, bone grafting will be done. If, however, the fracture gap is larger or arthritis or avascular necrosis is observed, then complete sesamoidectomy will be done. Finally, if the fracture fragment is small, then a partial sesamoid excision with repair of the flexor hallucis brevis will be recommended.

Postoperatively, athletes are kept non–weight bearing for 3 weeks after a complete sesamoid excision or 6 weeks for bone grafting. They are placed into a short leg splint for 2 weeks after surgery and a boot thereafter. Athletes are weaned out of the boot into a regular shoe with a full-length semi-rigid foot orthosis, with a 1st metatarsal pad and relief well at 6 weeks in patients with sesamoid excision and in 10 weeks for those treated with bone graft. High-impact activities including running, jumping, and cutting are restricted until 16 weeks after surgery for both excision and bone graft athletes.

The most common complication from nonoperative treatment is the long duration of symptoms athletes may have even after radiographic union of the fracture. The rates of persistent pain can range from 30% to 100%. In addition, 20% to 33% of patients may convert to operative management.[86,96,97]

The risks related to complete sesamoid excision are most commonly related to an increase in varus or valgus angle at the 1st metatarsophalangeal joint depending on whether the fibular or tibial sesamoid is excised. The great toe goes into a more valgus position with a tibial sesamoid excision and varus with fibular sesamoid excision. Risks are low for a symptomatic hallux varus or valgus deformity with rates of 4% for each.[98,99] Other risks of surgery include nonunion after bone grafting, postoperative scarring with neuroma symptoms at 8%,[98] transient paresthesia at 18%, and postsurgical continued pain at 18%.[99] A study by Anderson and McBryde found 10% of continued nonunion after bone grafting and 5% of neuropathic pain in their bone grafting patient group.[93] One of the most recalcitrant complications to treat is avascular necrosis of the sesamoids after a stress fracture. Kane et al. in their retrospective review of 37 patients with sesamoid fracture, either direct or stress related, found 9 cases of avascular necrosis of the sesamoids.[92] However, other studies evaluating sesamoid stress fractures did not observe avascular necrosis as a potential complication.

In summary, sesamoid BSIs have an insidious course with typically delayed presentation. Localized pain to the plantar distal 1st metatarsal head is the most common symptom. The majority of these fractures will heal with conservative care and return to sport; however, symptoms can be present for a much longer period of time even after radiographic union of the fracture. Nonoperative care should be continued for up to 6 months before considering surgical intervention. Although many surgical techniques have been described, the most optimal technique is yet to be identified. Sesamoidectomy offers the earliest return to play; however, athletes can lose some push-off strength, and in a setting of baseline hallux valgus deformity, their deformity can worsen with tibial sesamoidectomy. The decision to operate should be made cautiously.

CONCLUSION

BSIs in the foot and ankle are a common cause of injuries in the athlete. Many of these are low-risk injuries and can be treated conservatively with activity modification and a short period of immobilization. However, some of these stress fractures can occur in bones that require very specific treatments such as at the navicular and 5th metatarsal. BSIs in these high-risk areas require very specific treatments such as extended non–weight bearing, and, in some situations, surgery may be needed to increase the healing rate. As a result, physicians must have astute knowledge of the foot and ankle to be able to differentiate between the two types of injuries. Understanding the mechanics of the foot and ankle along with knowing the key surface anatomy is critical so that correct diagnosis can be made to provide optimal and timely treatment. Failure to identify these high-risk injuries can result in not only incorrect diagnosis but also a delay in the proper treatment, which can have profound results in the athlete's ability to return to play. Finally, regardless of the type of injury, high-risk versus low-risk by anatomy it is important to identify and correct any biological and biomechanical risk factors for stress injuries to improve the healing rate and reduce future recurrences.

KEY REFERENCES

Only key references appear in the print edition. The full reference list appears in the digital product found on http://connect.springerpub.com/content/book/978-0-8261-4424-9/part/sec02/chapter/ch10

11. Anderson RB, Cohen BE. Stress fractures of the foot and ankle. In: *Mann's Surgery of the Foot and Ankle*. 9th ed. Elsevier Inc; 2014:1688–1722.

15. Torg JS, Moyer J, Gaughan JP, Boden BP. Management of tarsal navicular stress fractures: conservative versus surgical treatment: a meta-analysis. *Am J Sports Med*. 2010;38:1048–1053.

17. Mallee WH, Weel H, Dijk CN, et al. Surgical versus conservative treatment for high-risk stress fractures of the lower leg (anterior tibial cortex, navicular and fifth metatarsal base): a systematic review. *Br J Sports Med*. 2015;49:370–376.

49. Kavanaugh J, Brower T, Mann R. The Jones fracture revisited. *J Bone Joint Surg*. 1978;60:776–782.

65. Kerkhoffs GM, Versteegh VE, Siervelt IN, et al. Treatment of proximal metatarsal V fractures in athletes and non-athletes. *Br J Sports Med*. 2012;46:644–648.

72. Den Hartog BD. Fracture of the proximal fifth metatarsal. *J Am Acad Orthop Surg*. 2009;17:458–464.

78. Coughlin MJ. Sesamoids and accessory bones of the foot. In: *Mann's Surgery of the Foot and Ankle*. 9th ed. Elsevier Inc; 2014:492–568.

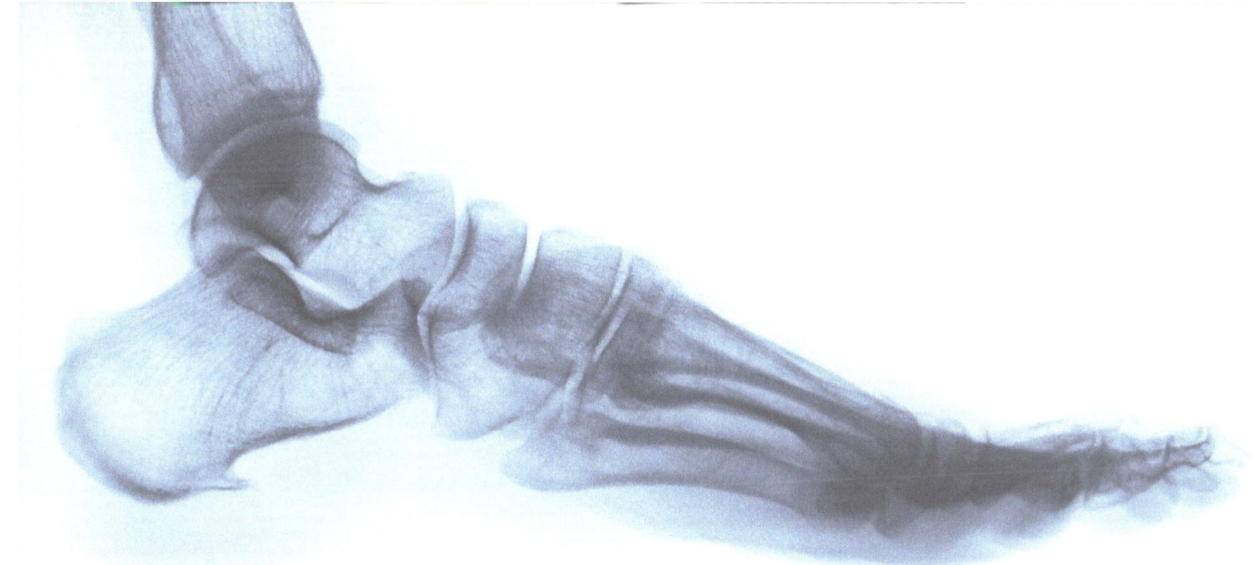

PART III

SPECIAL POPULATIONS

CHAPTER 11

Pediatric Athletes

Stephanie DeLuca and Emily Kraus

INTRODUCTION

As participation in organized sports increases in the pediatric population, so does the prevalence and incidence of bone stress injury (BSI).[1] BSIs are classified as overuse injuries in this patient population. BSIs typically result from accumulated microtrauma to the bone due to the bone's inability to accommodate repetitive, submaximal, cyclic loading forces and inadequate time for recovery. There is a spectrum of BSIs that ranges from stress reactions to stress fractures. The clinical presentation for BSIs can vary significantly in the pediatric population depending on the athlete's skeletal maturity, site of injury, and respective sport. This can make diagnosing BSIs in the pediatric athlete particularly challenging. BSIs can have significant detrimental effects on one's bone health, growth, and optimal skeletal maturity. Adolescent years are a critical time to achieve peak bone mass.[2,3]

Sport participation provides athletes, particularly those under the age of 18, with an opportunity to develop their physical and social skills. Unfortunately, BSIs force athletes to take time away from sport to allow for healing. As many athletes strongly identify with their respective sport, such time away from sport can be particularly challenging.

The high prevalence and potential long-lasting complications related to BSIs in this population prompt a need to further educate and guide clinicians on how to promptly identify and treat BSIs, as well as effectively educate athletes and parents on appropriate preventative measures. This chapter aims to highlight the epidemiology of BSIs in the pediatric population, identify risk factors associated with increased risk of BSI, and address specific considerations for evaluation and management of BSIs in this unique population, with the ultimate goal of implementing preventive strategies to allow for safe participation in sports.

BONE HEALTH, GROWTH, AND DEVELOPMENT

Before discussing the details pertaining to BSI, it is important to understand growth and development in the pediatric population. On average, peak bone mass is achieved early in the third decade of life.[4] During adolescent years, individuals acquire about 40% to 60% of their peak bone mass.[5,6] About 90% of peak bone mass is achieved by the age of 18 in girls and 20 in boys.[5-7] The highest rate of bone mass accrual takes place during puberty at an average age of 12.5 years for girls and 14 years for boys.[8] Interestingly, peak bone mass accrual occurs on an average of about 6 to 12 months after peak height velocity, which is defined as the maximum rate of growth in height.[9-11] During this period of rapid linear growth where bone mineral density (BMD) lags behind, there is potentially heightened risk for bony injury, making childhood and adolescent years critical for bone development.[12]

EPIDEMIOLOGY OF BONE STRESS INJURIES IN THE PEDIATRIC POPULATION

Bone Stress Injury by Age

The incidence of BSI in the pediatric population varies by age. In a large, national epidemiological study on high school athletes participating in 22 sports from 2005 to2006 through 2012 to 2013, 0.8% of injuries were stress fractures with an overall stress fracture rate of 1.54 per 100,000 athletic exposures (AEs).[13] While the literature on BSIs in the pediatric population is limited to high school athletes, one large epidemiological study raises awareness regarding the distribution of all sports injuries in younger children aged 5 to 12 years versus older children aged 13 to 17 years. Younger children were more likely to endure traumatic injuries and fractures compared to adolescents, who were more likely to develop overuse injuries including BSIs.[14] This is potentially due to the increased intensity of sports with age as well as biological factors. It is important to note that the dearth of literature on the prevalence of BSIs in younger children highlights the need for further understanding of BSIs in this younger population.

Bone Stress Injuries in Girls and Boys

Similar to female adult athletes, the female sex is a well-known risk factor for BSIs in pediatric athletes. A prospective cross-sectional study of 748 competitive high school runners identified that while both genders are at risk for BSIs, female runners had a nonstatistically significant greater rate of stress fractures compared to their male counterparts (5.4% vs. 4%).[15] Nonetheless, the predilection of BSIs for female athletes is not limited to runners. Such gender differences exist in other sports as well. In a descriptive epidemiologic study that evaluated data on high school athletes through the National High School Sports-Related Injury Surveillance System from 2005 to2006 through 2012 to 2013, 63% of the reported stress fractures endured by athletes affected girls, while 37% of fractures impacted boys in sex-comparable sports, including cross-country, soccer, volleyball, basketball, lacrosse, swimming and diving, softball, and baseball.[13] In the prospective Growing Up Today Study, which consisted of a cohort of about 7,000 preadolescent and adolescent females, 3.9% of the participants sustained a BSI over 7 years of observation.[16] Differences with injury rate between female and male youth athletes may be related to gender-related factors, which are discussed in the section titled Risk Factors and Preventive Strategies for Bone Stress Injuries.

Bone Stress Injury by the Sport

Certain sports are more commonly linked to the prevalence of BSIs in the pediatric population. Running is commonly associated with increased rates of injury. A previously mentioned national epidemiologic study found that stress fracture rates per 100,000 AEs were highest in both girls' and boys' cross-country as well as gymnastics.[13] Aesthetic sports, including gymnastics and dance, may be viewed as high-risk sports for BSIs. In a study on adolescent runners, participation in dance or gymnastics was associated with a four-times greater risk for stress fractures.[15] Despite the potential benefits related to the high-impact weight-bearing nature of gymnastics and dance, as discussed in prior investigations, such sports may demonstrate an elevated risk for BSIs due to their emphasis on leanness. Such a focus can lead to poor behaviors with negative health consequences.[15,17]

Studies have shown that certain sports can positively influence bone geometry and strength. Ferry et al. compared the impact of sport on bone geometry patterns in 26 female swimmers (average age 15.9 ± 2 years) and 32 female soccer players (average age 16.2 ± 0.7 years) to that in a control group. Swimmers demonstrated a significantly higher lean body mass in their upper extremities, whereas soccer players had a higher lean body mass in their lower extremities. In comparison to swimmers, soccer players had a higher bone mineral content (BMC) and BMD at nearly every observed bone site, while there was no significant difference between swimmers and the control. Through hip structural analysis (HAS) that involved utilization of BMD to determine bone strength, bone geometry at the hip was improved in soccer players and diminished in swimmers compared to the control.[18] These findings highlight the enhanced effect of participation in impact-loading sports on muscle mass, BMD, and bone geometry. While the hypogravity nature of swimming may enhance upper body muscle mass, it may not positively impact bone health.[18]

Anatomical Distribution of Bone Stress Injuries

BSIs are more likely to develop in the lower extremities and is best explained due to the level of repetitive weight bearing placed on the lower extremities during land-based sports. However, the anatomical distribution of BSIs is typically multifactorial and varies with sport. An epidemiological study showed that the most commonly injured sites in high school runners in descending order included the lower leg (tibia, fibula), foot (metatarsals, sesamoid bones), and lumbar spine/pelvis.[13] A study on adolescent runners reported greater involvement of the tibia in girl runners, while boy runners were more likely to endure injury at metatarsals.[15] An Japanese study analyzed the characteristics of stress fractures in 208 athletes (100 girls, 108 boys) with an average age of 14.2 ± 2.2 years. In this particular population, the most common anatomical regions in the lower extremity to sustain a stress fracture in descending order were the tibia, metatarsals, pars interarticularis, fibula, femur, and tarsal bones.[19] On the contrary, in a 2-year retrospective review on athletes between the ages of 7 to 18 years who suffered a trunk or lower extremity BSI, the lumbar spine emerged as the most common location for BSIs followed by the foot and then the tibia.[20] Of note, these athletes participated in a wide range of sports including gymnastics, football, cross-country/track and field, and/or soccer.[20]

BSI to the lumbar spine, specifically a spondylolysis stress fracture to the pars interarticularis, is commonly associated with athletic activities that put athletes into repetitive, hyperextended positions with increased force on the lumbar spine. An example of such a sport is gymnastics. A retrospective, randomized case comparison study with two cohorts consisting of 100 adolescent athletes (ages 12–18 years) and 100 adults (ages 21–years) who all presented with a chief complaint of acute low back pain showed that 47% of the adolescent group endured a stress fracture of the pars interarticularis compared to 5% of the adults. Interestingly, all the adolescent athletes reported training in a sport with repetitive hyperextension movements, such as gymnastics.[21] Among another cohort study on 200 youth athletes (144 boys, 56 girls, average age of 14.1 ± 1.5 years) with low back pain, 48.5% of the participants suffered a pars interarticularis fracture that was confirmed on imaging, with most cases related to baseball, soccer, and basketball.[22] Therefore, such findings emphasize the point that the anatomic location of a BSI may be influenced by the nature of the athlete's sport of choice.

BSIs are less common in the upper extremity and trunk. Athletes who sustain these injuries include overhead athletes such as baseball, softball, football, and lacrosse players.[11] On the contrary to BSIs, physeal stress injuries, unique to pediatric athletes, can inflict both the upper and the lower extremities. The physis is particularly susceptible to injury due to its relative weakness. Adolescents are at increased risk for physeal stress injuries for a multitude of reasons. The most commonly referenced risk factors for physeal stress injuries in the sports medicine literature include muscle imbalances, accelerated growth periods, flexibility, strength, training factors including volume and coaching styles, and history of previous injuries.[23,24] While the mechanism of a physeal stress injury relies on a traction-related stress, physeal stress injuries are considered to be overuse injuries, similar to BSIs.[24] BSIs do not typically impact the upper extremity and trunk; however, physeal stress injuries occur at major tendon insertion sites of the upper and lower extremities.[11,21] Common sites for physeal stress injuries are the proximal tibial tubercle, distal femur, pelvic apophyses, proximal and distal humerus, and calcaneus.[24,25]

While we discussed earlier the specific bones commonly involved in BSIs, it is important to highlight the different bone microarchitectures impacted by BSIs. Both cortical-rich (tibia, metatarsals, fibula, femoral shaft, sesamoid, navicular) and trabecular-rich (pelvis, femoral neck, sacrum) bones are susceptible to BSIs. Injuries to such microstructures may be associated with negative health consequences. In a cohort study of 28 male athletes (mostly runners) ages 14 to 36 years, 43% of the athletes who suffered trabecular-rich BSIs also met the diagnostic criteria for low BMD. Those athletes who suffered trabecular-rich BSIs had a 4.6-fold increased risk for low BMD compared to those who suffered cortical-rich BSIs.[26] Therefore, clinicians shoulder consider a bone health workup, including a BMD assessment, for athletes with trabecular-rich BSIs.

RISK FACTORS AND PREVENTIVE STRATEGIES FOR BONE STRESS INJURIES

Risk factors for BSIs are best divided into two categories (Table 11.1): biological and biomechanical.

TABLE 11.1

RISK FACTORS FOR BONE STRESS INJURY IN PEDIATRIC ATHLETES DIVIDED BY BIOLOGICAL AND BIOMECHANICAL ETIOLOGIES

BIOLOGICAL	BIOMECHANICAL
Low EA	Anatomic variants
Menstrual irregularities (primary or secondary amenorrhea, oligomenorrhea)	Training intensity and volume
Low BMD	Sports specialization
Low BMI	
Family history of osteoporosis/osteopenia	
Inadequate calcium, dairy, vitamin D intake	
Prior injuries	

BMD, bone mineral density; BMI, body mass index; BSI, bone stress injury; EA, energy availability.

Biological Factors

Low Energy Availability

Energy availability (EA) is defined as the difference between the energy intake and exercise energy expenditure per fat free mass per day.[27] When the energy utilized exceeds the amount of energy consumed, there are inadequate stores available for the body's metabolic processes to maintain optimal health and performance.[27,28] Contrary to adult athletes, there are no specific parameters for adequate EA in the pediatric population, which highlights the need to develop thresholds that can be identified through a standardized measurement tool for the purpose of detecting individuals at risk.[27,29] Low EA is a key component of the female athlete triad and relative energy deficiency in sport (RED-S).[27,29]

Low EA may be inadvertent due to high exercise needs not met through adequate caloric intake, although low LA may also result from intentional restriction of intake to achieve a certain physique for their respective sport, unhealthy dietary patterns including disordered eating, or eating disorder patterns.[28] There are certain sports that emphasize a lean body appearance. In an Australian study that assessed eating disorders in a population of adolescents and adult elite athletes compared to nonathlete controls, the athletes at greatest risk for eating disorders were those who participated in sports that placed the greatest emphasis on leanness. In all, 31% of the female athletes and 6% of the male athletes involved in "thin-build" sports, including gymnastics, ballet, light-weight rowing, diving, swimming, and long-distance running, endorsed a history of an eating disorder compared to 5.5% of the female control group and 0% of the male control group.[30] Not only are eating disorders more prevalent in athletes, particularly those who participate in aesthetic, endurance, or weight-class sports, they are also more common in female athletes. In a two-stage study conducted on athletes, ages 15 to 39 years, the diagnostic criteria for subclinical and clinical eating disorders were met by 20% female athletes compared to 8% male athletes.[31]

It is critical that clinicians assess eating behaviors in athletes during well visits and preparticipation physical evaluations (PPEs) to identify those individuals at risk for low EA. Of note, it is important to keep in mind that athletes with eating disorders or disordered eating habits may not self-report such behaviors. It is critical for clinicians to gain their athletes' trust to elicit such behaviors that may jeopardize their development. Such treatment may include mental health referrals for cognitive behavioral, group, and family-based therapy. It is recommended to have increased family involvement, especially in younger pediatric athletes.[31,32] Furthermore, it is important to be able to identify risk factors for eating disorders. In a large randomized cohort study over 3 years, dieting and psychiatric illness were the most sensitive, independent predictors for development of an eating disorder.[33] Therefore, this places the task upon clinicians to inquire about psychiatric comorbidities through the appropriate screening models and treat associated behaviors including disordered eating behaviors. Nutritional counseling and education are critical for optimization of nutritional status. All in all, it is clear that management of low EA is best achieved through a multidisciplinary approach in youth athletes.

Menstrual Dysfunction

The female athlete triad refers to a spectrum of diseases that involves the interplay between low EA, menstrual dysfunction, and low BMD in female athletes.[34]

Menstrual dysfunction ranges from primary amenorrhea (no onset of menses by age 15 years) to secondary amenorrhea (absence of menstrual cycles for 3 or more consecutive months in the past year) to oligomenorrhea (after onset of menses by age 15 years, cycles occur at intervals of greater than 35 days in the past year).[16,32] The proposed mechanism of action in which regular menses offers protection against BSI is through the association between improved BMD and endogenously produced normal levels of estrogen.[16,35] Rauh et al. performed a cohort study on 89 female cross-country and track-and-field athletes with a mean age of 15.5 ± 1.3 years in which a history of oligomenorrhea or amenorrhea was significantly associated with increased risk for general musculoskeletal injuries, including bone injuries.[36] Meanwhile, Tenforde et al. conducted a prospective study on high school runners that confirmed the association between menstrual history factors and increased risk for BSI. Athletes with amenorrhea had a twofold increase in development of stress fractures. Fewer number of periods in a year was associated with an increased risk for BSI. There was a four times increased risk for stress fractures in girls who experienced menses at the age of 15 years or older.[15] In a prospective cohort study including 6,831 girls ages 9 to 15 years from the Growing Up Today Study conducted by Field et al., the older the age of the athlete at menarche, the greater the risk for stress fracture; specifically, there was approximately a 30% increase in risk with every 1-year delay in menarche.[16]

These findings highlight the need to specifically discuss menstrual history with young female athletes as bone mineralization in part depends on normal menstrual function. It is important to modify questions pertaining to menstrual history on an individual basis. For instance, with regards to the topic of hormonal therapy (oral contraception pills, intrauterine device, injections), it is key to ask such athletes the reasoning for such treatment. Menstrual dysfunction is sometimes treated with hormone treatment, and clarifying use may lead to understanding triad risk factors.[35,37]

Low Bone Mineral Density

Low BMD is the final component of the female athlete triad that is associated with increased risk for BSI. In athletes with low BMD, there is diminished ability to withstand increased mechanical stresses, and thereby there is increased risk for fractures.

While there are several factors involved in the optimization of bone health, the American College of Sports Medicine focuses on BMD due to its use in screening and diagnosis of bone disease, regardless of the limited data on BMD in youth athletes.[32] It is challenging to utilize BMD in the pediatric population due to a lack of standards that adjust for bone size, pubertal stage, skeletal maturity, and body composition in the pediatric population. The International Society for Clinical Densitometry (ISCD) recommends utilization of z-scores to characterize BMD.[29,32] "Low bone density for chronological age" in female and male youth athletes is defined as a dual energy x-ray absorptiometry (DXA) BMD z-score <-1.0.[29,32,35,38] While osteoporosis is diagnosed solely on BMD in adults, this is not the case in pediatrics. Per the ISCD, the diagnosis of osteoporosis includes (1) the presence of ≥1 vertebral compression fracture without a history of trauma or local disease, (2) the presence of low BMC or BMD for a given chronological age (z-score <-2), and (3) a history of long bone fractures (≥2 fractures by 10 years old or ≥3 fractures by 19 years).[29,32,39,40]

BMD can vary among pediatric athletes depending on their respective sport. For instance, in a cohort study of 161 female high school athletes, BMD was greater in those who participated in multidirectional sports including soccer, softball, volleyball, tennis, lacrosse, tracking sprinting and jumping events versus repetitive/nonimpact sports such as swimming, cross-country, and track distance running.[41] Similarly, a cohort study on 28 male runners ages 14 to 36 years with a history of ≥1 BSI demonstrated an association between trabecular-rich BSIs and increased risk for low BMD.[26]

In order to prevent low BMD, it is imperative that clinicians provide athletes with education regarding healthy lifestyles including regular physical activity, a healthy, balanced diet with adequate calcium and vitamin D, and avoidance of tobacco products.[39,42]

Vigorous, high-impact, weight-bearing loads that include jumps are effective in order to improve peak bone mass in adolescence.[43] Bone strength depends on a number of factors, including mechanical loads that result in remodeling and increased bone strength. Muscles generate the largest mechanical strain on bone;[44,45] hence, sports that require maximum muscle force put the greatest stress on the bone.[44,45] Sports that involve high/odd impact, multidirectional movements, weight bearing, and quick changes in speed and direction put peak strains on the bone in various planes that allow for increased strength, particularly at regions most stressed in the sport. Examples of such sports include ball sports (basketball, soccer), gymnastics, and martial arts.[45,46] In fact, Fredericson et al. conducted a retrospective cohort study on 106 elite female and 118 elite male distance runners that showed that ball sports in one's youth reduced the risk for BSI later in life.[47]

Aside from the previously mentioned sports, running may also be associated with increased BMD due to the weight-bearing nature of the sport that places substantial ground reaction forces on the bone as shown in a study on female athletes (swimmers, cyclists, runners, triathletes).[48] On the contrary, sports such as cycling and swimming inflict minimal stress on the bone and thereby have minimal influence on BMD.[49] In fact, in a cohort study that compared adolescent swimmers and soccer players to nonathletes, swimmers demonstrated lower BMD than not only soccer players but also the control group.[18] Therefore, such findings emphasize that the nature of the sport can impact BMD.

The timing of exposure to sports associated with increased BMD can impact the effect on bone health. The literature varies in terms of a specific age at which one should participate in such sports to receive the beneficial impact on bone health; however, the general consensus among experts is that such participation should occur when peak bone mass accrual rates take place during adolescent years.[50]

Nonetheless, participation in such protective sports earlier in life may also benefit an athlete. For instance, in a retrospective study on elite runners, male runners experienced an even greater benefit if they began such sports before the age of 10 years;[47] however, such a correlation was not evident in female athletes. Meanwhile, in a cross-sectional study on elite female athletes, there was greater impact on BMD for those who participated in sport before or at menarche, opposed to after menarche.[51] Therefore, the consensus is that participation in such high/odd impact, multidirectional sports should be initiated during early adolescence at the latest to maximize bone health and reduce risk for BSI. Physical activity in youth should be encouraged for lifelong bone health due to long-term benefits on bone size and strength.[52]

In addition to weight-bearing sport participation, resistance training may be an effective strategy to increase BMD in adolescence, particularly using moderate- to high-intensity exercises.[43,53] A pilot study on adolescent females found significant improvements in lumbar spine BMC and BMD after a school-based resistance training intervention consisting of body weight exercises, handheld weights, and resistance bands.[54]

The literature demonstrates a cumulative effect of risk factors for the development of BSI. In a prospective cohort study involving female athletes, the risk for BSIs increased in individuals with multiple female athlete triad risk factors.[55] Likewise, a similar relationship has been demonstrated in male distance runners.[38,56]

Low Body Mass Index

An additional risk factor for BSI includes low body mass index (BMI). A prospective cohort study on 748 competitive high school runners (442 girls and 306 boys), ages 14 to 18 years, demonstrated that a BMI <19 kg/m^2 was independently associated with a three times greater risk for BSI in female runners compared to those individuals with a BMI >19 kg/m^2.[15] A cross-sectional study of 69 male adolescent athletes (51 runners,

18 non-runners) ages 13 to 19 years showed single-variable risk factors associated with low BMD to include low body weight (<85% of expected weight) and low BMI (BMI z-score <−1.0).[38]

It is critical to educate athletes, parents, and coaches on proper nutrition; healthy BMI values for pediatric athletes; and the negative health consequences associated with low BMI. It is important to educate parents and coaches as they are in the most ideal situation to identify behaviors that may be associated with low BMI. In addition, such knowledge may influence how parents and coaches speak with the highly impressionable pediatric population.

Family History of Osteopenia/Osteoporosis

In the pediatric population, it is important to consider the potential influence of genetics on risk for BSI. Two prospective cohort studies demonstrate such findings. A study on 168 active females ages 13 to 22 years presenting with their first stress fracture found that such athletes had three times the odds of having a family history of osteopenia or osteoporosis.[57] A much larger study on 6,831 girls ages 9 to 15 years demonstrated that girls with a family history of osteoporosis or low BMD were twice as likely to endure a BSI.[16]

Regardless of the potential challenges that may arise in obtaining a family history from a pediatric patient, it is necessary to obtain such information as 60% to 80% of peak bone strength is dependent on genetics.[2,3] Such information can help identify potentially higher-risk athletes and allow for closer monitoring with the appropriate screening tests.

Calcium, Vitamin D, Dairy Intake

Nutritional intake of calcium and vitamin D plays a key role in the optimization of bone health through bone mineralization and remodeling. Therefore, such bone-building micronutrients are perceived to play an important role in the prevention of BSIs.

In a prospective study on 39 adolescent female cross-country runners (mean age 15.7 ± 0.2 years), girls with an increased bone turnover consumed less than the daily recommended 1,300 mg calcium and had lower levels of 25-hydroxycholecalciferol,[58] highlighting the importance of vitamin D and calcium in achieving peak bone strength. Tenforde et al. identified that female adolescent athletes on calcium supplementation were three times more likely to have a history of BSI and endure a future BSI due to a preexisting deficiency. Unfortunately, a protective effect from increased calcium or dairy intake was not appreciated.[15] On the contrary, a prospective cohort study of 6,712 adolescent females ages 9 to 15 years did not demonstrate an association between calcium and dairy intake with increased risk for BSI,[59] as supported by prior studies in children and adolescents.[60,61] Similar to the previously mentioned Tenforde et al. study, higher calcium and dairy intake was not protective against BSI.[59]

Interestingly, in a randomized clinical trial that studied the effects of calcium supplementation in females with a mean age of 10.9 ± 0.9 years over 7 years, increased daily calcium intake of 1,500 mg was associated with increased bone mass acquisition during pubertal growth spurt.[62] Therefore, it is reasonable to suspect that the recommended calcium intake for adolescent athletes may exceed the American Academy of Pediatrics (AAP)–recommended calcium intake of 1,300 mg/day due to the increased demands on the skeletal system during this period of growth and development.[63] In terms of meeting adequate calcium intake, youth athletes should be able to obtain sufficient calcium through diet, specifically calcium-fortified foods such as dairy products; however, if necessary, supplementation can be considered.[42,63]

The literature on vitamin D intake and increased risk for BSI is more consistent compared to that on calcium and dairy intake. The already-discussed prospective cohort study of 6,712 girls ages 9 to 15 years demonstrated that girls with the highest intake of

TABLE 11.2

CALCIUM AND VITAMIN D RECOMMENDATIONS BY AGE IN PEDIATRIC ATHLETES

AGE (YEARS)	CALCIUM (MG)	VITAMIN D (IU)
1–3	500	600
4–8	800–1,000	600
9–18	1,300	600

vitamin D (600 IU) had a 50% reduction in risk for BSI compared to those with the lowest intake of vitamin D. This relationship was strengthened in those who performed ≥1 hour/day high-impact activity. It is important for clinicians to consider the developmental stage and activity level for each athlete when assessing for adequate nutritional intake.[59] This inverse relationship between vitamin D intake and risk for BSI can guide treatment recommendations. In a cross-sectional study on girls and boys ages 12 and 15 years, 25-hydroxycholecalciferol ≥29.64 ng/mL was associated with greater forearm BMD and reduction in bone turnover markers.[64] These findings suggest that it may be necessary to maintain vitamin D levels above the commonly accepted threshold of 20 ng/mL to optimize bone health in adolescents.[64] Vitamin D deficiency can be prevented through adequate intake of calcium-fortified foods as well as sun exposure. The AAP recommendations (Table 11.2) on daily vitamin D intake vary with age and development. For instance, the standard recommendation for adolescents is 600 IU of vitamin D/day.[65] Higher intake of vitamin D may be necessary for pediatric patients at risk for vitamin D deficiency, including those with malabsorption, with limited sun exposure, and on medications that impair vitamin D metabolism.[66]

Prior Injury History

A history of prior injury has been linked to increased risk for BSI in pediatric athletes. Barrack et al. observed that when combined with other factors such as an average weekly mileage >30 miles and <85% of expected weight, a history of stress fracture increased the risk for low BMD in an adolescent male runner.[38] Traumatic fractures are also associated with increased risk for BSI. In 748 competitive high school runners (442 girls, 306 boys), a history of fracture, which included stress and traumatic fractures, put adolescent girl athletes at a sixfold increased risk for BSI and adolescent boys at a sevenfold increased risk.[15]

Biomechanical Factors

Anatomic Variants

There are anatomical features that may predispose an athlete for increased risk of BSI. Yagi et al. conducted a 3-year prospective study of 230 high school runners (137 boys, 97 girls), which showed that limited hip internal rotation in female athletes increased their risk for development of medial tibial stress syndrome (MTSS); meanwhile, reduced straight leg raise in male athletes was associated with increased risk for stress fractures.[67] This highlights the potential association between hip range of motion and flexibility and increased risk for BSI.

Foot mechanics are commonly studied in runners. There is conflicting data regarding the degree of foot pronation that may increase one's risk for BSI. In a predictive correlational study of 125 high school cross-country runners (68 girls, 57 boys), results demonstrated that athletes with increased navicular drop, a measure utilized to assess the degree of pronation at the subtalar joint, were more likely to sustain MTSS.[68] However, in a prospective cohort of 105 cross-country high school runners (46 girls, 59 boys), there was no association between the degree of navicular drop and MTSS.[69] Step rate, or the total number of steps per minute, has also been implied in the development of tibia BSIs. Luedke et al. conducted a study of 68 high school cross-country runners (47 girls, 21 boys), which demonstrated a greater likelihood of shin injury in those athletes with a step rate <166 steps/min. Reduced step rate is inversely associated with step length, which results in increased ground reaction forces and shock attenuation.[70]

Running assessments can help physical therapists and clinicians identify movement patterns that put athletes at a higher risk for BSI and can lead to earlier intervention to potentially correct such biomechanical abnormalities.

Training: Intensity, Volume, and Sports Specialization

A number of training factors, including intensity, volume, and patterns, have been considered when assessing for BSI risk. In the 2016 cross-sectional study by Barrack et al. that evaluated male adolescent athletes and predictors for low BMD, an average weekly mileage >30 in the past year was associated with increased risk for low BMD. The greater the number of risk factors associated with low EA, the stronger the association.[38] A prospective cohort study of high school girls observed that girls who participated in ≥8 hours of activity/week had a twofold increased risk for stress fracture compared to those girls who did <4 hours of activity/week.[35]

Youth sports have dramatically changed with a shift toward sports specialization, which is defined as a focus on one sport, usually year round with exclusion of other sports.[71] A case–control study of 1,214 athletes ages 7 to 18 years demonstrated that sports specialization serves as an independent risk factor for overuse injury in a dose-dependent manner.[72] Similarly, two additional studies of high school athletes showed that the incidence of lower extremity overuse injuries was greater in those athletes with higher levels of sports specialization as defined by the researchers.[73,74] A case–control study of 2,011 youth athletes (989 girls, 1,022 boys) ages 12 to 18 years revealed that youth athletes who participated in a single sport for >8 months/year or trained for more hours per week than their age in years were more likely to suffer an overuse injury.[75]

Experts recommend that athletes delay sports specialization until after puberty to minimize the physiologic and psychological effects of sports specialization.[71] It is recommended that weekly training hours do not exceed the athlete's age in years.[71–73] Furthermore, athletes should not participate in >8 months per year of participation in a single sport.[71–73] There are no recommendations on when athletes can increase training volume and intensity safely, but one must consider the athlete's stage in development as well as the nature of their respective sport. It is essential for clinicians to provide such guidance to athletes, parents, and coaches.

CLINICAL EVALUATION

History and Physical Exam

BSIs and associated risk factors are assessed for during PPEs and annual health visits. One should obtain a detailed medical history including injury history as well as sports history focusing on changes in training intensity and volume, changes in training terrain, shoe type, frequency of competition, and any recent changes in running mechanics. For female athletes, you should assess for the presence of triad risk factors. For male athletes, providers should assess for factors related to low EA including symptoms of low testosterone status that can manifest through absence of morning erections or loss of libido. You should also ask athletes about medication use including hormonal therapies, vitamin supplementation, oral contraception, and oral steroids. It is essential to obtain a detailed dietary history, specifically identifying any avoidance or restricted eating behaviors and eating disorders. A family history of osteoporosis or osteopenia can help identify high-risk athletes.

On physical exam in those athletes in whom a BSI is suspected, range of motion (ROM) and muscle strength and bulk are usually preserved. Edema may be present. When performing a physical exam on a patient with suspected BSI, the affected location will guide the clinician's exam maneuvers. For instance, if tibial injury is suspected, direct percussion may elicit tenderness and pain.[39,76] The single hop test may also reproduce index pain; however, one can defer such a test if concerned for higher-risk BSI.[39,77] It is also important to assess for other physical exam findings that can be associated with pathological behaviors.[77] Classic physical exam findings in patients with eating disorders include skin abnormalities such as facial lanugo, dry mucous membranes, decreased subcutaneous tissue, skin discoloration, hair loss, evidence of self-harm, and callus formation on the proximal interphalangeal joints.[77]

Diagnostic Testing

Diagnosis of BSI is paramount in pediatrics given the significant long-term effects on bone health that can arise from inappropriate treatment and management. There are various types of imaging for evaluation of BSI, but we will just highlight those specific to pediatrics.

MRI is the gold standard for diagnosis of BSI in youth athletes. CT scan is typically deferred due to the high level of ionizing radiation and reserved for surgical planning.[39] Bone scintigraphy can be a helpful diagnostic tool when standard radiographs are inconclusive; however, interpretation of such a test in pediatric athletes can be challenging. Increased radiotracer uptake is not specific to BSI as such findings may be normal as the physis and apophysis typically have high uptake compared to nonossified structures.[78]

DXA screenings should be performed on athletes with multiple risk factors associated with low EA.[39,42] Such studies should be conducted at centers with pediatric expertise. The preferred skeletal sites per ISCD recommendations include the lumbar spine and total body, not the head.[42,79,80] The proximal femur is challenging in pediatrics due to improper positioning from lack of developed bony landmarks and extensive normative data.[79,81] While DXA is commonly utilized in pediatric patients due to low levels of ionizing radiation and availability of normative measures, interpretation of such studies can be challenging in the pediatric population. Sex-specific reference standards must be utilized to prevent misdiagnosis of low BMD in boys who historically experience puberty and skeletal maturity later compared to girls.[82] To diminish the effect of bone size in pediatric patients on DXA measurements, BMC can be adjusted for height or estimated bone volume.[82] To accommodate for skeletal and pubertal maturity, BMD findings can be adjusted for Tanner stage or chronological bone age.[82] However, for individuals with delayed skeletal maturity or puberty, bone age, opposed to chronological bone age, better correlates with pubertal maturation, thus making it a better tool for analysis of DXA scans.[79,80,82] When utilizing bone age to interpret DXA readings, it is important to recalculate z-scores using bone age.[80] Contrary to adults, T-scores are not utilized in pediatrics and are inappropriate to use during times of skeletal maturation.[81]

TREATMENT OF BONE STRESS INJURY

Due to the multifactorial nature of BSIs, they are best managed through a multidisciplinary team of a pediatric sports medicine physician, an endocrinologist, a radiologist, a dietician, a mental health specialist, a physical therapist, coaches, athletic trainers, and parents.[40]

BSIs are managed either conservatively or surgically depending on the location and severity of injury. Conservative management involves activity modification and reduced weight bearing. Historically, for high-risk fractures, noncompliant patients, or patients in whom symptoms persist, immobilization and strict non–weight bearing are recommended.[83–85] They can be achieved through controlled ankle motion (CAM) boots and casting. While CAM boots are adjustable, removable, and lightweight, they may not be ideal for younger athletes due to potential difficulties with compliance.[86] In such patients, casting may be preferred to keep the affected limb in a fixed position. Orthopedic consultation is indicated for high-risk fractures (femoral neck, patella, anterior tibial diaphysis, medial malleolus, lateral process of the talus, and navicular), complete fractures, and fractures that fail to achieve union.[87]

CONCLUSION

BSIs are highly prevalent overuse injuries in the pediatric population. Youth athletes are particularly vulnerable to BSIs during their adolescent years due to the lag in time between linear growth and accrual of BMD. Most BSIs are seen in adolescent children due to biological factors and increased intensity in sport. Similar to adult counterparts, girls are more likely to endure BSIs. Aesthetic sports and running were most commonly associated with increased risk for BSI in this population. In pediatric athletes, BSIs typically occur in the lower extremities, but can also occur in the lumbar spine in sports that put the athlete into repetitive lumbar extension. For both girl and boy athletes with BSI, it is crucial to screen for the appropriate risk factors to reduce future injuries and optimize long-term bone health. Girls and boys should be screened for triad risk factors minus menstrual history in boys. Assessing for low BMD is critical in such a population as BSIs may hinder skeletal maturity. Both sexes should be screened for biomechanical factors including training and anatomic factors. When assessing youth athletes for BSIs, it is pivotal for clinicians to perform a thorough history, physical exam, and diagnostic workup, as inappropriate management can lead to significant sequelae. Prevention of BSIs largely involves addressing the identified risk factors through a multidisciplinary approach consisting of multiple health specialists, parents, and coaches.

With the rising prevalence of sports specialization, there is increased interest in BSIs in pediatric athletes. Most investigations focus on high school athletes, raising the need for further studies on middle school-aged athletes. Future research domains include development of BSI risk assessment tools to incorporate in the PPE or annual health visit to better identify athletes at high risk; standardized educational programs for coaches, athletic trainers, parents, and athletes; and further data on the epidemiology and risk factors in younger pediatric athletes.

KEY REFERENCES

Only key references appear in the print edition. The full reference list appears in the digital product found on http://connect.springerpub.com/content/book/978-0-8261-4424-9/part/sec03/chapter/ch11

13. Changstrom BG, Brou L, Khodaee M, et al. Epidemiology of stress fracture injuries among US high school athletes, 2005–2006 through 2012–2013. *Am J Sports Med.* 2015;43(1):26–33. doi:10.1177/0363546514562739

15. Tenforde AS, Sayres LC, McCurdy ML, et al. Identifying sex-specific risk factors for stress fractures in adolescent runners. *Med Sci Sports Exerc.* 2013;45(10):1843–1851. doi:10.1249/MSS.0b013e3182963d75

27. Mountjoy M, Sundgot-Borgen JK, Burke LM, et al. IOC consensus statement on relative energy deficiency in sport (RED-S): 2018 update. *Br J Sports Med*. 2018;52(11):687–697. doi:10.1136/bjsports-2018-099193

35. De Souza MJ, Nattiv A, Joy E, et al. 2014 female athlete triad coalition consensus statement on treatment and return to play of the female athlete triad: 1st international conference held in San Francisco, California, May 2012 and 2nd international conference held in Indianapolis, Indiana, May 2013. *Br J Sports Med*. 2014;48(4):289. doi:10.1136/bjsports-2013-093218

39. Kraus E, Bachrach LK, Grover M. Team approach: bone health in children and adolescents. *JBJS Rev*. 2018;6(10):e6, 1–10. doi:10.2106/JBJS.RVW.17.00205

55. Barrack MT, Gibbs JC, De Souza MJ, et al. Higher incidence of bone stress injuries with increasing female athlete triad-related risk factors: a prospective multisite study of exercising girls and women. *Am J Sports Med*. 2014;42(4):949–958. doi:10.1177/0363546513520295

81. Bachrach LK, Gordon CM; Section on Endocrinology. Bone densitometry in children and adolescents. *Pediatrics*. 2016;138(4):e2016–e2398. doi:10.1542/peds.2016–2398

CHAPTER 12

Male Athletes

Andrea Kussman

INTRODUCTION

Bone stress injuries (BSIs) represent an overuse injury among male athletes. These injuries occur when a bone is unable to withstand the repetitive submaximal forces to which it is exposed and occur on a continuum ranging from stress reactions to stress fractures. The majority of the research on BSIs in male athletes has involved distance runners and military recruits, but male athletes in a wide range of sports are also susceptible, depending on the specific demands of their sport. A BSI can cause significant time lost from training and competition and can also be the initial presenting symptom of impaired bone health. This chapter explores what is known regarding sex-specific considerations in the evaluation and management of BSIs in male athletes.

EPIDEMIOLOGY OF BONE STRESS INJURIES IN MALE ATHLETES

A Comparison of Bone Stress Injury Rates Among Male and Female Athletes

Two large epidemiological studies give us insight into rates of injury within athlete populations and suggest that this form of injury may occur less often in men than in women. One study evaluated data from a national sports injury surveillance program at the high school level; in that study, it was found that in sex-comparable sports (such as basketball, soccer, or volleyball), 36.7% of stress fractures occurred in male athletes.[1] A similar study at the collegiate level analyzed data from the National Collegiate Athletic Association (NCAA) injury surveillance program and found that in sex-comparable sports females sustained stress fractures at a rate of 9.13 per 100,000 athlete exposures (AEs), as compared to 4.44 stress fractures per 100,000 AEs in males.[2] In a study of collegiate track and field athletes, 35% of BSIs occurred in male athletes.[3] A systematic review of BSI in athletes reported incidences of 6.5% in males and 9.7% in females.[4] Studies in military populations provide similar information and indicate a lower frequency of BSI among male recruits when compared to females.[4-6] Interestingly, the racial differences in stress fracture incidence among men mirror those seen in women: In one military study, non-Hispanic black men had the lowest incidence of stress fracture, while Hispanic men had a 19% increase in risk and white men had a 59% increase in risk.[6] Although the overall rates of BSI differ between men and women, there do not appear to be significant differences in the rates of recurrent BSI.[2]

Locations of Bone Stress Injury in Male Athletes

The majority of BSIs in male athletes occur in the lower extremities. However, athletes in some sports may sustain BSIs in other areas due to the specific demands of their sport. For example, throwing athletes may develop BSIs of the upper extremity,[7] and rowers are prone to developing stress fractures of the ribs.[8] It is likely that the anatomic distribution of BSIs also differs between males and females, although studies have not demonstrated a consistent pattern. In a military study, male cadets sustained over 90% of their stress fractures in the tibia, as compared to female cadets, who had 51% of their stress fractures in the pelvis and only 39% in the tibia.[5] Studies in track-and-field athletes have found that women sustain more pelvic and metatarsal stress fractures and less fibular stress fractures than men.[9] In contrast, in a study across multiple sports, men were more likely to have stress fractures affecting the back, lumbar spine, and pelvis (12.8%) compared to women (6.9%), and women were more likely to have stress fractures of the femur (12.2%) compared to men (4.4%).[2] The anatomic distribution of BSIs in male and female athletes likely differs, but the exact nature of these differences is challenging to fully elucidate due to the heterogeneity of studies on the subject, particularly with regard to the sports or activities included.

A Comparison of Bone Stress Injury Severity Between Male and Female Athletes

Thus far, the literature does not suggest a significant difference in the severity of BSIs sustained by male and female athletes. A population of cross-country runners demonstrated similar return-to-sport times for both male and female athletes with a BSI.[10] Time lost to stress fracture was also relatively similar in military recruits (4.5 weeks for males and 4.9 weeks for females).[5] Likewise, in a study of collegiate track and field athletes, although females trended toward higher-grade injuries, this difference was not statistically significant.[3] Among sex-comparable sports, male and female athletes also had a similar proportion of stress fractures that were season ending.[2]

Sports Associated With Higher Rates of Bone Stress Injury

As is clear from the studies cited earlier, the majority of the research on BSIs in men has been performed in the military or on runners. We can turn to large epidemiological studies of stress fractures to shed some light on which sports are associated with higher rates of stress fracture in male athletes. At the collegiate level, the male sport with the highest rate of stress fracture per AE was cross-country, followed in descending order by basketball, outdoor track, indoor track, soccer, lacrosse, and football.[2] Similarly, in a high school population, the male sports with the highest rates of stress fracture per AE were, in descending order, cross-country, track and field, soccer, football, lacrosse, and basketball.[1] Of note, football did have the most absolute stress fractures reported for high school athletes but a lower rate of injury per AE.[1]

TREATMENT OF BONE STRESS INJURY IN MALE ATHLETES

As in female athletes, the mainstay of treatment for BSIs in male athletes is rest (often while cross-training to maintain cardiovascular fitness), followed by a gradual return to sport. The degree and duration of rest recommended should be guided primarily by anatomic location (high-risk versus low-risk bony sites), type of bone involved (primarily trabecular versus cortical), and severity of injury[11,12] and is not dependent on sex. This approach is supported by research that demonstrates that higher MRI grades and injuries in sites with increased trabecular bone were associated with longer return-to-sport time for both male and female athletes.[3]

Aside from the immediate management of the BSI, both male and female athletes with BSIs should have a thorough risk assessment performed.[13] Research has demonstrated that history of prior stress fracture increases the risk for future BSIs in both males and females, which emphasizes the importance of addressing these risk factors proactively.[11] As will be explored further in the following, male athletes have unique risk factors. Addressing these risk factors not only optimizes healing from the current injury but also reduces future risk of injury and improves long-term health outcomes.

RISK FACTORS FOR BONE STRESS INJURY IN MALE ATHLETES AND STRATEGIES TO MODIFY RISK

Cumulative Effect of Risk Factors

There is evidence that risk factors for BSI are cumulative in female athletes.[14] Similarly, evidence now suggests that risk factors for BSI are also cumulative in male athletes. In male adolescent runners, an increased number of risk factors (including weight <85% of expected, weekly running mileage >30, history of prior stress fracture, and obtaining less than one serving of calcium-rich food per day) are associated with increased risk of having low bone mineral density (BMD).[15] Another study of collegiate male runners found that each additional risk point (assigned for low body mass index [BMI], low energy availability [EA], prior history of low BMD, and prior BSI) increased an athlete's risk for BSI by 27%.[16] Since the effect of these risk factors is cumulative, it is especially important to identify as many risk factors as possible in male athletes with a BSI.

Extrinsic Risk Factors

As in female athletes, extrinsic risk factors may contribute to the development of BSIs in male athletes. These factors have been studied in both male and female populations and include modifiable training variables such as the type of running surface, age of running shoes, use of shoe inserts, or the training schedule followed by the athlete.[12,17,18] When training errors are identified, they represent an easy behavioral modification that may help prevent future injuries.

Low Energy Availability

The female athlete triad, which consists of the interrelated conditions of low EA (with or without disordered eating [DE]), menstrual dysfunction, and impaired bone health, has been well documented.[19,20] There is an increasing body of literature on a similar entity in male athletes, consisting of low EA, hypogonadotropic hypogonadism, and impaired bone health.[21-24] As is noted in the female athlete triad, the underlying cause of this male athlete triad appears to be low EA, which has led to the development of a new term by the International Olympic Committee—relative energy deficiency in sport.[23,24] The evidence for low EA in male athletes, the important effect this has on bone health, and strategies to improve EA in male athletes are reviewed in the following.

Male athletes may have unintentional low EA if they are not aware of their increased metabolic demands during training. However, low EA may also be intentional, due to either a drive to conform to the demands of their sport or DE or an eating disorder (ED). Male athletes are less likely to have an ED than female athletes but more likely to have an ED compared to nonathletes.[25–27] One study reported a higher rate of EDs in female athletes compared to male athletes (20% vs. 8%) and a higher rate in athletes compared to controls (9% and 0.5% in women and men, respectively).[26] Even in the absence of a formal ED diagnosis, numerous studies have found high rates of DE among male athletes.[28–32]

Low EA is most common among male athletes in "lean sports" such as endurance sports, anti-gravitational sports, and weight class sports.[26,33] There are extensive examples of low EA and DE behaviors among cyclists and runners.[32,34–38] In combat sports with weight classes, athletes will often engage in DE behaviors in an effort to "make weight."[30,31,36] A similar phenomenon is seen in lightweight rowing[28,36,39] and in jockeys.[36,40–42]

Athletes in lean sports also tend to have lower BMD. For example, distance runners have been shown to have lower BMD when compared to athletes in ball sports or non-athlete controls.[15,43,44] Similarly, elite cyclists were found to have lower BMD when compared to both physically active controls and sedentary controls.[45–47]

Several studies have directly demonstrated the effect that these low EA states have on bone health in male athletes. In two studies of cyclists, those with lower EA also had lower BMD.[34,48] Proxy markers of low EA, such as lower percent body fat or BMI, have also been associated with impaired bone health.[49,50] Two studies looked specifically at changes in bone metabolic markers in response to low EA states in men: The first found changes in bone metabolic markers among males at low EA states, while the second study found changes in bone metabolic markers among female participants but not among male participants.[51,52] These differing findings may be related partially to different methods of calculating the energy restriction and also pose the question of whether male athletes exhibit physiologic changes at a different EA cutoff than female athletes.

Given the important impact low EA has on bone health, all male athletes should be screened for low EA annually and more frequently if they present with a BSI or with other medical concerns, such as mood changes, fatigue, or illness.[21,22] Because it can be clinically challenging to accurately determine EA, it may be helpful to refer to a sports dietitian for a more complete assessment.[24,53,54] Additional proxy indicators that might suggest a low EA state include BMI <17.5 kg/m^2 or weight less than 85% of expected, as well as significant changes in weight compared to prior. However, it is important to keep in mind that a stable weight does not rule out low EA, since this may be achieved by suppression of normal physiologic functions.[19] Adaptation to chronic low EA may be suggested by a reduced resting metabolic rate (RMR), low T3 levels, and a ratio of measured RMR/predicted RMR that is less than 0.90.[55–60]

If low EA is identified, it is important to optimize nutrition.[22,23,61] This is usually best accomplished with the help of a multidisciplinary team, which should include a physician, a sports dietitian, and, if DE or ED is present, a mental health provider.[25,53] The multidisciplinary team may also include additional members, such as an athletic trainer or consultants, depending on the case. Optimizing nutrition often involves increasing energy intake, decreasing energy expenditure, or some combination of these. However, it may also require addressing the macronutrient composition of an athlete's diet and increasing the frequency of meals and/or snacks in order to minimize within-day energy deficits. Evidence has shown that male athletes with within-day energy deficits had a suppressed RMR and changes in catabolic markers even if their overall 24-hour EA was adequate.[62] In a study of competitive cyclists who received an educational intervention designed to increase their EA, the main barriers cited by participants were psychological factors,[63] which highlights the importance of using a multidisciplinary team.

Awareness of low EA in male athletes is increasing, but further educational efforts are necessary. There are minimal studies that investigate the impact of education interventions in male athlete populations, but this is a promising area for future study. Some sports federations have also explored regulatory changes to encourage healthier nutrition. For example, the International Ski Federation changed the rules for ski jumping to reduce incentives for athletes to achieve a lower BMI, which resulted in a significant reduction in the number of underweight ski jumpers.[64] NCAA wrestling also successfully changed their weigh-in practices in an effort to curb unhealthy weight-cutting strategies.[65] Sports federations and governing bodies are encouraged to explore ways that they can promote an increased emphasis on health and performance rather than on weight or appearance, particularly in lean sports or sports with weight classes.

Hypogonadotropic Hypogonadism

In the female athlete triad, functional hypothalamic amenorrhea is known to result from low EA.[19] The study of hypothalamic–pituitary–gonadal (HPG) axis dysfunction in male athletes is more challenging given that amenorrhea and oligomenorrhea are generally easier to monitor; however, several studies document alterations in testosterone, luteinizing hormone (LH), follicle-stimulating hormone, or sperm profiles in male endurance athletes engaged in high training volumes.[66–85] Interestingly, many of these studies do not directly measure EA, although most of them occur in settings that one could expect are likely associated with low EA. The few studies that have directly examined the role of EA suggest that there is a link between low EA states and hypothalamic hypogonadism in men.[48,86,87] For example, in one study, male Army Rangers underwent an extreme training program that involved physical activity and an energy deficit. In the group that did not receive supplemental nutrition partway through the protocol, there were severe reductions in testosterone and mean LH levels, while the group that received nutritional supplementation did not demonstrate these changes.[88]

Given the associations between low EA, impaired bone health, and hypogonadotropic hypogonadism, if any one of these three conditions are identified, male athletes should also be screened for the other two. Further research is needed regarding the optimal method of screening for hormonal dysfunction in male athletes. We suggest that men should be asked about symptoms including decreased libido, an absence of morning erections, or a history of low testosterone. In addition, it may also be helpful to obtain free and total testosterone levels.[21,89] It is important to note that in the majority of studies, athletes with suppressed testosterone levels often do not meet clinical criteria for low testosterone (<8 nmol/L) and instead fall into the "gray zone" range where levels are lower than expected for age but do not meet formal diagnostic cutoffs (8–12 nmol/L).[82,89,90] Even in these cases, it can be useful to track testosterone levels longitudinally.

If hypogonadism is identified, athletes should be screened for other potential causes, such as the use of medications like selective serotonin reuptake inhibitors (SSRIs), illicit drug use, or other endocrine conditions. Provided no other causes are identified, the mainstay of treatment should be a nonpharmacologic approach that focuses on restoring EA.[21,22] Several studies that documented hormonal perturbations in male athletes also demonstrated resolution of these abnormalities when EA was optimized,[78,85,88] and a case report illustrates the success of this approach in a clinical setting.[91]

Pharmacologic treatment for hypogonadotropic hypogonadism in male athletes is not routinely recommended for a couple of reasons. First, as noted earlier, the majority of male athletes with decreased testosterone levels do not meet clinical cutoffs for hypogonadism. Second, the use of testosterone therapy or medications such as clomiphene citrate is currently prohibited by the World Anti-Doping Agency (WADA).[89] Third, although there have been some studies on the use of testosterone, clomiphene citrate, or pulsatile gonadotropin-releasing hormone (GnRH) in hypogonadal males, most of these were not performed in athletes, and many did not focus on bone health as the clinical end point.[92–97] There have been isolated case reports of using these treatments in hypogonadal male athletes, but there is a lack of more rigorous scientific data to support the efficacy and safety of this approach.[98] Similar to treatment of female athletes with functional hypothalamic amenorrhea,[19] experts recommend addressing hypogonadism in male athletes with nonpharmacologic approaches, focusing on optimizing energy balance and nutrition.[24]

Low Bone Mineral Density

Low BMD is a significant concern in many male athletes who present with a BSI. In some cases, the BSI is the initial presenting symptom of impaired bone health. Men who sustained stress fractures in the military were found to have low BMD, low bone mineral content (BMC), or smaller bone dimensions.[99,100] Clinicians should not miss this opportunity to screen for low BMD in young men, because it is crucial to optimize bone health during periods of peak bone accrual. Bone accrual is greatest in the 4 years surrounding puberty corresponding with time of peak height velocity, which occurs on average around age 13.5 years in males.[101] Total body peak bone mass is achieved around age 20.5 years in men, although at some bony sites, such as the lumbar spine, total hip, and femoral neck, peak bone mass occurs even earlier.[101] Other studies also confirm that male athletes reach peak bone mass during the third decade of life.[102–104] If men miss these key windows for bone accrual, they may not achieve their ideal peak BMD and may be at a higher risk for osteoporosis in the future.

Athletes at an increased risk for BSI should be screened for low BMD with dual-energy x-ray absorptiometry (DXA). The 2014 Female Athlete Triad Consensus Statement provided a risk stratification system to guide clinicians.[19] A similar risk assessment tool (minus the questions regarding menstrual history) was found to predict risk for future BSI in male athletes as well.[16] Based on this information, it is suggested that males with two or more moderate-risk factors or one or more high-risk factors should receive a DXA (see Table 12.1).[16,21,22] This is supported by data that showed that male athletes with a history of trabecular BSI (including the pelvis, femoral neck, and calcaneus) had a 4.6-fold increased risk of having low BMD when compared to athletes with a cortical BSI.[105]

When interpreting a DXA scan, clinicians should use age- and sex-specific standards for patients under the age of 50.[22] The International Society for Clinical Densitometry (ISCD) defines osteoporosis in men <50 years of age as a clinically significant fracture history (a long bone fracture of the lower extremities, a vertebral compression fracture, or two or more long bone fractures of the upper extremities) and low BMC or BMD, as defined by a Z-score less than or equal to −2.0.[106] The American College of Sports

TABLE 12.1

MODERATE- AND HIGH-RISK FACTORS FOR BONE STRESS INJURY IN MALE ATHLETES

MODERATE-RISK FACTORS	HIGH-RISK FACTORS
Some dietary restriction or DE	Current or past history of ED
BMI <18.5 or weight <90% of expected	BMI <17.5 or weight <85% of expected
Prior Z-score <−1.0	Prior Z-score <−2.0
One prior BSI	Two BSI or one BSI in a trabecular bone

BMI, body mass index; BSI, bone stress injury; DE, disordered eating; ED, eating disorder.

Source: Data from Kraus E, Tenforde AS, Nattiv A, Sainani KL, Kussman A, Deakins-Roche M, et al. Bone stress injuries in male distance runners: higher modified Female Athlete Triad Cumulative Risk Assessment scores predict increased rates of injury. *Br J Sports Med*. 2019;53(4):237–242.

Medicine (ACSM) defines low BMD in weight-bearing sports as a BMD or BMC Z-score of less than −1.0, because athletes in weight-bearing sports should generally have higher than average BMD.[20] Although this definition has been primarily used in female athletes, some suggest applying the same guidelines to male athletes.[15] According to the ISCD, Z-scores reported for male athletes older than age 20 should include weight-bearing sites such as the spine, total hip, and femoral neck. For athletes less than age 20, BMD should be reported as the BMC in the lumbar spine and areal BMD, and whole body less head BMC and BMD.[106]

Any men with low BMD should be screened for additional contributing causes, such as medical conditions, vitamin D deficiency, or medication use (including glucocorticoids). In the absence of alternative causes for low BMD, most cases will be due to low EA. Thus, the primary treatment approach should be nonpharmacologic and should seek to optimize EA.[21,22] Although much of the research into nonpharmacologic treatment for low EA has been conducted in women, there is some emerging evidence in male athletes as well. For example, one study of competitive cyclists found that if EA increased, BMD also increased by 2.2%, while decreases in EA were associated with a 2.3% decrease in BMD over a 6-month period.[63]

Another interesting strategy for improving BMD is participation in multidirectional sports such as basketball, soccer, or volleyball. Studies have demonstrated that athletes in sports with multidirectional loading tend to have higher BMD as compared to non-athletes.[43,107–110] In contrast, athletes in low- or nonimpact sports, such as cycling or swimming, have decreased BMD.[107,111–115] Participation in weight-bearing physical activity improves bone mineral accrual across all stages of pubertal development in male athletes,[116] and these effects may persist for years. A randomized controlled trial (RCT) followed children who performed a jumping activity 3 times per week for 7 months; they found increased BMC when compared to the control group, and this difference persisted even 8 years after stopping the intervention.[117]

Thus, if undertaken in childhood or adolescence, participation in ball sports or other impact activities may actually help prevent BSIs. In studies performed on military recruits, participation in a ball sport for at least 2 years prior to basic training significantly reduced the incidence of stress fracture.[118] A study in male adolescent runners also found that prior participation in basketball was associated with a lower incidence of stress fractures.[119] Similarly, another study of elite male distance runners found a dose-dependent response, where each additional year of playing a ball sport reduced future risk of stress fracture by 13%.[120] These data suggest that male athletes should be encouraged to participate in multiple sports at younger ages and that, in keeping with other recommendations from the sports medicine community, early sports specialization should be discouraged.[22,121–124] Although athletes with low BMD may not be able to alter their prior history of sports participation, they may benefit from the addition of resistance training or other impact exercise. In studies of male cyclists or runners, athletes who engaged in resistance training had higher BMD or showed improvements in BMD compared to athletes who did not.[63,114,125]

In some cases, when male athletes fail nonpharmacologic treatment, pharmacologic treatment for low BMD may be considered. There is some evidence for the use of parathyroid hormone or parathyroid hormone related-protein analogs such as teriparatide and abaloparatide to treat decreased BMD in aging males. There is some limited evidence for use in female athletes, but currently evidence for their use in male athletes is very limited.[126,127] In addition, these medications have been associated with an increased risk of osteosarcoma. Romosozumab is a monoclonal antibody that inhibits sclerostin, and although it was approved for use in older men to increase BMD and decrease fracture risk, unfortunately there is minimal evidence for its use in male athletes.

TABLE 12.2

INSTITUTE OF MEDICINE GUIDELINES FOR RECOMMENDED DAILY ALLOWANCE OF CALCIUM IN MEN

	<19 years old	19–70 years old	>70 years old
Daily calcium	1,300 mg	1,000 mg	1,200 mg

Source: Data from Institute of Medicine. *Dietary reference intakes for calcium and vitamin D*. The National Academies Press; 2011.

TABLE 12.3

INSTITUTE OF MEDICINE GUIDELINES FOR RECOMMENDED DAILY ALLOWANCE OF VITAMIN D IN MEN

	9–70 years old	>70 years old
Daily vitamin D	600 IU	800 IU

Source: Data from Institute of Medicine. *Dietary reference intakes for calcium and vitamin D*. The National Academies Press; 2011.

Bisphosphonates have improved BMD in older men, but evidence for their use in male athletes is unfortunately also very limited.[128,129] If pharmacologic treatment is considered, the prescribing physician should be familiar with the use of these agents or should consider consulting an endocrinologist.

Calcium and Vitamin D

Studies have shown that military recruits with below-median vitamin D levels are at an increased risk of stress fractures, and among collegiate distance runners with a BSI, higher vitamin D levels were inversely related to time lost to injury.[130,131] Given the important role that calcium and vitamin D both play in bone health, there have been some prospective studies examining the impact of calcium and vitamin D supplementation in male athletes. In jockeys, supplementation with calcium and vitamin D improved bone metabolic markers and peripheral quantitative computed tomography (pQCT) measurements.[132,133] Similarly, an RCT of male army recruits found that calcium and vitamin D supplementation improved volumetric BMD, cortical BMC, and bone thickness.[134] Further research in this area is needed to confirm that these bony changes correlate with a reduction in BSI risk.

Male athletes should follow the Institute of Medicine (IOM) guidelines for daily calcium and vitamin D intake.[11,21,135] See Tables 12.2 and 12.3 for specific recommendations by age. Whenever possible, an athlete should strive to obtain their daily calcium requirements from their diet; however, patients may need vitamin D supplementation in order to meet their daily recommended intake.[22] Since many patients require higher doses of vitamin D to achieve adequate levels, men with high-risk BSIs should be screened for vitamin D deficiency and supplemented accordingly.[21] The optimal serum vitamin D level to ensure adequate bone health in male athletes has not yet been fully elucidated and warrants further study.

CONCLUSION

Although less common than in female athletes, BSIs represent an important overuse injury in male athletes. Rates of BSI are particularly high among cross-country and track-and-field athletes, as well as in the military, but may occur in a range of weight-bearing sports. Most BSIs in men occur in the lower extremity, and the exact location is influenced by the particular demands of an athlete's sport. Treatment for BSIs in male athletes is similar to treatment for female athletes and should be guided by the severity and location of the injury. As in female athletes, it is crucial to screen male athletes with a BSI for underlying risk factors. These factors should be proactively addressed, in order to improve the rate of healing, reduce risk of future injury, and promote long-term bone health. Risks to consider in male athletes include extrinsic factors such as footwear and training pattern, micronutrient intake (including calcium and vitamin D), low EA with or without DE, hypogonadotropic hypogonadism, and low BMD. Since a BSI may be the initial presenting symptom for a male athlete with impaired bone health, it is of vital importance to screen for low BMD. Especially since peak bone accrual in male athletes occurs by the third decade of life, every effort should be made to identify and correct underlying risk factors. The primary treatment to many of these risk factors includes a nonpharmacologic approach that focuses on improving nutrition and EA. As awareness of these risk factors in male athletes improves, clinicians can hopefully intervene earlier to decrease future injury, prolong participation in sport, and improve long-term health outcomes.

Historically, much of the research on BSI prevention and risk factors has been done on females. However, as was explored in this chapter, there is increasing interest in BSIs among male athletes. Promising areas for future research include exploring the EA levels at which men develop endocrine or hormonal adaptations, investigating the physiologic mechanisms that link low EA to hormonal disturbances in male athletes, studying the efficacy of nonpharmacologic approaches to treatment in male athletes, and evaluating the potential role for pharmacologic treatments of hypogonadism, low BMD, or delayed fracture healing in men. In addition, there is a need for evidence-based guidelines regarding screening for hypogonadism in male athletes and for effective educational or preventive programs for male athletes.

KEY REFERENCES

Only key references appear in the print edition. The full reference list appears in the digital product found on http://connect.springerpub.com/content/book/978-0-8261-4424-9/part/sec03/chapter/ch12

2. Rizzone KH, Ackerman KE, Roos KG, et al. The epidemiology of stress fractures in collegiate student-athletes, 2004–2005 through 2013–2014 academic years. *J Athl Train*. 2017;52(10):966–975.

15. Barrack MT, Fredericson M, Tenforde AS, Nattiv A. Evidence of a cumulative effect for risk factors predicting low bone mass among male adolescent athletes. *Br J Sports Med*. 2017;51(3):200–205.

16. Kraus E, Tenforde AS, Nattiv A, et al. Bone stress injuries in male distance runners: higher modified Female Athlete Triad Cumulative Risk Assessment scores predict increased rates of injury. *Br J Sports Med*. 2019;53(4):237–242.

21. Tenforde AS, Barrack MT, Nattiv A, Fredericson M. Parallels with the Female Athlete Triad in Male Athletes. *Sports Med*. 2016;46(2):171–182.

22. Tenforde AS, Nattiv A, Ackerman K, et al. Optimising bone health in the young male athlete. *Br J Sports Med*. 2017;51(3):148–149.

36. Burke LM, Close GL, Lundy B, et al. Relative energy deficiency in sport in male athletes: a commentary on its presentation among selected groups of male athletes. *Int J Sport Nutr Exerc Metab*. 2018;28(4):364–374.

CHAPTER 13

Female Athletes

Megan Roche, Emily Miller Olson, and Emily Kraus

INTRODUCTION

Bone stress injuries (BSIs) are among the most common chronic sports medicine injuries in female athletes and are often season-ending injuries.[1] Sex-specific risk factors for BSIs in female athletes are well defined in the literature and are important to address in BSI management.

The female athlete triad (triad) is defined as the interrelationship of energy availability (EA), menstrual function, and bone health.[2] Female athletes may suffer negative health consequences from a spectrum of any of the three individual components.[3] A cohort study on adolescent and young adult females found that the cumulative risk for BSI increases as the number of triad-related risk factors increase.[4] Overall, the triad is a result of low EA from an underlying energy imbalance between dietary intake and energy expenditure. Relative energy deficiency in sport (RED-S) is caused by low EA and describes possible health and performance influences that include the triad and expand to describe effects of low EA, to gastrointestinal, metabolic, endocrine, cardiovascular, and immunologic abnormalities.[5]

Female athletes participating in sports emphasizing leanness are at a higher risk for low EA and impaired bone health. A study of National Collegiate Athletic Association (NCAA) Division I female athletes found that athletes participating in cross country, gymnastics, lacrosse, and swimming/diving have a high risk of low EA.[6] Female athletes participating in sports in which leanness is emphasized, such as ballet, figure skating, and cheerleading, are also at high risk.[1,2]

This chapter reviews evidence-based medicine and rehabilitation principles for management of BSIs in female athletes. Within this framework, the epidemiology, risk factors, clinical evaluation, and overall management of BSIs in female athletes are discussed.

EPIDEMIOLOGY

In a systematic review of BSI incidence, female athletes had an average incidence of 9.7%, which was higher than the 6.5% average BSI incidence in male athletes.[7] A study in collegiate athletes used in the systematic review found a higher incidence of stress fractures in females compared to males in every sport except for soccer.[8] Sports emphasizing leanness and/or involving repetitive movement patterns involve higher risk for BSI.

In female athletes, the most common injury sites are the tibia, metatarsals, femur, and calcaneus.[7] A study of NCAA athletes found sex-specific difference in injury site, with larger proportions of stress fractures to the femur in female athletes and the lumbar spine/pelvis in male athletes.[9]

Overall, BSIs occur with higher intensity and duration of sports participation. Female athletes who participated in sports for 8 or more hours per week had twice the number of stress fractures compared to female athletes engaged in 4 or fewer hours per week.[10] Collegiate athletes have a higher incidence of BSI than high school athletes, which can be attributed in part to higher-intensity training levels and additional years of cumulative training.[9]

The higher BSI incidence in female athletes compared to male athletes may not be due to sex itself; it is more likely due to higher rates of underlying low EA in female athletes.

In a systematic review by Gibbs et al. on female athletes with a mean age of 21.8 (± 3.5 year), the prevalence of any two or one of the triad components in female athletes ranged from 2.7% to 27% and 16% to 60%, respectively.[11]

The prevalence of disordered eating behaviors in adolescent and young female athletes ranged between 18% and 35% using the Eating Disorder Examination Questionnaire.[12] In the high school population, the prevalence of menstrual dysfunction (excluding the initial 2 years after menses) ranged between 18% and 54%.[13] Finally, a study of 170 high school athletes found a 21.8% prevalence of low bone mass.[14]

Taken together, epidemiological studies indicate that healthcare practitioners need to have a high index of clinical suspicion for BSI in the evaluation of a female athlete presenting with insidious onset of pain particularly localized to bone. Screening for triad components can help guide management and prevent subsequent BSI.

BONE STRESS INJURY RISK FACTORS IN THE FEMALE ATHLETE

Identification and modification of risk factors can help prevent BSI, improve return-to-play duration when a BSI does occur, and optimize overall bone health of female athletes. Warden et al. group BSI risk factors into two categories: (1) factors modifying load applied to bone and (2) factors influencing the ability of bone to resist load and prevent accumulation of damage.[15]

Factors that modify the load applied to bone include biomechanical factors and training patterns. Factors that influence the ability of bone to resist load include EA, calcium and vitamin D status, and past medical history. This chapter focuses on risk factors unique to female athletes. Risk factors common to male and female athletes are covered in other chapters and are briefly mentioned.

FACTORS THAT MODIFY BONE LOAD

Biomechanical Risk Factors

Biomechanical risk factors involve anatomic features that impact static alignment and dynamic biomechanical loading patterns. Anatomic features reported to be related to BSI common to male and female athletes include leg length discrepancy and pes planus or pes cavus feet.[16] The research on biomechanical risk factors primarily originates from studies on military recruits, while studies on runners are limited to case series, thus limiting the ability to properly compare injured and uninjured runners. Each anatomic feature has variable impact on BSI risk based on degree of pathology, with evidence on female runners limited to tibial BSI.[17,18] Further, evidence is variable and often based on the interplay between an athlete's pathology and individual characteristics.

Training Patterns

Increases in velocity, duration, or frequency of training can increase bone stress in male and female athletes. The impact of modifying court surface, running surface, or hill work is complex and subject to debate; changes should still be assessed for potential BSI risk.[16]

FACTORS THAT ENABLE BONE TO RESIST LOAD AND PREVENT ACCUMULATION OF DAMAGE

Athletic History and Past Medical History

Studies show that adolescent participation in high-impact and multidirectional loading sports may improve bone density and bone geometry. In adult male and female distance runners, participation in ball sports such as basketball and soccer during adolescence was protective against BSIs.[19]

Resistance training can provide an osteogenic stimulus that can lead to improvements in bone mineral density (BMD) and/or BSI risk. Kelley et al. found that premenopausal females participating in ground reaction force and joint reaction force exercise experienced small but statistically significant improvements in femoral neck and lumbar spine BMD.[20] More research is needed to examine the impact of resistance training on BMD in female athletes, particularly while controlling for EA.

In both male and female athletes, prior fracture is a risk factor for development of subsequent BSI.[6,21,22] Medications such as steroids, anticonvulsants, antidepressants, and antacids can impact risk of BSI.[23] In addition, consuming more than 10 alcohol-containing drinks per week increases risk of BSI.[10] Female athletes with a family history of BSI or osteoporosis/osteopenia may have increased risk of BSI. Studies indicate that genetics impact BMD with estimates of heritability of 0.45 to 0.82.[24]

Calcium and Vitamin D Status

Calcium is part of the mineralized matrix that gives strength to bone, and vitamin D promotes absorption of calcium to enable bone remodeling and growth. A study of female runners aged 18 to 26 found that females who consumed less than 800 mg of calcium a day had nearly 6 times the stress fracture rate than females who consumed more than 1,500 mg of calcium.[25]

Triad and Relative Energy Deficiency in Sport

Both the triad and RED-S reflect underlying low EA that can impair bone health in female athletes. Barrack et al. studied a group of female adolescent and young athletes participating in competitive or recreational exercise and found that the cumulative risk for BSI increased as the number of triad-related risk factors accumulated. Specifically, the risk of BSI increased from 15% to 20% for single risk factors to 30% to 50% for combined triad-related risk factors.[4]

Low EA has been shown to cause estradiol suppression, which increases bone resorption and decreases bone formation.[26] A recent randomized clinical trial on transdermal estradiol administration use in athletes with oligomenorrhea showed that it may be a useful adjunct therapy to enhance bone health in female athletes, likely by restoring more physiological estradiol status.[27] Combined oral contraceptives (COCs) should not be used to improve bone health.

CLINICAL EVALUATION

During BSI evaluation, health practitioners should inquire about triad and RED-S risk factors when eliciting a female athlete's history and past medical history. Questions should address nutrition status, menstrual function, BSI history, contraceptive use, and exercise habits. Questionnaires can more specifically address individual components of the triad and can group female athletes into low-, moderate-, and high-risk triad groups. We provide examples of evidence-based questionnaires that can be incorporated into clinical practice in our diagnostics section.

General questions common to male and female athletes should evaluate onset/quality of pain, training patterns including any change in volume or intensity, biomechanical risk factors, footwear, calcium and vitamin D status, family history of low BMD, and past medical history.

The physical exam may be unremarkable in female athletes presenting with the triad. However, in some circumstances, particularly in athletes with disordered eating or eating disorders, clinical signs may be apparent. Bradycardia, orthostatic hypotension, low body weight (<85% expected for body weight), or low body mass index (BMI; less than 5th percentile) can occur in athletes with the triad. Fluctuations in body weight, including weight loss, in the presence of normal BMI may be seen in athletes with the triad. Athletes with eating disorders may present with lanugo hair and parotid gland enlargement.[28] Physical examination assessments of BSI are reviewed in Chapter 1.

DIAGNOSIS OF TRIAD/RELATIVE ENERGY DEFICIENCY IN SPORT

Guidelines for diagnosing BSIs by anatomical locations have common features in both male and female athletes. Here, we focus on sex-specific guidelines for diagnosing the triad and RED-S in female athletes. Early detection of athletes at risk for the triad can help prevent BSI.[6] According to the Female Athlete Triad Coalition Consensus Statement, screening for the triad should occur as part of the annual preparticipation physical examination (PPE) in high school and collegiate female athletes.[2]

Determining an Athlete's Risk for the Triad

The Female Athlete Triad Coalition developed a cumulative risk assessment (CRA) tool that can be used to help group athletes into low-, moderate-, and high-risk groups (Table 13.1). Sports participation and return-to-play decisions can be evaluated based on an athlete's risk category. The six risk categories in the CRA tool include low EA with or without disordered eating, low BMI, delayed menarche, oligomenorrhea and/or amenorrhea, low BMD, and stress reaction/stress fracture history.[2]

A four-year prospective study at one NCAA Division I institution used the CRA tool to predict female runners' risk of sustaining a BSI. Female runners in the moderate- and high-risk categories had a 4-fold and 5.7-fold increased risk of sustaining a BSI

TABLE 13.1

CUMULATIVE RISK ASSESSMENT TOOL

RISK FACTORS	MAGNITUDE OF RISK		
	LOW RISK = 0 POINTS EACH	**MODERATE RISK = 1 POINT EACH**	**HIGH RISK = 2 POINTS EACH**
Low EA with or without DE/ED	☐ No dietary restriction	☐ Some dietary restriction[‡]; current/past history of DE	☐ Meets *DSM-5* criteria for ED[*]
Low BMI	☐ BMI ≥18.5 or ≥90% EW[**] or weight stable	☐ BMI 17.5 <18.5 or <90% EW or 5 to <10% weight loss/month	☐ BMI ≤17.5 or <85% EW or ≥10% weight loss/month
Delayed menarche	☐ Menarche <15 years	☐ Menarche 15 to <16 years	☐ Menarche ≥16 years
Oligomenorrhea and/or amenorrhea	☐ > 9 menses in 12 months[*]	☐ 6–9 menses in 12 months[*]	☐ <6 menses in 12 months[*]
Low BMD	☐ Z-score ≥–1.0	☐ Z-score –1.0[***] <–2.0	☐ Z-score ≤–2.0
Stress reaction/ fracture	☐ None	☐ 1	☐ ≥2; ≥1 high risk or of trabecular bone sites[†]
Cumulative risk (total each column, then add for total score)	_____ **points +**	_____ **points +**	_____ **points =** _____ **total score**

[‡]Some dietary restriction as evidenced by self-report or low/inadequate energy intake on diet logs; [*]current or past history; [**]≥90% EW66; absolute BMI cut-offs should not be used for adolescents. [***]Weight-bearing sport; [†]high-risk skeletal sites associated with low BMD and delay in return to play in athletes with one or more components of the Triad include stress reaction/fracture of trabecular sites (femoral neck, sacrum, pelvis).

BMD, bone mineral density; BMI, body mass index; DE, disordered eating; *DSM-5, Diagnostic and Statistical Manual of Mental Disorders, Fifth Edition*; EA, energy availability; ED, eating disorder; EW, expected weight.

Source: Reproduced with permission from Joy E, De Souza M, Nattiv A, et al. 2014 Female Athlete Triad Coalition Consensus Statement on treatment and return to play of the female athlete triad. *Nutr Ergogenic Aids*. 2014;13(4):219–232.

compared to low-risk runners.[6] Kussman et al. found that each 1-point increase in the CRA score predicted a 13% increased risk for BSI.[29]

The Female Athlete Triad Coalition Consensus Statement provides guidelines for diagnosing low EA, amenorrhea, and low BMD with screening questions to be asked at sport preparticipation evaluation outlined in Box 13.1. Overt signs and measured data can inform a diagnosis, but a female athlete's honesty in answering triad-related questions is key for understanding the spectrum of the diagnosis. It is important to develop a therapeutic alliance with a female athlete to foster compliance and honesty.

Diagnosing Low Energy Availability

Physical signs of low EA include a BMI <17.5 kg·m^{-2} or <85% of expected body weight in adolescents.[2] Other quantitative signs of low EA include reduced resting metabolic rate and low triiodothyronine (T3) measurements.

Box 13.1 Triad Consensus Panel Screening Questions

- Have you ever had a menstrual period?
- How old were you when you had your first menstrual period?
- When was your most recent menstrual period?
- How many periods have you had in the past 12 months?
- Are you presently taking any female hormones (oestrogen, progesterone, birth control pills)?
- Do you worry about your weight?
- Are you trying to or has anyone recommended that you gain or lose weight?
- Are you on a special diet or do you avoid certain types of foods or food groups?
- Have you ever had an eating disorder?
- Have you ever had a stress fracture?
- Have you ever been told you have low bone density (osteopenia or osteoporosis)?

Note: The Triad Consensus Panel recommends asking these screening questions at the time of the sport preparticipation evaluation.

Source: Reproduced with permission from Joy E, De Souza M, Nattiv A, et al. 2014 Female Athlete Triad Coalition Consensus Statement on treatment and return to play of the female athlete triad. *Nutr Ergogenic Aids.* 2014;13(4):219–232.

Studies show an association between low fat mass, low leptin, and increased ghrelin in adolescent and young amenorrhoeic athletes.[30] Leptin and ghrelin are hormones that inhibit and upregulate hunger respectively. Levels of leptin are low in conditions of low-fat mass, whereas levels of ghrelin are high in conditions of low-fat mass. More research is needed to examine how leptin and ghrelin may be used in the clinical evaluation of low EA in female athletes. Further, more research is needed to evaluate the clinical utility of insulin-like growth factor-1 (IGF-1), a metabolic biomarker responsible for mediating metabolic cellular response during altered energy states, in low EA.[31]

Assessments for dietary intake and energy expenditure can be estimated by a sports dietitian. An index of daily EA can be calculated by energy intake (kcal) minus energy expenditure (kcal) divided by fat-free mass (FFM) or lean body mass (kg). Energy intake and energy expenditure can be calculated by 3-, 4-, and 7-day dietary logs, 24-hour dietary recall, or food frequency questionnaires. A limitation of exercise expenditure estimates is the reliance on athlete self-report.[2]

Given that many practices lack the resources to have their own sports dietitian, other qualitative questionnaires can be administered in clinical practice to assess EA. The Low Energy Availability in Females Questionnaire (LEAF-Q) is a 25-item questionnaire, which showed a 78% sensitivity and 90% specificity in correct classification of current EA, and/or reproductive health, and/or bone health.[32] Further, the Eating Disorders Examination-Questionnaire (EDE-Q) can be used to understand eating attitudes and behaviors.

Diagnosing Menstrual Dysfunction

The spectrum of menstrual dysfunction includes primary amenorrhea, secondary amenorrhea, and oligomenorrhea. Primary amenorrhea is the absence of menarche by 15 years, and secondary amenorrhea is the cessation of regular menses for 3 months or cessation of irregular menses for 6 months in a female after menarche. Oligomenorrhea is considered infrequent menstruation, with cycles longer than 35 days. Anovulation and luteal phase deficiency are also elements of menstrual dysfunction but are difficult to diagnose based on history alone.

An energy deficit (which can occur independently of body weight) appears to be the critical factor in both weight-loss and exercise-induced forms of functional hypothalamic amenorrhea (FHA). Stress may also play a role. FHA is presumed to occur from a disruption of pulsatile hypothalamic gonadotropin-releasing hormone (GnRH) secretion, which causes low serum estradiol concentrations and anovulation as a result of absent midcycle surges in luteinizing hormone (LH).[33,34] This state of estrogen deficiency may compromise peak bone mass attained in adolescent females.[35]

The diagnosis of FHA in female athletes is a diagnosis of exclusion. Laboratory assessments for other causes of amenorrhea/oligomenorrhea including pregnancy, polycystic ovarian syndrome, and endocrinopathies such as prolactinoma and thyroid dysfunction should be completed (Figure 13.1).[28]

Hypothalamic or pituitary dysfunction can be determined from the following laboratory tests: serum LH, follicle stimulating hormone, prolactin, total and free estradiol, total and free testosterone, thyroid stimulating hormone (TSH), free T3, prolactin, and dehydroepiandosterone and its sulfate (DHEA-S).[5] After excluding other conditions, a diagnosis of FHA can be made in an athlete presenting with amenorrhea plus a precipitating factor including significant exercise, low body weight, or stress, as well as low serum gonadotropins and estradiol.

Diagnosing Impaired Bone Health

The Female Athlete Triad Coalition Consensus Statement outlines criteria for determining whether a female athlete should receive a dual-energy x-ray absorptiometry (DXA) scan for BMD assessment and provides considerations for selecting anatomical sites for measurement. Indications for DXA testing include one or more "high-risk" Triad risk factors, two or more "moderate-risk" Triad risk factors, or a history of one or more nonperipheral or two or more peripheral long bone traumatic fractures (Table 13.1).

Frequency of DXA evaluation will depend on the clinical status of the athlete. Athletes may need repeat DXA scans every 1 to 2 years to evaluate changes in bone health. Z-scores, as opposed to *T*-scores, should be used for evaluation in premenopausal female athletes. Female athletes aged 20 or older should be measured at weight-bearing sites including the posteroanterior spine, total hip, and femoral neck. Female athletes younger than 20 should be measured at the posteroanterior spine and whole body less head. When evaluating young athletes, it is important to use pediatric reference data and adjust for growth delay or maturational delay.[2]

Relative Energy Deficiency in Sport Evaluation

RED-S is an alternative way of characterizing physiological end points as a result of low EA. The RED-S clinical assessment tool (RED-S CAT) was designed to assist in clinical evaluation, management, and return-to-play decisions in athletes. RED-S CAT was developed from the 2014 International Olympic Committee Consensus Statement on RED-S.[36]

In the RED-S CAT, athletes are grouped into three categories: "red light (high risk)," "yellow light (moderate risk)," and "green light (low risk)." These categories correspond to sports participation and return-to-play guidelines.[36]

In addition to screening for EA, menstrual dysfunction, and bone health, the RED-S CAT addresses psychologic, cardiovascular, and hormonal conditions in evaluation of health status. These conditions include depression, anxiety, cardiac arrhythmia, electrolyte abnormalities, and abnormal metabolic function.[36]

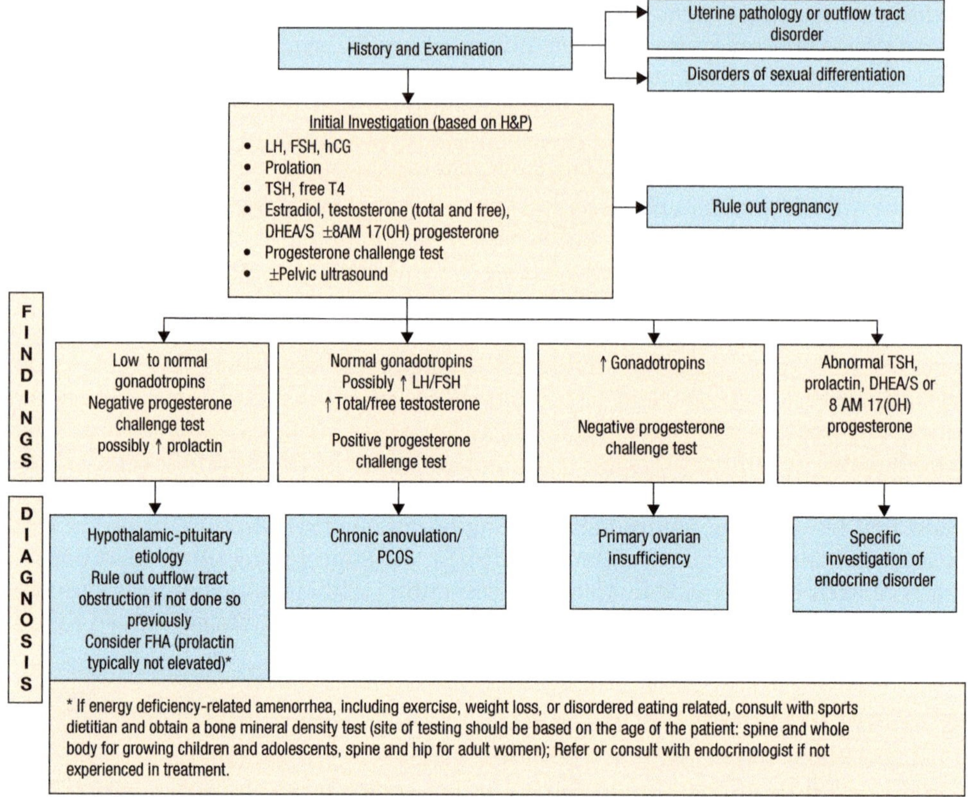

FIGURE 13.1 Amenorrhea algorithm from the Female Athlete Triad Coalition Consensus Statement.

Source: Reproduced with permission from Joy E, De Souza M, Nattiv A, et al. 2014 Female Athlete Triad Coalition Consensus Statement on treatment and return to play of the female athlete triad. *Nutr Ergogenic Aids*. 2014;13(4):219–232.

MANAGEMENT OF THE TRIAD/RELATIVE ENERGY DEFICIENCY IN SPORT

Early diagnosis of the triad or RED-S can improve bone health outcomes. When working with a female athlete with the triad or RED-S, the benefits of a multidisciplinary team cannot be overstated. A sports nutritionist and/or sports psychologist can be essential in guiding the athlete and discussing mental health. An endocrinologist may provide further insight into the diagnostic workup regarding specific hormonal imbalances that may be contributing to the overall picture. An athletic trainer, if available, may already have an established relationship with the athlete, enabling trust and more consistent interaction.

Management of Low Energy Availability

Treatment for low EA is focused on increasing energy intake to match or exceed energy requirement. Depending on the severity of low EA, decreasing exercise energy expenditure may also be necessary. Treating low EA is essential in athletes with other components of the triad as normalization of body weight is the best strategy for restoration of menses and for improving BMD.[2,37]

The treatment strategy for low EA is based on the underlying etiology. The goal of treatment is adequate weight gain to achieve restoration of menses and maintenance of BMI >18.5.[2] Of note, dietary changes should be gradual. As shown in the following, treatment requires management by a multidisciplinary team:

1. For female athletes with low EA due to either inadvertent undereating or weight loss without disordered eating, referral to a sports dietitian for nutrition education and planning is likely sufficient. For further information, an exercise physiologist could complete an assessment of energy expenditure and EA in order to further tailor nutrition recommendations to the individual athlete.
2. For female athletes with disordered eating, a referral to a sports psychologist or other mental health practitioner may be beneficial in addition to the previously mentioned recommendations. A sports psychologist can help modify unhealthy attitudes and emotions related to food and body image.
3. Female athletes with a clinical eating disorder will need to be evaluated and followed by a physician, a sports psychologist or other mental health practitioner, and a sports dietitian. For these athletes, a certified psychiatrist will be beneficial if conditions including depression or anxiety coexist. A psychiatrist may prescribe medications including antidepressant medications for bulimia nervosa.[2]

The 2014 Coalition Statement provided a stepwise approach to treatment:[2]

1. Perform assessment of baseline energy intake using dietary logs and energy expenditure. Energy expenditure can be estimated by determining the resting metabolic rate and multiplying by an activity factor, which will account for exercise energy expenditure.
2. Develop an individualized meal plan with an adequate balance of macronutrients and micronutrients, especially calcium, vitamin D, iron, zinc, and vitamin K. Real foods should be prioritized over supplements. Nutrient dense foods should be emphasized.
3. Monitor body weight regularly, depending on the severity of the energy deficiency and other factors. In order to promote a healthy relationship with body weight, body weight monitoring should be performed by a healthcare professional as opposed to female athletes themselves. Weekly monitoring may occur at initiation of treatment.
4. Cognitive behavioral therapy is effective in athletes with eating disorders and disordered eating and can be incorporated to improve compliance as athletes increase energy intake.[2]

Management of Functional Hypothalamic Amenorrhea and Menstrual Dysfunction

Exercise-related menstrual dysfunction, usually due to FHA, has been shown to have wide-reaching overall health disruptions and is best treated through early intervention.[38] Menstrual dysfunction leads to chronically low levels of estrogen. Low levels of estrogen are associated with greater muscle damage and oxidative stress after running as well as slower muscle strength recovery after stretch-shortening exercise loads.[39–41] Amenorrhea is also linked to endothelial dysfunction, which can cause cardiovascular impairment.[42]

Current treatment models focus on dietary interventions guided by certified nutritionists. Several small case–control studies and published case series have demonstrated that focused dietary interventions can restore menses.[2,43] Interventions need to be tailored to the individual athlete based on specific deficits and should focus on increased overall food intake and/or adjustments to food choices to meet nutrient goals.[31] If menses do not resume with dietary interventions, it may be necessary to temporarily decrease exercise. In these studies and in a retrospective analysis of collegiate athletes, restoration of menses was closely tied to adequate weight gain in the range of 1 to 4 kg.[2,44] Resumption of menses through nonpharmacologic modalities is associated with improvement of low BMD and endothelial function.[37,42]

Many physicians prescribe COCs to treat menstrual dysfunction and/or low BMD, despite inconclusive evidence to support this decision.[45,46] Lack of efficacy of oral estrogen is attributed to (1) hepatic first-pass effects that downregulate IGF-1, an important bone-trophic hormone, and (2) ethinyl estradiol, the most common form of estrogen in COCs, being nonphysiological, with a dose-dependent effect on sex hormone-binding globulin, which may lower bioavailable estradiol.[47,48]

The Coalition Statement states that the use of COCs for menstrual regulation is not recommended and may have a detrimental effect on BMD.[2] Athletes who are using COCs for other reasons should be counseled that COC use may mask menstrual dysfunction, which is often the first sign of low EA.[36] A randomized clinical trial by Ackerman et al. found that transdermal estradiol administration, given as an adjunct therapy with nutritional improvements and training modifications, improved bone health in oligoamenorrheic athletes.[27]

Management of Low Bone Mineral Density

The 2007 ACSM Position Stand on the Triad defined low bone mass as BMD or BMC Z-scores of less than −1.0.[49] For female athletes, the development of low BMD is intricately related to menstrual dysfunction and subsequent low estrogen levels. Therefore, the main treatment target, as discussed earlier, is restoring adequate EA.

In patients with anorexia nervosa, restoration of menses and weight gain are associated with significant improvements in lumbar spine (3.1%) and hip (1.8%) BMD.[50] Weight gain alone, independent of restoration of menses, has also been shown to have a positive effect on BMD. Both nutritional and hormonal recovery are necessary for optimal improvement in BMD.[37] To date, there are no prospective randomized controlled trials with large samples of exercising women with menstrual irregularity and low BMD to confirm the benefit of menses restoration and weight gain to understand association to changes in bone health.[37,51] More research is needed in this area.

When athletes have low BMD, especially in the setting of a prior BSI, calcium and vitamin D status should also be addressed. Both calcium and vitamin D supplementation have been found to decrease the incidence of BSI.[52] Deficiency is especially common during the winter and/or in northern latitudes. In addition, adequate vitamin D has been shown to have a positive effect on femoral and hip BMD.[53] Adequate calcium intake (1,500 mg/day for athletes) also may decrease the risk of BSI.[54]

Additionally, weight-bearing exercise is key for increasing and maintaining BMD. A meta-analysis demonstrated significant improvements in femoral neck and lumbar spine BMD in premenopausal women following weight-bearing exercise training.[20] Eumenorrheic weight-bearing endurance athletes have significantly greater BMD and favorable adaptations to bone microarchitecture compared to nonathlete controls; however, these effects are lost in amenorrheic weight-bearing athletes.[55,56] While treatment of low EA may demonstrate alterations in hormone profiles within weeks and cause restoration of menses within months, improvements in BMD take place over several years. It is unclear whether BMD can ever be fully restored to levels appropriate for age and training status in at-risk female athletes.[57]

Recombinant parathyroid hormone (PTH[1,34]) has been shown to improve BMD in anorexia nervosa patients. Short-term use could be considered in the setting of delayed

TABLE 13.2

FEMALE ATHLETE TRIAD: CLEARANCE AND RETURN-TO-PLAY GUIDELINE BY MEDICAL RISK STRATIFICATION

	CUMULATIVE RISK SCORE	LOW RISK	MODERATE RISK	HIGH RISK
Full Clearance	0 – 1 point	☐		
Provisional/ Limited Clearance	2 – 5 points		☐ Provisional Clearance ☐ Limited Clearance	
Restricted from Training and Competition	≥ 6 points			☐ Restricted from Training/ Competition-Provisional ☐ Disqualified

Source: Reproduced with permission from Joy E, De Souza M, Nattiv A, et al. 2014 female athlete triad coalition consensus statement on treatment and return to play of the female athlete triad. *Nutr Ergogenic Aids.* 2014;13(4):219–232.

fracture healing or very low BMD, though this should be done in consultation with an endocrinologist as it is on off-label use and there are potential side effects with the medication if used inappropriately.[58] Bisphosphonate treatment is typically used in older women with osteopenia or osteoporosis with risk factors. However, bisphosphonates are stored in bone for prolonged periods of time and are known to be teratogenic; therefore, they are contraindicated in women of reproductive age.[59] For postmenopausal female athletes, bisphosphonates can be more safely used for the treatment of osteopenia or osteoporosis. In general, however, nonpharmacologic treatments should be used for 1 year prior to switching to pharmacologic options except in the cases of severely low BMD or fracture during the period of nonpharmacologic management.[2]

Return to Play

The triad CRA tool and the RED-S CAT classify athletes into low-, moderate-, or high-risk categories. Low-risk athletes can return to play without restrictions (Table 13.2). Moderate-risk athletes can return to play contingent on their adherence to the management plan designed by the multidisciplinary team. For moderate-risk athletes, training hours may be restricted on a case-by-case basis. High-risk athletes should be held out of competition and training during initial management, with a plan for reevaluation to determine when the athlete may begin a gradual return to activity. Restrictions for the high-risk athlete are a matter of safety given the increased risk of BSI and health consequences from severe low EA.[2]

CONCLUSION

BSIs occur as a result of repetitive, mechanical loading and are common in female athletes. The triad and RED-S are caused by low EA and can occur in female athletes of all levels and across all sports. Early identification and proper management of low EA decreases risk of BSI and triad- or RED-S-associated negative health outcomes. Use of the triad CRA tool and/or the RED-S CAT tool can assist in identification of at-risk athletes, even prior to BSI occurrence.

Management of the triad and RED-S requires a multidisciplinary approach. An optimal multidisciplinary team includes dietitians, psychologists, athletic trainers, exercise physiologists, physicians, and, potentially, endocrinologists and/or psychiatrists, depending on the specific needs of an athlete. While management is primarily nonpharmacologic, treatment plans should be individualized, taking into account sport requirements, dietary limitations, and need for psychiatric care. There are pharmacologic options for athletes who are not progressing despite adequate nonpharmacologic management. Pharmacologic management should be judiciously used and initiated under the supervision of an endocrinologist.

In summary, assessing and then maintaining or restoring adequate EA is critical for BSI management in female athletes. A multidisciplinary team focused on practicing evidence-based medicine and establishing trust with a female athlete is integral in the prevention and management of both low EA and BSI.

KEY REFERENCES

Only key references appear in the print edition. The full reference list appears in the digital product found on http://connect.springerpub.com/content/book/978-0-8261-4424-9/part/sec03/chapter/ch13

2. De Souza MJ, Nattiv A, Joy E, et al. 2014 female athlete triad coalition consensus statement on treatment and return to play of the female athlete triad: 1st international conference held in San Francisco, California, May 2012 and 2nd international conference held in Indianapolis, Indiana. *Br J Sports Med*. 2014;48(4):289.

6. Tenforde AS, Carlson JL, Chang A, et al. Association of the female athlete triad risk assessment stratification to the development of bone stress injuries in collegiate athletes. *Am J Sports Med*. 2017;45(2):302–310.

16. Tenforde A, Kraus E, Fredericson M. Bone stress injuries in runners. *Phys Med Rehabil Clin N Am*. 2016;27(1):139–149.

21. Tenforde AS, Sayres LC, McMurdy ML, et al. Identifying sex-specific risk factors for stress fractures in adolescent runners. *Med Sci Sports Exerc*. 2013;45(10):1843–1851.

22. Kelsey JL, Bachrach LK, Proctor-Gray E, et al. Risk factors for stress fracture among young female cross country runners. *Med Sci Sports Exerc*. 2007;39(9):1457–1463.

36. Mountjoy M, Sundgot-Borgen J, Burke L, et al. IOC consensus statement: beyond the triad—RED-S in sport. *Br J Sports Med*. 2014;48:491–497.

49. Nattiv A, Loucks AB, Manore MM, et al. American College of Sports Medicine position stand: the female athlete triad. *Med Sci Sports Exerc*. 2007;39(10):1867–1882.

CHAPTER 14

Military Stress Fractures

Charles Milgrom

INTRODUCTION

Since the first description of a metatarsal stress fracture in the Prussian Army in 1855, the nature of military service and the structure of armies have undergone continual change.[1] Today, only a minority of those who serve in the military are those whose "boots are on the ground" and therefore most susceptible to sustain stress fracture. While the goal of all military training is to produce soldiers, the methods of recruit training, length of training, and the recruit populations vary widely between countries. It is during such recruit training that there is historically a high incidence of stress fractures.[2] Some armies are composed entirely of volunteers, while in others there is selective or universal conscription. In the U.S. Army, all new recruits are required to complete basic combat training, while in the Israeli Defense Forces (IDF), basic training is customized according to a new recruit's future role in service.

Training programs generally try to balance, producing the best possible soldier while minimizing the attrition rate, which has reached 29.7% at 36 months in the U.S. Army.[3] One of the reasons for attrition is stress fracture, which has been termed an unwanted side effect of military combat training.[4] This has served as an incentive for many armies to study the etiology of military stress fractures and develop programs to prevent their incidence and improve diagnosis and treatment. The purpose of this chapter is to present from a perspective of military medicine recent military stress fracture knowledge that reflects the experience of 21st-century Western armies and military service.

RISK FACTORS

Risk factors for military stress fractures can be either physiologically intrinsic to the trainee or a function of the training program or equipment. Determining risk factors intrinsic to trainees has proven to be somewhat of an academic exercise and not of real practical value to Western armies. This is because most of these armies are made up of volunteers and are faced with a shortage of high-quality candidates. Without a surplus of candidates, selection is not possible. The U.S. Army has missed its recruiting goals for several years and been forced to continually lower its minimum recruiting standards.

Several intrinsic risk factors for military stress fracture have been identified, but for many it is not known if they are universal to all armies. Female gender, poor physical fitness, and those with slender bones and low area moment of inertia are probably universal risk factors.[5-8] Other risk factors such as high external rotation of the hip, recruit age, and recruit ethnic group may not be universal.[8-10] Attempts to find a genetic link to stress fractures have been unsuccessful.[11]

It is inherent in military culture that every officer training recruit, be it on the squad, platoon, or company level, wants to make his unit the best. This leads to a tendency of officers to add additional elements to the training above and beyond the formal training program. Sometimes, these additional elements include punishments. A 32-year IDF longitudinal study of stress fractures in a single elite infantry unit analyzed what factors were important in lowering the incidence of stress fracture. By multivariable analysis, it was found that not allowing officers to make their own additions to the prescribed training schedule was the most important factor in lowering the incidence of stress fractures.[4] This is probably the most valuable controllable military stress risk factor available. Simple solutions to stress fracture incidence, such as shoe orthotics and shoe modifications, have not proven to be silver bullets.

ETIOLOGY OF MILITARY STRESS FRACTURES

Recently reported in vivo tibial strain gauge studies have helped to further elucidate the mechanism of tibial stress fracture in the military. Intuitively, one would think that recruits who had participated in long-distance running before induction would be protected from stress fracture, but this has not been found to be the case.[12] The study of Milgrom et al. offers a possible mechanistic explanation for this observation.[13] During in vivo tibial strain gauge measurements, the angle of the principal strain during running and ordinary civilian activities performed on engineered surfaces was found to vary little and be in the range of +5.40° to +2.75°. In activities that mimicked those performed by infantry recruits on a dirt hill, at the points of change of direction during zig-zag running uphill, the range of the angle of the principal strain was between −115° and 123° when running downhill and in the range of −32.8° to −51° when running uphill. The authors hypothesized that exposure to unusual angles of the principal strain may initiate the bone remodeling response in an attempt to strengthen the tibia to a new stress pattern. The first state of this bone adaptive strengthening response is reabsorption of old bone. If excessive cyclical loading continues during the reabsorption phase of remodeling, when bone is transitorily weakened, a stress fracture may result. If the remodeling response is completed uneventfully, stronger bone is produced. Running, with its repetitive cyclical pattern and uniform angle of principal strain, according to this hypothesis would not produce bone accommodated to the bone stresses of military training.

Another recent in vivo tibial strain gauge study assessed the mechanism of the most common stress fracture in the military: the medial tibial stress fracture.[14,15] In previous in vivo tibial strain gauge recordings, tibial compression and tension forces were not found to exceed 1,000 microstrain during running.[16] Ex vivo experiments have shown that this level of strain is below the threshold value needed to cause cortical bone fatigue even in millions of loading cycles.[17,18] Typically, medial tibial stress fractures occur at the posteromedial border of the tibia, and oblique fracture lines are observed when they are visible on plain x-rays. Such a fracture line represents failure in shear. In the Milgrom et al. study, tibial shear strains approaching 5,000 microstrain were recorded during stair jumping and vertical standing jumps, while shear strains were only slightly above 1,250 microstrain during runs up and down stadium steps.[14] Ex vivo studies show that more than a threshold of 2,500 microstrain cyclical loading can result in cortical bone failure.[17] The authors concluded that during stair and vertical jumping, tibial shear strain was high enough to potentially produce tibial stress fracture subsequent to repetitive cyclic loading without the necessity of an intermediate remodeling response that transitorily weakens bone.

CLINICAL DIAGNOSIS OF MILITARY STRESS FRACTURES

Stress fracture clinical diagnosis in the military can be challenging. A recent prospective military study provides evidence-based guidelines for the clinical diagnosis of tibial stress fracture.[19] Prior to that study, it was considered that a band of tibial tenderness <5 cm was consistent with medial tibial stress fracture and that a band of tenderness ≥5 cm was consistent with medial tibial stress syndrome.[19] Yates et al. reference this convention to a prior article of Batt et al.[20,21] However, there is no scientific source data provided in the Batt et al. study for the 5-cm threshold value.[21] The Milgrom et al. prospective study was conducted during the basic training of five successive elite infantry induction companies.[19] It was found that medial tibial stress fractures occurred when the band of tibial tenderness was ≤10 cm. At above 10 cm, stress fracture did not occur. Figure 14.1 is based on their study data.

The study also assessed the accuracy of other elements of the medial tibial stress fracture physical examination. It was found that if a recruit with tibial exertional pain and focal tibial tenderness had a positive hop test, the sensitivity for predicting medial tibial stress fracture was 100%, the specificity was 45%, the positive predictive value was 74%, and the negative predictive value was 100%.[21] Without the presence of a positive hop test, the positive predictive value decreased to 25%.

The same study also evaluated recruits' self-estimation of their tibial pain as a predictor of the presence of medial tibial stress fracture. The evaluation was made on a 1 to 10 scale for pain at rest, during walking, during exertion, and post exertion. Table 14.1 is

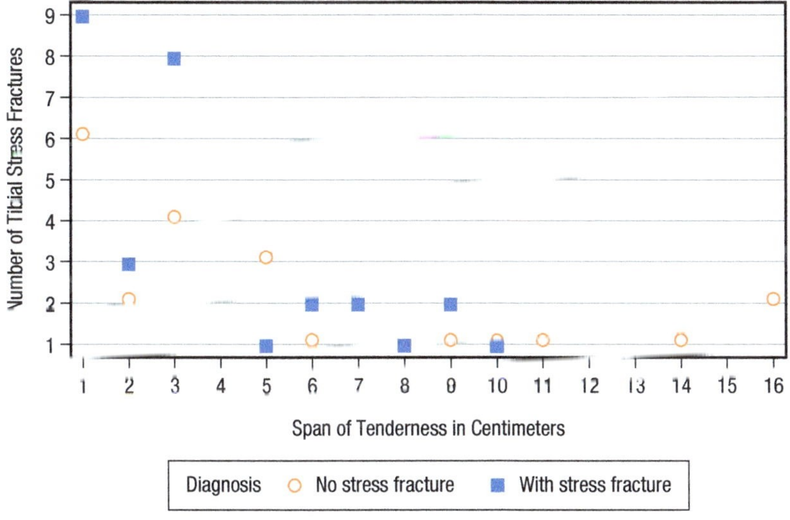

FIGURE 14.1 The presence or absence of medial tibial stress fracture versus the span of tibial tenderness.

TABLE 14.1

SUBJECTIVE RECRUIT ASSESSMENT OF THEIR MEDIAL TIBIAL PAIN VERSUS ACTIVITY

	MEAN MAXIMUM PAIN SCORE ±SD		
ACTIVITY	**TIBIAL SF**	**NO TIBIAL SF**	*P* **VALUE**
Rest	3.0 ± 2.9	2.84 ± 3.0	0.9
Walking	4.9 ± 2.7	5.0 ± 2.6	0.9
Exertion	7.2 ± 3.0	6.3 ± 3.4	0.4
Post exertion	7.0 ± 2.5	6.7 ± 3.1	0.8

SF, stress fracture.

based on the data presented in their study. From this, it can be concluded that taking a detailed pain history is of little or no value in predicting the presence of medial tibial stress fracture.

IMAGING IN MILITARY STRESS FRACTURES

It should be noted that in the military, unlike in sports medicine, the presence of medial tibial pain in itself is not of great concern to the medical staff unless it represents stress fracture or a precursor to stress fracture. Combat recruits are trained to perform in adverse conditions carrying heavy loads. They need to have the ability to ignore or tolerate the pain associated with these conditions and still perform. Military recruits are also on tight training schedules that have little flexibility. If they lose too much training time, they will be attriters.[3]

Both bone scan and MRI have been used for the early detection of tibial stress fracture before it is evident on plain x-ray.[22,23] Because of radiation concerns, MRI has replaced the use of bone scan in many Western armies.[24,25] For bone scan, there is a defined correlation between the grades and the presence of stress fracture on plain x-ray. Zwas et al. reported that for 4% of grade 1 lesions, 21% of grade 2 lesions, 76% of grade 3 lesions, and 100% of grade 4 lesions, plain radiographs were positive for stress fracture.[22] The MRI grading system for evaluating medial tibial pain first presented by Fredericson et al. and subsequent systems by Nattiv et al. and Kijowski et al. are presented in Table 14.2.[24,26,27]

No good correlations with the presence of stress fracture on plain x-rays have been established for any of these MRI grading systems, with the exception of grade 4 lesions, where a clear fracture line is visible on MRI. Medial tibial stress fractures occur in cortical bone. MRI has an inherent weakness in evaluating medial tibial cortical bone because the cortical bone has short-lived proton nuclear magnetic resonance signals. This gives cortical bone a dark signal.[28] Therefore, MRI evaluation of medial tibial stress syndrome is primarily based on noncortical findings, such as periosteal and bone marrow edema. Only in grade 4 lesions where a cortical fracture line is present is there direct MRI information from the cortex.

All of these MRI medial tibial stress syndrome grading systems assume that medial tibial stress fracture is at the end of the spectrum of the medial tibial stress syndrome. This however is not consistent with the clinical finding that tibial tenderness below a certain boundary value is consistent with tibial stress fracture and that above is not.[18,19] Studies that have attempted to show that medial tibial stress fracture is part of the medial tibial stress syndrome continuum have had equivocal findings.

TABLE 14.2

TIBIAL STRESS REACTION GRADING SYSTEMS

GRADE	FREDERICSON	NATTIV	KIJOWSKI
1	Mild to moderate periosteal edema on T2; normal marrow on T2 and T1	Mild marrow or periosteal edema on T2; T1 normal	Periosteal edema with no associated bone marrow signal abnormalities
2	Moderate to severe periosteal edema on T2; marrow edema on T2 but not T1	Moderate marrow or periosteal edema plus positive T2; T1 normal	Periosteal edema and bone marrow edema visible only on T2-weighted images
3	Moderate to severe periosteal edema on T2; marrow edema on T2 and T1	Severe marrow or periosteal edema on T2 and T1	Periosteal edema and bone marrow edema visible on both T1-weighted and T2-weighted images
4	Moderate to severe periosteal edema on T2; marrow edema on T2 and T1; fracture line present	Severe marrow or periosteal edema on T2 and T1 plus fracture line on T2 or T1	4a. Multiple focal areas of intra-cortical signal abnormality and bone marrow edema visible on both T1-weighted and T2-weighted images 4b. Linear areas of intra-cortical signal abnormality and bone marrow edema visible on both T1-weighted and T2-weighted images

Winters et al. analyzed six tibial bone biopsy specimens taken from the painful area in athletes with medial tibial stress syndrome to see if there was targeted remodeling.[29] No diffuse microdamage and only a single potential remodeling front was observed in the specimens. Only in three of the specimens were linear microcracks found. These findings do not support the concept that medial tibial stress syndrome is related to a bone remodeling response to stress. In another study, Winters et al. used ultrasound to assess whether medial tibial stress syndrome is related to periosteal, bony, or tendinous abnormalities of the leg.[30] They found no difference in the periosteal and tendinous findings between athletes with and without medial tibial stress syndrome.

The IDF study of Hadid et al. showed the problems related to the use of MRI criteria in evaluating exertional medial tibial pain in military recruits.[31] Their study, done among new special forces recruits, found that 26 of 55 of the recruits had tibial MRI stress reactions before the onset of formal training. The study used a 0.5 Tesla extremity scanner. In a subsequent IDF study, also done among new special forces recruits at the beginning of their training (unpublished data), using a 3 Tesla scanner and a T2 Dixon sequence, it was found that 15 of 60 recruit tibias had isolated periosteal edema. In clinical follow-ups, during subsequent demanding training, none of the 15 tibias developed exertional tibial pain. Figure 14.2 shows the tibia of a recruit from that study who had isolated bilateral periosteal edema. At the time of the MRI and in subsequent training, the recruit had no tibial pain or tenderness. Isolated periosteal edema is considered by all three of the major MRI grading systems shown in Table 14.2 to represent a grade 1 tibial stress reaction. Bergman et al. observed a parallel finding among runners.[32] In their study, 43% of asymptomatic runners had MRI signs of tibial stress reaction.

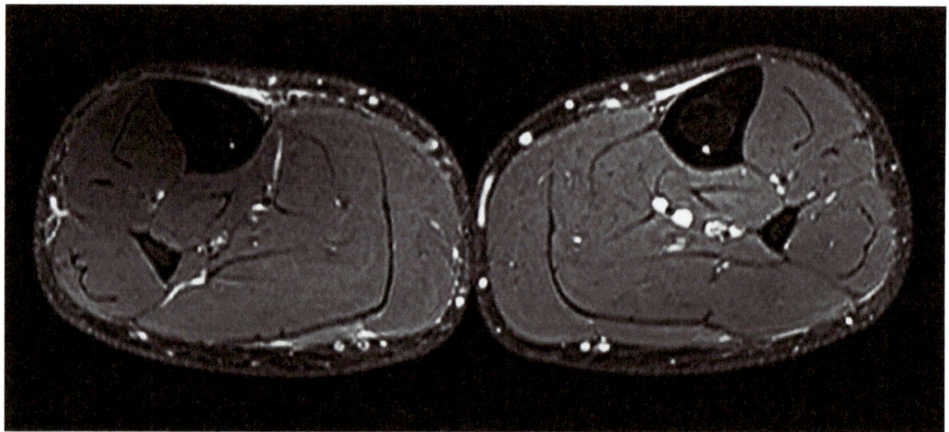

FIGURE 14.2 Pre-training tibial MRI of special forces recruit.

TREATING SUSPECTED TIBIAL STRESS FRACTURES WITHOUT IMAGING

Because of the problems associated with both MRI and bone scan in determining the presence of tibial stress fracture, the IDF developed an alternative approach to the problem, which minimizes the use of imaging. This approach is presented and validated in the study of Milgrom et al.[19] The protocol assumes that a recruit who has exertional medial tibial pain, medial tibial tenderness less than 10 cm in length, and a positive hop test has a high probability of having a grade 1 or grade 2 lesion by MRI or bone scan evaluation. Such lesions may represent either a normal bone adaptation to physiological stress or an early stage of stress fracture. They are treated initially without imaging, as if a positive bone scan or MRI lesion were present, with 10 to 14 days of rest. Recruits who have exertional tibial pain and tibial tenderness >10 cm continue training, as do recruits whose tibial tenderness is ≤10 cm but have negative hop tests. In 69% of the cases, this initial rest regimen resulted in disappearance or marked improvement in symptoms, and the recruits returned to duty never having been imaged. Only those who did not respond to this initial treatment are sent for imaging. The current IDF protocol for treating those with medial tibial pain is presented in Figure 14.3.

BEWARE OF THE FEMORAL STRESS FRACTURES IN THE MILITARY

The hallmark of tibial and metatarsal stress fractures is pain. The presence of pain serves as a warning flag of possible danger and as a protective factor against progression to frank fracture. This is not the case for stress fractures of the femoral shaft or neck. They may be accompanied by little or no pain. If pain is present, it may be hard to differentiate from muscle pain. The problem is increased because military recruits are in subordinate and vulnerable positions. They may be unwilling to complain, lest they may be seen as weak by their superiors. The femoral stress fracture physical exam is also difficult and inaccurate because the femur is a deep structure surrounded by much soft tissue. Its periosteum is less sensitive than that of the tibia. Therefore, the military treatment of a suspected femoral stress fracture may be summarized in one word: stop. A recruit

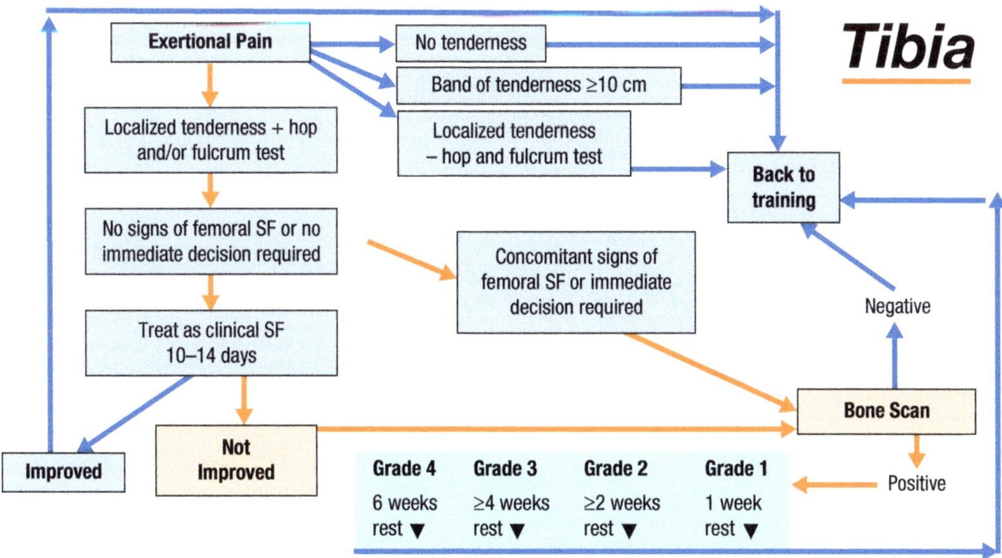

FIGURE 14.3 Israeli Defense Forces' painful medial tibia management protocol.

SF, stress fracture.

with a suspected femoral stress fracture needs to be grounded until imaging, whether MRI or bone scan, is done and results received. A metatarsal stress fracture that progresses to a frank fracture requires only conservative treatment, and clinical results can be expected to be good. Medial tibial stress fracture does not progress to complete displaced fracture because it involves only one cortex and the level of associated pain does not allow the recruit to continue training. The femur is different. A complete femoral shaft fracture requires major surgery and a rehabilitation period. A displaced femoral neck fracture can result in a lifelong medical disability. Therefore, it is better to always err on the safe side.

FEMALE SOLDIERS

Female gender has been found to be a risk factor for stress fracture in the military. Females doing the same training as males sustain higher rates of stress fractures than males.[5] Pelvic stress fractures occur more frequently in female than in male recruits.[33] Accurately differentiating a pubic stress fracture from that of a femoral neck stress fracture is difficult on physical examination, so the same *stop* training rule needs to be applied to both when they are suspected. Because of the high risk of stress fracture in female recruits, their stress fracture surveillance by the training and medical staff needs to be high.

WHEN DO MILITARY STRESS FRACTURES OCCUR

The accepted dogma is that stress fractures occur when subjects are suddenly exposed to new or higher levels of bone stress. Most military stress fracture data are from military basic training. This is because for most armies, follow-up of recruits once they have completed their basic training is difficult because they subsequently go on to a variety

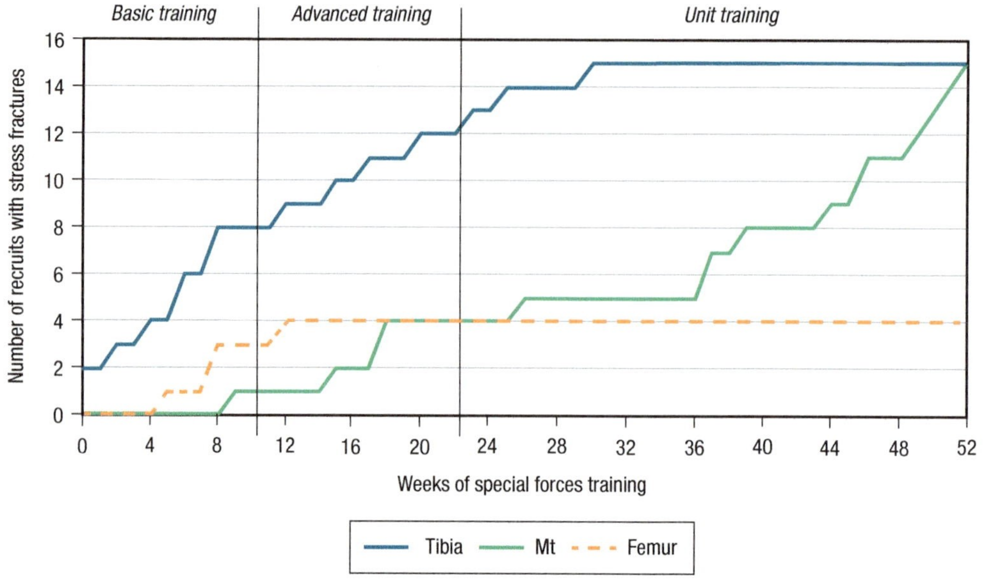

FIGURE 14.4 Incidence of stress fracture over 1 year of training.

of different units that are geographically dispersed. Long-term follow-up in the IDF is easier because the role and units of new recruits are largely determined before their induction. The study by Milgrom et al. tracked the incidence of stress fracture over the course of 1 year of training in a special forces unit.[34] An adaptation of their data is presented in Figure 14.4.

Their data indicate that in the military, tibial and femoral stress fractures have a different epidemiology than metatarsal stress fractures. After week 12, there was no femoral stress fracture occurrence, and after week 30 there was no tibial stress fracture occurrence. Metatarsal stress fractures, however, occurred throughout the entire year's monitoring period. This continual risk for metatarsal stress fractures needs to be remembered by military physicians.

LONG-TERM MANIFESTATIONS OF STRESS FRACTURES

In 1986, an editorial appeared in the *Lancet* about stress fractures.[35] It noted the report of an extremely high, 31%, incidence of stress fractures in the IDF.[2] It hypothesized that those recruits who sustained stress fractures might be found in middle life to have weaker bone. They asked the authors to follow the recruits long term. A 25-year follow-up assessment of the bone strength using quantitative computed tomography (QCT) was performed on a cohort of the recruits from the original study who sustained and did not sustain stress fractures.[36] No difference in any of the bone strength parameters were found between the cohorts.

CONCLUSION

Demanding military training is associated with recruit musculoskeletal pain, which is commonly referred to as "infantry pain." Fortunately, in most cases, the pain does not reflect the presence of serious pathology and really is simply infantry pain. The approach and attitude toward musculoskeletal pain are different in military medicine than in sports medicine. Stress fracture, unlike infantry pain, is of major concern in military medicine. There is no single magic bullet to prevent its occurrence. In the military, musculoskeletal stress cannot be lowered beyond the level that compromises the training goals. Stress fractures in the military can be best managed by the awareness that identifies them while they are still in the micro stage and not in the more dangerous macro stage. This requires stress fracture education and awareness to be given to the recruit training staff and to the recruits themselves.

KEY REFERENCES

Only key references appear in the print edition. The full reference list appears in the digital product found on http://connect.springerpub.com/content/book/978-0-8261-4424-9/part/sec03/chapter/ch14

19. Milgrom C, Zloczower E, Fleishmann C, et al. Medial tibial stress fracture diagnosis and treatment guidelines. *J Sci Med Sport*. 3 Dec 2020; [Epub ahead of print] PMID: 33298373

29. Winters M, Burr DB, van der Hoeven H, et al. Microcrack-associated bone remodeling is rarely observed in biopsies from athletes with medial tibial stress syndrome. *Bone Miner Metab*. May 2019;37(3):496–502.

32. Bergman AG, Fredericson M, Ho C, et al. Asymptomatic tibial stress reactions: MRI detection and clinical follow-up in distance runners. *Am J Roentgenol*. 2004;183(3):635–638.

34. Finestone A, Milgrom C, Wolf O, et al. Epidemiology of metatarsal stress fractures versus tibial and femoral stress fractures during elite training. *Foot Ankle Int*. Jan 2011;32(1):16–20.

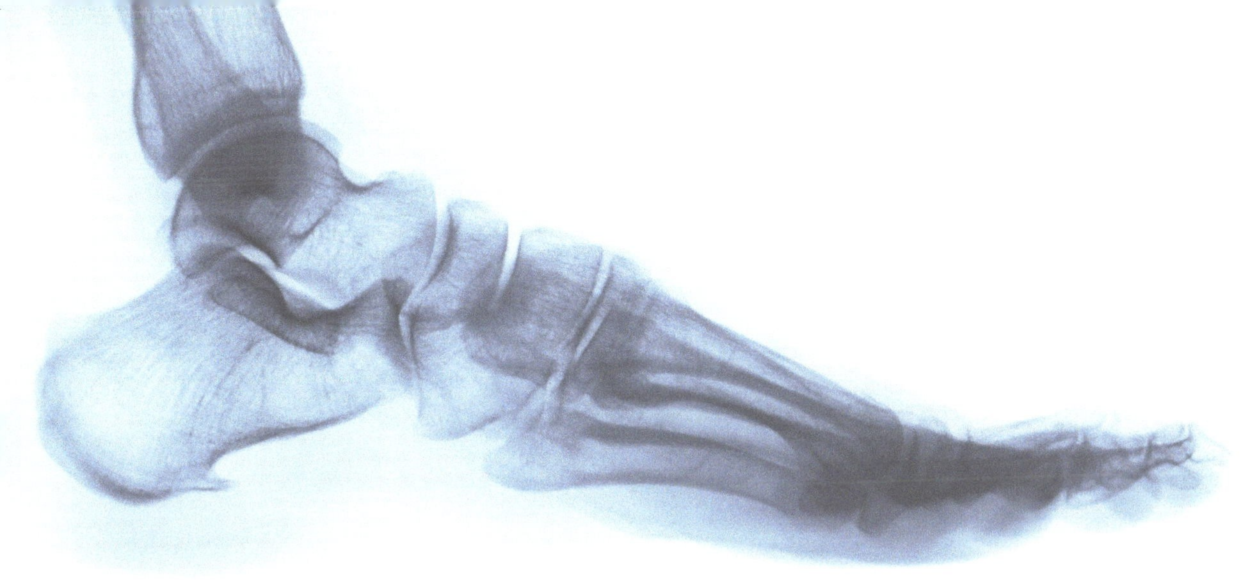

PART IV

SPECIAL CONSIDERATIONS

CHAPTER 15

Prevention of Bone Stress Injuries

Kenneth Vitale, Adam S. Tenforde,
and Michael Fredericson

INTRODUCTION

The commonly used term "stress fracture" is one point on a spectrum of injury that includes bone strain, stress reaction, and stress fracture.[1] The term "bone stress injury" (BSI) is used hereafter to describe this continuum of injury. Originally described in military recruits by Breithaupt in 1855,[2,3] BSI can often occur in athletes (e.g., runners, dancers). Traditionally, stress fractures were thought of as "abnormal stress on normal bone" (normal in terms of bone mineral density [BMD] and elastic resistance).[3] However, there is growing concern that children and adolescents may not optimize bone health, placing this population at risk for future injury. With the increasing participation in youth sports, these athletes are especially at risk for BSI. While the incidence of BSI in the general population is less than 1%,[4] it can be much higher in specific populations, such as collegiate athletics (1%–8%), military recruits (1%–31%), and runners (13%–52%).[5] Although the incidence varies according to the type of athlete, it is commonly reported that BSI may account for 20% of all sports medicine injuries.[6] Further, adults who have reached peak bone mass may require strategies to maintain optimal skeletal health. As such, BSI prevention strategies can significantly influence management of athletes and active individuals presenting to a sports medicine practice. Additionally, knowledge on BSI prevention may influence recommendations for school, collegiate, and professional sports teams as well as the general exercising population.

This chapter reviews the literature on BSI prevention, with a focus on athletes and endurance sports. Risk factors for BSI are examined, and approaches regarding prevention are discussed. Several strategies are introduced, including the roles of nutrition, sleep, training, and biomechanics on reducing risk of BSI. The concept of exposure to multiple sports during youth and adolescence (such as early participation in ball sports or "cross-training" with ball/power/loading sports) is also discussed as a way to reduce and possibly prevent BSI.

NUTRITION

Diet and exercise have long been considered the foundations of well-being,[7] and these lifestyle modifications may also positively impact bone health. Studies, however, assessing the impact of dietary factors on BSI (especially in female athletes) have remained limited and inconsistent.[8] Three main aspects of nutrition that may have the greatest impact on bone include energy availability (EA), calcium, and vitamin D.

Energy Availability

Low EA is the key cause of the female athlete triad (triad)[9] and relative energy deficiency in sport (RED-S). EA is the difference in energy intake to exercise energy expenditure, standardized to fat free mass,[10] and the threshold of low EA is commonly defined at below 30 kcal/kg fat free mass per day.[11] EA represents the energy remaining after accounting for demands of exercise to support physiological function. The updated position stand by the American College of Sports Medicine (ACSM)[9] defines the triad as a spectrum of three interrelated conditions of EA, menstrual function, and BMD. EA (defined as the difference between dietary intake and exercise energy expenditure standardized to fat free mass per day) affects BMD both directly and indirectly (including effects on menstrual and hormone function). Presence of combined or even single triad risk factors are associated with increased BSI risk in females[12,13] and males.[14] In 2014, the International Olympic Committee updated their 2005 triad consensus statement by introducing a broader term "relative energy deficiency in sport," to further expound upon the potential effects of low EA on decrements in physiology and performance may be caused by low EA in RED-S model includes several features not limited to just the triad, such as metabolic rate, menstrual function, bone health, immunity, protein synthesis, and cardiovascular health.[15]

Optimizing EA is critical to ensuring appropriate bone mass accumulation and maintenance. Screening for triad and RED-S includes evaluating dietary, physical activity, and behavioral patterns along with menstrual function and risk factors for low BMD. Detecting at-risk individuals (e.g., young female runners) especially during adolescence is key to ensuring that they achieve adequate bone formation during this critical window of growth and maximize chances of avoiding not only BSI but the additional systemic complications of low EA.

Calcium

A recent position statement by the American Association of Clinical Endocrinologists and the American College of Endocrinology (AACE/ACE) summarized the current understanding of optimizing vitamin and mineral intake to maximize bone gain, minimize bone loss, and reduce fracture risk.[16] Calcium at 2 to 3 servings a day is recommended, in doses of 400 to 500 mg totaling 1,200 to 1,500 mg/day (higher doses exceeding 2,500 mg/day may increase cardiovascular disease risk).[16,17] In terms of reducing BSI, an earlier Cochrane review in 2005[18] yielded insufficient evidence to support calcium supplementation offers added protection from BSI (although tibia only assessed). More recent studies also have had mixed results but appear to show a beneficial effect, especially if calcium is combined with other nutrients. A 2008 study by Lappe et al. suggests that calcium supplementation of 2,000 mg daily with 800 international units (IU) vitamin D reduces stress fracture incidence in female Navy recruits.[19] In female runners ages 17 to 26, calcium, vitamin D, and protein (major components in milk) were each associated with greater bone gains and a lower rate of future stress fracture.[8] There is also limited evidence suggesting that calcium intake (500–1,000 mg) prior to or during exercise may even prevent calcium bone resorption that occurs in the setting of calcium sweat losses.[20] A 2010 review by Tenforde et al. importantly pointed out study design limitations. Although calcium intake improves BMD and fracture risk at all ages, the data are conflicting with respect to younger athletes (ages 18–35 years), and males and non-whites are poorly represented. The authors suggested that 1,500 mg may potentially reduce stress fracture particularly in at-risk populations for impaired bone health and BSI (e.g., young female distance runners).[21]

Vitamin D

Calcium alone is not sufficient; calcium given with vitamin D reduces vertebral and non-vertebral fracture risk, as vitamin D improves gastrointestinal (GI) absorption of calcium and ensures adequate bone mineralization.[16] Vitamin D plays a major role in active GI transport of calcium and may improve muscle function and balance, thereby reducing fall risk and potential injury.[16] Defining adequate intake versus "vitamin D inadequacy" however is controversial, and the recommended dose varies significantly according to clinician, patient (e.g., obesity, malabsorption, and sun exposure all affect vitamin D levels), and geographic location. In the Lappe study, calcium plus vitamin D at 800 IU/day appeared to lower stress fracture incidence.[19] In a review comparing calcium, vitamin D, and dairy intake, it was found that vitamin D may confer the most protection against BSI.[22] AACE/ACE guidelines recommend adjusting vitamin D dosing by checking vitamin D blood levels; a minimum of 30 nmol/mL is considered sufficient in terms of preventing disease (based on an increased prevalence of secondary hyperparathyroidism below this level).[16] Ruohola et al. found that insufficient vitamin D levels in male military recruits had a greater risk of BSI.[23] However, *sufficient* versus *optimal* vitamin D levels remain unknown. Furthermore, the upper limit of normal is also controversial. Since highly sun-exposed adults reach vitamin D levels of 50 to 60 nmol/mL, this may be considered a safe upper limit.[16] McCabe et al. suggest that higher doses at 800 to 1,000 IU (and even up to 2,000 IU/day) should be considered in at-risk individuals, with a goal range of at least 50 nmol/mL (and up to 90–100 nmol/mL, due to relative safety and high therapeutic index).[24]

Other Vitamins and Minerals

Other micronutrients have unclear evidence, but magnesium and vitamins A, K, and C may play supportive roles in skeletal health.[16] The AACE/ACE[16] provided recommendations on other micronutrients. Magnesium is a cofactor for numerous enzymes and metabolic pathways in the body and necessary for both calcium and potassium homeostasis. Although found widely in foods, 48% of the U.S. population consume less than the recommended daily amount (RDA) of magnesium. Hypomagnesemia (low magnesium) may impair osteoblast function, decrease parathyroid hormone and vitamin D production and/or action, and increase osteoclast activation; all of these pathways weaken bone. Magnesium may therefore impact skeletal health, but its role is unclear. Vitamin A does influence bone content, although studies are uncertain how it may regulate osteoclastogenesis. Vitamin K is a cofactor for γ-carboxylation of osteocalcin, one of the major proteins for bone mineralization. Undercarboxylated osteocalcin binds poorly to bone; however, currently, there is no clear beneficial evidence on vitamin K supplements for bone health. Studies on vitamin C generally show either positive trends or significant effects on bone. Vitamin C plays a role in collagen formation, bone matrix development, osteoblast differentiation, and limiting bone resorption. However, the exact effect it may have on bone density is presently unknown. Finally, at present, there is no clear evidence on fluoride, strontium, boron, phosphate, vitamin E, flavonoids, or trace element (zinc, copper, iron) supplementation for optimal bone health.[16]

In summary, calcium plus vitamin D may primarily influence bone health, magnesium may be helpful if deficient, and there are possible but unclear roles for vitamins A, K, and C supplementation. A proper balanced diet is recommended prior to considering supplements for micronutrient deficiency.

Protein

Regarding macronutrients, protein is a major macronutrient essential for bone collagen synthesis. The Iowa Women's Health Study and the Canadian Multicentre Osteoporosis

Study report a decreased hip fracture risk with increasing animal protein intake, and low protein intake was associated with increased fracture risk.[16] Higher dairy protein intake compared to plant protein was associated with higher BMD and animal protein intake compared to vegetable protein lowered fracture risk.[16] In the Nieves' study, higher intakes of skim milk, dairy foods, and animal protein were associated with greater BMD and lower BSI risk.[8] Lower overall protein intake has been associated with increased BSI risk.[25,26]

It has been hypothesized that a high-protein (i.e., acid-based) diet is associated with calcium urinary excretion (hypercalciuria) from bone resorption, but AACE/ACE concluded that this hypothesis is not supported by current evidence.[16] Additionally, a protein and calcium interaction has been identified: Increased protein intake decreased fracture incidence if calcium intake is >800 mg/day, whereas the effect reverses with lower calcium intake.[16] Therefore, the current body of evidence suggests that adequate protein intake is an important risk factor associated with reduced fracture risk.

EXERCISE AND THE CROSS-OVER INFLUENCE OF BALL/LOADING SPORTS

Adequate weight-bearing exercise is well recognized as beneficial in youth for bone mass accumulation,[27] and in older adults for prevention and treatment of bone loss.[28] Active youth and adolescents are known to have higher bone mass than comparable inactive controls.[29,30] Weight-bearing exercise is preferred for its bone-building properties compared to non–weight-bearing activities, as swimmers and cyclists are known to have lower bone mass than athletes in ball and power sports, sometimes even lower than nonathlete inactive controls.[34]

Early participation in ball sports may serve as a potential strategy to prevent BSI.[32] Per Wolff's law,[31] bone adapts to mechanical loading by optimizing its structure to withstand the demand of the load placed upon it. Bone responds to increased magnitude and rate of loading, shorter intermittent durations of load, and distribution and novelty of load (odd-impact activities being favorable). High-impact, odd-impact, multidirectional, and/or jumping activities (ball sports are a good example of these) promote greater gains in BMD and favorable bone geometric properties compared to repetitive or low-impact sports (e.g., endurance running) or nonimpact/non–weight-bearing sports (e.g., cycling, swimming).[34]

This concept introduces the approach of a "pretraining" or "cross-training" program, which has been investigated by Milgrom et al. showing that preseason simulation of the loading forces occurring in basketball may help athletes in reducing BSI risk.[35] This is supported in a later study showing that ball sport participation in childhood/adolescence is associated with a significant (almost half) reduction in BSI incidence in runners later in life.[33] According to a 2011 review, both young men and women who engage in high-impact or odd-impact sport display the best BMD gains.[34] Furthermore, in a prospective longitudinal study of adolescent male athletes, the PRO-BONE study showed that bone acquisition over 1 year of participation in osteogenic sport (soccer) is clearly higher than nonosteogenic sports (swimming and cycling, which showed similar findings to controls).[36,37,38] These findings have been reproduced in other studies by the same group, also demonstrating more favorable bone geometrical and stiffness properties with osteogenic sports.[39] Moreover, a progressive countermovement jumping program when used as an intervention in the PRO-BONE swimmer and cyclist cohort improved bone mineral content and trabecular bone scores and reduced bone biochemical turnover markers.[39] These studies highlight the importance of osteogenic sports on bone acquisition at a critical time in adolescence and furthermore that participation only in nonosteogenic sports is not enough to induce positive bony adaptations. This may represent not only an ideal "prehabilitation" strategy to promote optimal bone health later in life but also a primary prevention strategy to avoid BSI altogether.[32]

SLEEP

Although diet and exercise are considered the two fundamentals of health and longevity, some consider the "3 pillars of health" include diet, exercise, and sleep.[40] The three pillars are interrelated, as ignoring one may negatively impact the other two. Sleep is an essential body function and often does not get sufficient attention. The detrimental effects of sleep deprivation are well studied in the general population. Inadequate sleep is associated with a multitude of negative effects spanning neurocognitive, metabolic, immunologic, and cardiovascular dysfunctions.[41] Furthermore, elite athletes are known to get less total sleep than nonathletes.[42,43] In a review on the effects of sleep deprivation and sleep extension in athletes, even as few as 2 hours less sleep/night resulted in a variety of impairments, from strength to power to cognitive function including reaction time, judgment, and decision-making.[40] Conversely, sleep extension can improve both physical and cognitive performance in athletes.[40]

Sleep disturbance may also affect bone physiology and metabolism.[44] Few studies exist on the specific effect of sleep on BSI risk, and results are mixed. In a review of successive military basic training recruits over several years, the introduction and enforcement of a 7-hour/day sleep regimen did not appear to decrease stress fracture incidence.[45] However, an earlier study by the same group showed that the combined effect of a minimum nightly sleep requirement (6 hours/night) combined with a decrease in recruits' cumulative marching and running did reduce BSI compared to prior year recruits.[46] In runners, a retrospective survey on an elite cross-country team failed to demonstrate sleep to be a significant risk for BSI.[47] However, in an epidemiological study examining BSI in adolescent high school sports, individuals with BSI slept significantly less than noninjured athletes (7.2 vs. 7.95 hours) and girls slept significantly less than boys (7.2 vs. 7.63 hours).[48]

There are ample studies however on the more clear effects of obstructive sleep apnea syndrome (OSAS) and bone loss. Obstructive sleep apnea is a sleep disorder resulting in upper airway collapse during sleep, frequent hypoxia, and sleep disturbance.[49] It results in bone loss via various mechanisms. In common with obesity, causes may include altered adrenergic tone, inflammation, oxidative stress, hypogonadism, diabetes, and vitamin D deficiency, while others are specific to OSAS, including hypoxia and altered glucocorticoid regulation.[50] Although increased fracture rate has not yet been demonstrated with OSAS, it is now recognized as a risk factor for osteoporosis.[49] However, Eimar et al. challenged in a systematic review and meta-analysis that while an association between sleep apnea and low bone mass is plausible, many supporting studies have risk of bias and are inconsistent.[51]

However, there is growing evidence that sleep abnormalities in general, and sleep duration in specific, are associated with low BMD.[52] Further supporting this finding are studies showing that circadian rhythm disruption is associated with increased fracture risk.[53] Swanson et al. showed that sleep restriction with circadian disruption alters bone turnover biomarkers and leads to an uncoupling of bone turnover; that is, bone formation decreases while bone resorption remains unchanged.[52] This uncoupling effect persists even when controlling for adequate energy balance, macronutrient distribution, and meeting the recommended dietary allowance for calcium.[54] For a more extreme example, US Army Ranger Training, an 8-week physically demanding program with energy expenditure 2,500 to 4,500 kcal/day, energy restriction deficit 1,000 to 4,000 kcal/day, and sleep deprivation <4 hour sleep/night showed increased bone resorption and suppressed bone formation.[55]

Therefore, sleep has positive impacts on health and should be a central focus to athletes. Sleep abnormalities, sleep deprivation, and even sleep apnea can occur in athletes and based on the previously mentioned factors have negative influence on bone mass. However, further studies are needed to better define the effects of impaired sleep specifically on BSI risk.

TRAINING

Although numerous studies have outlined various extrinsic and intrinsic risk factors for BSI,[6,56,57] the topics of training modifications including biomechanics, orthotics use, and running gait analysis are still contested.[58] In one study, it was felt that intrinsic factors other than gender played little role in BSI risk in military cadets (maximum variance explained by all risk factors was less than 10%).[59] In another military study, the only training change associated with decreased BSI incidence was simply restricting training to the authorized training protocol.[45] In theory, modifiable risk factors are a target for prevention; however, the influence of individual risk factors is difficult to precisely determine for risk of BSI. Methods have been proposed to prevent BSI, but few have been validated in studies of adequate power to make definitive recommendations.

Risk Factors

Traditionally, many refer to some alteration in training program as one of the most significant risk factors for BSI (other than history of a prior BSI).[60,61] This classically includes an abrupt change in volume, intensity, and/or frequency in training; new training format (e.g., hills, sprints, changes in shoes, surface camber or hardness without adequate acclimation time); or inadequate rest (altering hard/easy training on successive days or lack of "off" days).[6] In runners, prior work has suggested higher volume of training may contribute to BSI such as exceeding, previously >64 kilometers/week[62] however, other reports suggest elevated risk exceeding 32 kilometers[63] to 40 kilometers/week.[64] Training time, for example, >5 hours/day (in ballet dancers), is also a known BSI risk.[65] Repetitive single-plane primarily sagittal loading in running may also increase BSI risk compared to multidirectional sport (e.g., soccer) due to unfavorable asymmetric bone geometry.[66] Smaller calf girth and fatigued calf and lower leg muscles may also increase BSI risk.[64,67] As ultimately BSI is likely multifactorial, targeting as many of these factors as feasible in a training regimen and modifying training to avoid multiple risk factors may be a potential prevention strategy. According to the Cochrane review, modification of training schedules and ensuring adequate rest "may" reduce BSI incidence, but there is no definitive evidence and specific training regimens require individualization.[18]

Footwear

Footwear and orthotics also have mixed results. Change of footwear while modifying biomechanics of the foot has been reported to increase BSI risk;[68] however, other studies show that adjusting footwear (e.g., more comfortable boots during military basic training) does not alter BSI risk.[45] In the Cochrane review, the only intervention strategy that reduced BSI was the use of shock-absorbing inserts, which was found to "probably" reduce the incidence of BSI in military personnel based on limited evidence, although there was insufficient evidence to determine the best design.[18]

Gait Modification

Runners who exhibit higher vertical ground reaction forces, vertical loading rate, and peak acceleration rate have higher BSI incidence.[69,70] Therefore, these biomechanical parameters have been investigated in an attempt to prevent BSI. Gait retraining can reduce loading and vertical ground reaction forces, although it is unknown if this translates into reduced BSI risk.[71] Another study demonstrated that increasing cadence beyond preferred running cadence helps to optimize running biomechanics and reduce lower extremity loading.[72] Again, it is only postulated that this may reduce BSI risk.

Traditional Advice

In the absence of clear evidence, many turn to some of the more traditional axioms of sports medicine for guidance on injury prevention. Commonly handed-down adages include the three "golden rules of running": the "pain rule" (if the pain is 1–3, you may continue training; if 4–6, modify training until it is 1–3 again; if 7–10, you must stop running), the "no limping allowed" rule (if you are clearly altering your gait to run, something is wrong), and the commonly referenced "10% rule" (increase weekly training parameters by only 10% at a time; author's experience, unpublished). Also, some of the other published "universal truths of running" may offer practical advice that in theory could reduce BSI risk. These include the "2 day rule" (if something hurts for 2 days while running, take 2 days off), the "race-recovery rule" (for every one mile raced, take 1 day of recovery from hard training), the "sleep rule" (sleep 1 extra minute every mile run per week, more important in long-distance running), and the "hard/easy rule" (alternate hard and easy workouts).[73] In recent years, as the overreaching and overtraining syndromes have become more recognized, the old saying "it's better to be 10% undertrained than 1% overtrained when you step up to the start line"[74] may also be a reasonable maxim not only for BSI prevention but also for reduced EA and Triad/RED-S.

Single Sport Specialization

Furthermore, another potential contributor to overtraining, early single-sport specialization, may also play a role. Single-sport athletes may train almost twice as many hours/week compared to multisport athletes, according to a study by Sugimoto et al.;[75] increased training volume was associated with a greater likelihood of lower extremity overuse injury in the study. These findings are supported by another study[76] and may explain why high single-sport specialization increases lower extremity injury risk.

If returning an athlete from overtraining syndrome or steering an athlete away from single-sport specialization overuse, a brief rest and recovery period may be useful to prevent BSI. Athletes should start with light activity and follow a graded return to play based on their response. Often used for medical illness (e.g., pneumonia), in the author's clinical experience (K.V.), the general rule is for every day missed due to illness or overtraining, the athlete needs 2 to 3 days of graded return. Typically, the sequence of training increments should be increasing *frequency* first, then *duration*, and finally *intensity* of exercise. These rules would also appear relevant when assessing BSI risk and training progression.

Recently, a very practical "Four Pain Rules to Running Participation"[77] was formally published, giving clinicians (and athletes) four very sensible rules to follow: "(1) Pain that increases or changes from dull to intense (or achy to sharp) during running should be avoided, and the activity should be reduced or stopped immediately; (2) Joint pain should not persist or increase by 24 hours after exercise, indicating the musculoskeletal system was not prepared for that session; (3) If preexisting mild joint pain is present (<3 out of a 10-point scale), the pain should not worsen during the exercise session or last into the next day; (4) If the pain causes a limp or a compensatory gait change, the exercise volume must be reduced or stopped until a normal gait pattern occurs, as persistence of asymmetric gait due to pain interferes with normal tissue healing and may increase the risk for more injuries."[77] These easy-to-use, real-world rules can be applied to any runner, regardless of age, body habitus, experience, or training regimen and may help with a straightforward approach to BSI prevention strategies. These rules can help runners self-regulate their training progressions and determine if additional rest is necessary.

In summary, it is difficult to determine conclusively which training modifications may ultimately reduce BSI. Many clinicians use traditional common-sense rules when counseling athletes on training and modifications. Some studies show promise, whereas others conflict; more research is warranted to better assess individual and combined training modification effects on prevention of BSI.

CONCLUSION

BSI represents a spectrum of pathology characterized by an imbalance between modeling and remodeling and between stress and recovery. Its pathophysiology is complex but in essence can be summed up as an injury that occurs when bone is loaded beyond its capacity to bear the load and repair microdamage. Prevention of this injury is paramount by optimizing bone health. While the recognition of BSI may prompt further investigation into risk factors such as the triad and RED-S in order to prevent further BSI, primary prevention is key, especially in young athletes. Proper nutrition is essential, including adequate calcium, vitamin D, and adequate EA to meet the energy demand of athletics. Early participation in ball sports and avoidance of early single-sport specialization may represent a unique prevention strategy to optimally load the bone during youth and improve bone geometric properties. Quality sleep cannot be overstated to athletes; sleep provides a critical body function; lack of adequate sleep can have deleterious impact on skeletal health and put an athlete at a potential higher risk of BSI. Training modification strategies are perhaps the most enigmatic in terms of prevention with conflicting research, with studies on gait changes, orthotic use, and other modifications yielding unclear or conflicting results. Most agree that avoidance of an abrupt change in training regimen is critical to prevention. In the absence of conclusive data, the authors recommend a practical approach when counseling an athlete, a patient, a parent, or a coach on prevention of BSIs.

KEY REFERENCES

Only key references appear in the print edition. The full reference list appears in the digital product found on http://connect.springerpub.com/content/book/978-0-8261-4424-9/part/sec04/chapter/ch15

8. Nieves JW, Melsop K, Curtis M, et al. Nutritional factors that influence change in bone density and stress fracture risk among young female cross-country runners. *PM R*. 2010 Aug 1;2(8):740–750.

21. Tenforde AS, Sayres LC, Sainani KL, Fredericson M. Evaluating the relationship of calcium and vitamin D in the prevention of stress fracture injuries in the young athlete: a review of the literature. *PM R*. 2010 Oct 1;2(10):945–949.

32. Tenforde AS, Sainani KL, Sayres LC, et al. Participation in ball sports may represent a prehabilitation strategy to prevent future stress fractures and promote bone health in young athletes. *PM R*. 2015 Feb;7(2):222–225.

34. Tenforde AS, Fredericson M. Influence of sports participation on bone health in the young athlete: a review of the literature. *PM R*. 2011 Sep 1;3(9):861–867.

48. Nussbaum ED, Bjornaraa J, Gatt CJ Jr. Identifying factors that contribute to adolescent bony stress injury in secondary school athletes: a comparative analysis with a healthy athletic control group. *Sports Health*. 2019 Jan 1;11(4):375–379.

56. Chen YT, Tenforde AS, Fredericson M. Update on stress fractures in female athletes: epidemiology, treatment, and prevention. *Curr Rev Musculoskelet Med*. 2013 Jun 1;6(2):173–181.

CHAPTER 16

Medications

Madhusmita Misra

INTRODUCTION

Successful prevention and treatment of bone stress injuries (BSIs) requires a thorough understanding of factors that increase the risk for BSIs in athletes. In a prospective study, Barrack et al. demonstrated that in female athletes, a combination of lifestyle factors contributing to low energy availability, a history of oligo-amenorrhea, and low bone mineral density (BMD) conferred an increased risk for BSIs.[1] Similarly, in male athletes, Kraus et al. showed that a combination of low energy availability, low body mass index (BMI), a previous history of BSIs, and low BMD was associated with a prospective risk of BSIs.[2] These data suggest that the first line of management to prevent BSIs should be nonpharmacological and include steps to optimize energy availability in athletes[3] by increasing caloric intake, reducing exercise energy expenditure, or both.

However, if nonpharmacologic therapy is not successful, there may be a role for certain pharmacologic measures to optimize bone outcomes and reduce the risk for future BSIs. When considering pharmacological therapy, it is important to consider the mechanism targeted including the hormonal status of the athlete. Given that oligoamenorrhea is an important determinant of BSIs, reversing this hypogonadal state through lifestyle measures or replacing deficient reproductive hormones may be a useful strategy to optimize not just bone outcomes but also symptoms of hypogonadism or infertility. Because low BMD and impaired bone geometry are important determinants of BSIs,[1–5] other pharmacological measures that improve BMD may become necessary to prevent future BSIs, particularly when reproductive hormone replacement is not effective, not indicated (in the absence of hypogonadism), or not permitted (such as medications banned by the World Anti-Doping Agency for competitive athletes). A significant limitation in determining the best preventive or therapeutic strategy for BSIs is the paucity of good randomized controlled trials (RCTs) of potential pharmacological therapies in both male and female athletes. This chapter reviews available data for pharmacological measures to improve BMD measures in athletes and other populations. RCTs that demonstrate a reduction in BSIs as a study end point are lacking in athletes, and therefore, an improvement in BMD has been used in most available studies as a surrogate for improved bone health.

CALCIUM AND VITAMIN D SUPPLEMENTATION

Calcium and vitamin D intake through food and/or supplements should be optimized before initiating therapy with other pharmacological agents. Although data are currently lacking regarding a definitive 25-hydroxy vitamin D [25(OH)D] level below which BMD is compromised, a 25(OH)D level of 20 to 22 ng/mL or higher is typically sufficient to avoid deleterious effects on bone.[6,7] Other studies suggest that parathyroid hormone (PTH) levels start to rise and calcium absorption is lower, though still within the normative range, when 25(OH)D levels fall below 30 to 32 ng/mL.[8–10] Until more definitive data are available, we suggest maintaining 25(OH)D levels at or above 32 ng/mL, which may require supplemental vitamin D. 25(OH)D levels should not exceed the upper limit of the normal range (usually 80 ng/mL) given concerns of hypercalcemia. The recommended dietary allowance (RDA) for vitamin D is 600 IUs/day for most age groups and 800 IUs/day for those older than 70 years, per the Institute of Medicine.[11] The RDA for calcium intake is 1,300 mg/day for children and adolescents 9 to 18 years old, 1,000 mg/day for those 19 to 70 years old, and 1,200 mg/day for those >70 years old.[11] One study in young male athletes ages 13 to 18 demonstrated that receiving <1 serving of calcium-rich food per day was a risk factor for low BMD.[12]

Who Qualifies for Pharmacological Treatment for Low Bone Density?

In the female athlete, pharmacological treatment of low BMD may be considered after institution of at least a year of nonpharmacological therapy, if the athlete has a diagnosis of osteoporosis and/or a clinically significant fracture history *and* demonstrates lack of response to nonpharmacological therapy over this period.[3] Lack of response is a clinically significant reduction in bone mineral content (BMC) or BMD Z-scores after at least a year of nonpharmacological therapy *or* development of new fractures during such therapy.[3] Such individuals should be referred to a specialist in bone metabolic disorders or an endocrinologist for administration of pharmacological treatment to improve bone health. Similar guidelines may apply to the male athlete as well, but formal guidelines are currently lacking.

OPTIMIZING REPRODUCTIVE HORMONES IN FEMALE ATHLETES

Estrogen Replacement and Effects on Bone

In oligoamenorrheic female athletes, the next consideration is typically estrogen replacement therapy. In considering estrogen replacement therapy, it is important to consider the formulation, dose, and route of administration of estrogen. The greatest efficacy is observed with the physiologic (natural) form of estrogen that is, 17β-estradiol, a hormone that can be administered at a dose of 100 mcg daily as the transdermal patch. Randomized controlled studies in adolescent and adult amenorrheic women with anorexia nervosa (AN) and adolescent and young adult oligoamenorrheic athletes have demonstrated that estrogen administration as the combined oral contraceptive (COC) pill (containing 20–35 mcg of ethinyl estradiol and a progestogen) is not effective in improving BMD in these populations.[13–15] This has been attributed to (1) the insulin-like growth factor-I (IGF-I) suppressive effects of oral ethinyl estradiol (a synthetic form of estrogen) because of its hepatic first-pass metabolism, not observed with transdermal

17β-estradiol (IGF-I is an important bone trophic hormone), and (2) greater increases in sex hormone–binding globulin (SHBG; a binding protein of the sex hormones) with the ethinyl estradiol pill than the 17β-estradiol patch, resulting in lower bioavailable estrogen in COC pill users.

Consistent with this, significant reductions in IGF-I and increases in SHBG have been noted in adolescent and young adult oligoamenorrheic athletes receiving oral ethinyl estradiol versus transdermal 17β-estradiol or no estrogen.[15] Studies have also demonstrated significant increases in spine and femoral neck BMD and BMD Z-scores in oligoamenorrheic athletes receiving transdermal 17β-estradiol versus oral ethinyl estradiol or no estrogen,[15] and in total hip BMD and BMD Z-scores in adolescent girls with AN receiving the transdermal 17β-estradiol patch versus oral ethinyl estradiol.[16] Importantly, therapy with the patch does not have contraceptive efficacy, and alternate methods of contraception should be recommended when contraception is required. Those who use a COC pill for contraception should be cautioned that such therapy is unlikely to improve bone health. Of note, one RCT of a COC pill given with oral dehydroepiandrosterone (DHEA; 50 mg daily) versus double placebo showed maintenance of BMD Z-scores in those who received the COC with oral DHEA[17] versus a decrease over time in the placebo group, suggesting that administration of a COC (which is antiresorptive) may have beneficial effects on bone if given simultaneously with a bone anabolic agent (such as DHEA).

Estrogen replacement may be recommended to young athletes ≥16 and ≤21 years old if they have BMC or BMD Z-scores of ≤−2 even without a clinically significant fracture history and *if* they have ≥1 additional triad risk factors *and* demonstrate lack of response to nonpharmacological therapy for at least a year.[3] This is because adolescence is a very narrow window of time during which to optimize bone accrual, and deficits in bone accrual during this vulnerable period are likely to result in suboptimal peak bone mass, with long-lasting effects on bone strength and fracture risk. Thus, the criteria for providing estrogen replacement therapy are more lax in this younger population than in older adult women. The role of estrogen replacement is unclear in premenarchal athletes <16 years old and eumenorrheic athletes with low BMD.

All athletes receiving transdermal estrogen replacement therapy should receive cyclic progesterone/progestogen to avoid endometrial hyperplasia from unopposed estrogenic stimulation of the uterine lining, which predisposes the uterus to cancer in the long term. Options include 200 mg of micronized progesterone, 5 to 10 mg of medroxyprogesterone acetate, or 5 mg of norethindrone orally daily for 12 days of every month.

Because estrogen preparations increase the risk for blood clots, in athletes with a personal or family history of blood clots, estrogen replacement therapy should be instituted only after consultation with a hematologist regarding additional testing (e.g., through a hypercoagulation panel), and the preparation, dose, and route of administration of estrogen and progesterone/progestogen need to be considered. Of note, transdermal 17β-estradiol is less likely to cause thromboembolism than oral ethinyl estradiol because it does not undergo first-pass hepatic metabolism.[10]

Effects of Estrogen Replacement on Other End Points

Emerging data suggest that oligoamenorrheic young athletes have impaired cognitive function (verbal memory and executive function), greater anxiety levels, and a maintenance or worsening of disordered eating behavior compared with eumenorrheic women.[19,20] Small pilot studies have demonstrated that estrogen replacement therapy (as the 17-β estradiol patch) in these oligoamenorrheic women may improve cognitive function (verbal memory and executive function),[21] the tendency to be anxious,[22] and eating behavior (with improvement in drive for thinness and body dissatisfaction scores).[23] Topical estrogen administration is helpful in relieving symptoms of vaginal dryness and dyspareunia in hypogonadal women.

Testosterone Deficiency and Its Replacement in Females

Adult hypogonadal women with AN have low testosterone levels, which correlate with lower BMD measures.[24] However, a RCT of low-dose testosterone replacement in these women did not demonstrate a beneficial effect on BMD.[25] Low testosterone in females with AN has been linked to anxiety and depression scores, and an improvement in depression severity had previously been reported following testosterone replacement in these women.[26,27] However, a more recent study reported that 24 weeks of testosterone replacement therapy (versus placebo) led to less weight gain in women with AN and did not result in sustained improvements in depression, anxiety, or disordered eating symptoms.[28]

OPTIMIZING REPRODUCTIVE HORMONES IN MALE ATHLETES

Effects of Testosterone Replacement

Hormone therapy to normalize testosterone levels is fraught with challenges in male hypogonadal athletes given rulings of the World Anti-Doping Agency. Data are conflicting regarding associations of testosterone with bone end points. While some suggest a direct association of testosterone levels with bone outcomes, others suggest that it is estradiol (from aromatization of testosterone) that drives these outcomes.[29-31] Regardless, normalizing testosterone levels would be expected to improve BMD, sexual function, and quality of life in hypogonadal males. Consistent with this, studies in adult hypogonadal men indicate a beneficial effect of testosterone replacement on bone outcomes,[32-34] mostly related to its aromatization to estradiol.[35] In healthy adult men, an estradiol level above 10 pg/mL and a testosterone level above 200 ng/dL were noted to be sufficient to prevent an increase in bone resorption and a decrease in BMD.[36] However, data are lacking for effects of testosterone replacement on bone and other end points in specifically male athletes with hypogonadism.

Testosterone replacement therapy also has the potential to improve other outcomes such as muscle strength, impaired sexual function, mood, and quality of life.[37-39] However, studies assessing these end points in hypogonadal male athletes are currently lacking and logistically challenging.[40] Finally, studies of estradiol replacement are also challenging in men given difficulties attaining an estradiol level that is likely to optimize bone health without having deleterious effects on other systems (such as inducing gynecomastia and lipid abnormalities).

Effects of Clomiphene (Clomifene) Citrate Therapy

This selective estrogen receptor modulator stimulates gonadotropin-releasing hormone (GnRH) and therefore gonadotropin secretion and can increase testosterone secretion in males and induce ovulation in females with hypogonadotropic hypogonadism. In a study that compared testosterone replacement therapy to clomiphene (clomifene) citrate (CC) in men with symptomatic hypogonadism versus eugonadal men not on either medication,[41] both were effective at increasing testosterone. However, testosterone was more effective at raising serum testosterone and improving hypogonadal symptoms, while CC had a deleterious effect on libido.[41] In contrast, CC is less likely to cause secondary polycythemia than testosterone replacement (1.7% vs. 11.2%).[42] CC is banned by the World Anti-Doping Agency for use in male athletes.[40]

Other Therapies to Increase Testosterone Levels

In a case report of a male hypogonadal athlete treated with tamoxifen (an antiestrogenic drug) to increase gonadotropin production, and thus testosterone secretion, the treatment led to improved sexual drive, well-being, and reduction in muscle injury.[43] Aromatase inhibitors reduce aromatization of testosterone to estradiol and raise testosterone levels. However, this strategy is unlikely to benefit bone health, for which optimal estradiol levels are necessary.[35,44] Pulsatile GnRH therapy and gonadotropin administration can induce testosterone secretion and spermatogenesis in men with hypogonadotropic hypogonadism[45] and treat infertility in females with hypogonadotropic hypogonadism. Studies assessing the impact of such therapies to improve bone outcomes in hypogonadal athletes are lacking.

BONE ANABOLIC AND ANTIRESORPTIVE THERAPIES

Certain female athletes may meet criteria for pharmacological therapy but not estrogen replacement (e.g., eumenorrheic athletes/exercisers) *or* may have contraindications to or be resistant to estrogen replacement. Poor response or resistance to estrogen replacement therapy refers to a lack of response after ≥18 to 24 months of such treatment. In male athletes, lack of data supporting reproductive hormone replacement and the need to adhere to the tenets of the World Anti-Doping Agency limit the use of such therapy as a viable strategy to improve BMD and reduce risk of BSIs. If such athletes are in need of pharmacotherapy because of a significant history of BSIs, they should be referred to a specialist in metabolic bone disorders or an endocrinologist for consideration of other pharmacological treatments to improve bone health.

Bone Anabolic Therapies

Teriparatide and Abaloparatide

Teriparatide (a PTH analog; $rhPTH_{1-34}$) and abaloparatide (a parathyroid hormone-related protein [PTHrP] analog) are U.S. Food and Drug Administration (FDA)-approved bone anabolic agents for treatment of postmenopausal women with osteoporosis at high risk of fracture; teriparatide therapy is also approved to increase bone mass in men with primary or hypogonadal osteoporosis at high risk for fracture as well as men and women with glucocorticoid induced osteoporosis at high risk for fracture. Both are given as a subcutaneous injection (20 and 80 mcg daily for teriparatide and abaloparatide, respectively) and hold promise for athletes who qualify for pharmacological therapy, based on their effects in these other populations at a high risk for fracture.[46–53] These medications exert their effects through binding to the PTH/PTHrP receptor expressed on osteoblasts, osteocytes, renal tubule cells, and other tissues.[54] They improve trabecular bone mass and microarchitecture, increase bone strength, and reduce fracture risk despite an increase in cortical porosity. Recent data suggest that abaloparatide may be even more effective than teriparatide in this regard.[55,56]

One 6-month study of teriparatide (20 mg daily subcutaneous) verus placebo in older women with AN also showed a 6% to 10% improvement in lumbar spine BMD in those who received teriparatide.[57] However, both drugs have been associated with an increased risk of osteosarcoma in animal studies and are contraindicated in pregnancy. Further, they carry a black box warning for those at increased baseline risk for osteosarcoma, including children with open epiphyses and individuals with Paget's disease or a history of external beam radiation therapy or implant radiotherapy to the skeleton, and should not be given for any longer than 2 years over the lifetime of any individual. Studies have not examined the impact of teriparatide or abaloparatide on bone outcomes in male or female athletes. Reports of teriparatide use in athletes are limited to case reports and small trials[58,59] for healing of BSIs, for which its efficacy remains questionable.

Romosozumab

This is a monoclonal antibody that increases BMD and reduces fracture incidence in postmenopausal women and older men by inhibiting sclerostin,[60–62] and is now FDA approved for use in postmenopausal women with osteoporosis at high risk for fracture. Sclerostin is a protein that is secreted by osteocytes and inhibits osteoblast proliferation, differentiation, and survival by inhibiting the canonical *Wnt* signaling pathway and stimulates receptor activator of nuclear factor-κB ligand (RANKL), thus increasing osteoclastic activity and bone resorption. Romosozumab causes an initial increase in bone formation followed by a more prolonged decrease in bone resorption.[54] Importantly, the bone anabolic effect decreases after 12 doses (each dose includes two subcutaneous injections [total dose 210 mg] given once a month) and thus current recommendations are to stop the medication after 12 doses. Data are lacking for use of romosozumab in other populations including athletes.

Insulin-Like Growth Factor-I and Leptin

IGF-I is a bone anabolic hormone that is low in conditions of low energy availability compared with controls.[63,64] Administration of rhIGF-I increases bone formation markers in adolescents and adults with AN,[64,65] and when given with a COC pill, increases BMD at the spine and hip in adults with AN.[66] However, data are lacking regarding effects of rhIGF-I administration on bone in female or male athletes with low BMD or increased risk of BSIs. Further, normal-weight oligoamenorrheic athletes have some reduction in IGF-I levels compared with controls but not to the extent observed in AN.[67] Thus, effects of rhIGF-I administration on bone end points may differ in normal-weight athletes compared to low-weight athletes with disordered eating behavior. Most recently, the package insert of rhIGF-I has been modified to indicate that it is not intended for use in conditions of secondary IGF-I deficiency, including malnutrition (www.ipsen. com/websites/Ipsen_Online/wp-content/uploads/sites/9/2019/06/24180443/ Increlex_Full_Prescribing_Information.pdf).

Leptin is a bone anabolic hormone with stimulatory effects on GnRH secretion. Studies of metreleptin administration in adult women with functional hypothalamic amenorrhea have shown that metreleptin compared with placebo is effective in improving reproductive function,[68,69] increasing bone formation markers; one small study reported an increase in lumbar BMC (but not BMD) in women who received metreleptin versus placebo.[69] There are no studies to date that have examined the effects of metreleptin administration on bone outcomes in male athletes.

Antiresorptive Therapy

Bisphosphonates

Bisphosphonates may be effective in increasing BMD in those with evidence of increased bone resorption and have proven efficacy in improving BMD in postmenopausal women and older men.[70–72] One RCT of risedronate versus placebo in adult women with AN demonstrated a 2% to 3% increase in spine and hip BMD in those who received risedronate versus placebo,[25] although another RCT of alendronate versus placebo in adolescents with AN demonstrated no improvement in spine BMD and only a small improvement in femoral neck BMD in the alendronate arm.[73] The underlying state of increased bone resorption in adults versus suppressed bone resorption in adolescents with AN may explain why bisphosphonates were effective in improving BMD in young adult women but not in adolescents with this condition. Bisphosphonates have a very long half-life, and given concerns for potential teratogenic effects, this class of medication is rarely used in girls or in women of reproductive age. In limited cases of use, bisphosphonates should be prescribed with reliable contraceptive measures in those of reproductive age. Such therapy should be continued for a defined period before considering alternative measures to improve bone health.

Data are limited for bisphosphonate use in male athletes to optimize bone outcomes, with mostly case series and retrospective studies reported to date.[74,75] One retrospective study of intravenous bisphosphonates (ibandronate) and vitamin D to treat bone marrow edema in 22 male professional athletes reported pain reduction and improved mobility within the first 2 weeks after the first ibandronate infusion.[75] Time to return to competition was about 3.5 months. However, lack of a control group limited assessment of clinical efficacy of this intervention. One recent study of military recruits, who are at high risk for BSIs during basic training, randomized 324 recruits to 30 mg of risedronate or placebo daily for 10 doses during the first 2 weeks of training, followed by weekly maintenance dosing for 12 weeks.[76] The randomization groups did not differ for occurrence of BSIs at any site.

Denosumab

Denosumab (an inhibitor of RANKL) is a very effective medication for treatment of postmenopausal osteoporosis,[77] and studies are currently ongoing of denosumab versus placebo in adult women with AN. However, data are not available for the effects of denosumab on bone outcomes in male hypogonadal athletes. Of note, denosumab is the most rapidly acting antiresorptive agent currently in use, but its effects are rapidly reversible.[54]

COMBINATION THERAPY

Combination therapy using bone anabolic followed by antiresorptive medications may be more effective in improving BMD and reducing fracture risk than either therapy alone or use of antiresorptive therapies followed by bone anabolic therapy (summarized in Ref. 53). Studies are necessary to examine the effect of drug monotherapy as well as combination therapy in male athletes at risk for fracture.

CONCLUSION

The significant paucity of data around the use of pharmacological therapy in male and female athletes makes prescription of such therapy challenging. Until such data are available, providers must use their best judgment around determination for when to initiate and duration for pharmacological therapy and limited guidance has been published on the topic of best practices in males. Further, these decisions should be made in conjunction with a specialist in bone metabolic disorders and/or an endocrinologist.

KEY REFERENCES

Only key references appear in the print edition. The full reference list appears in the digital product found on http://connect.springerpub.com/content/book/978-0-8261-4424-9/part/sec04/chapter/ch16

3. De Souza MJ, Nattiv A, Joy E, et al. 2014 female athlete triad coalition consensus statement on treatment and return to play of the female athlete triad: 1st international conference held in San Francisco, California, May 2012 and 2nd international conference held in Indianapolis, Indiana, May 2013. *Br J Sports Med*. 2014;48:289.

14. Strokosch GR, Friedman AJ, Wu SC, Kamin M. Effects of an oral contraceptive (norgestimate/ethinyl estradiol) on bone mineral density in adolescent females with anorexia nervosa: a double-blind, placebo-controlled study. *J Adolesc Health*. 2006;39:819–827.

15. Ackerman KE, Singhal V, Baskaran C, et al. Oestrogen replacement improves bone mineral density in oligo-amenorrheic athletes: a randomized clinical trial. *Br J Sports Med*. 2019; 53(4):229–236.

16. Misra M, Katzman D, Miller KK, et al. Physiologic estrogen replacement increases bone density in adolescent girls with anorexia nervosa. *J Bone Miner Res*. 2011;26:2430–2438.

17. Divasta AD, Feldman HA, Giancaterino C, et al. The effect of gonadal and adrenal steroid therapy on skeletal health in adolescents and young women with anorexia nervosa. *Metabolism*. 2012;61:1010–1020.

CHAPTER 17

Gait Retraining

Irene S. Davis and Karen L. Troy

INTRODUCTION

Bone stress injuries (BSIs) are among the most serious of overuse injuries that a runner can sustain. Tibial BSIs are the most commonly sustained by runners. All BSIs require removal of impact loading as well as significant time for healing. The etiology of BSIs is multifactorial in nature, including bone structure and geometry, hormonal factors, diet, sleep, and training.[1] However, impact forces and faulty alignment have also been suggested to play a role. The purpose of this chapter is to describe the role these biomechanical factors play in the development of a tibial BSI and present a gait retraining intervention to address these factors.

INFLUENCE OF IMPACT LOADS ON BONE STRESS INJURIES

Ground reaction forces during heel-to-toe running typically include both an impact peak, which ranges from 1.5 to 2 bodyweights and occurs 15 to 50 ms after initial foot contact, and an active peak, which is usually larger and occurs around mid-stance.[2,3] Vertical instantaneous loading rate (VILR) and related measures describe how rapidly the impact peak is reached (and thus, how rapidly the musculoskeletal system is loaded during initial foot contact).[4] Loading rate–related measures have been associated with many running injuries including patellofemoral pain and BSI.[5-7] It is unclear whether high impact loading rates are the direct cause of injury or a surrogate measure for other mechanisms (e.g., fatigue-related changes in running biomechanics).

BSIs are thought to result from an accumulation of microdamage within bone, in combination with damage-associated bone remodeling.[8,9] When bone is loaded cyclically to subfailure levels, microdamage is generated within the tissue. In healthy physiologic situations, the damaged bone is removed and replaced through the coordinated action of osteoclasts and osteoclasts, termed "remodeling."[10] Typically, a full remodeling cycle takes 3 to 4 months to complete, during which cortical bone porosity is temporarily increased until the newly formed bone is fully mineralized.[11] In normal conditions, around 5% of cortical bone is being remodeled at any given time, so some level of

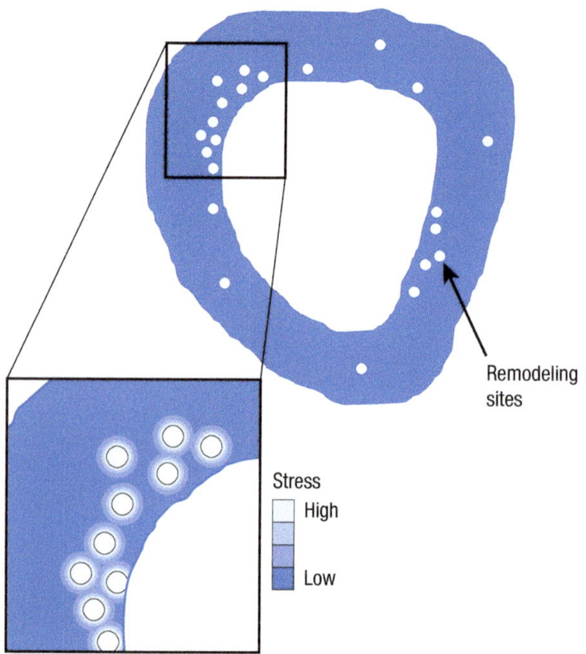

FIGURE 17.1 Remodeling temporarily introduces small pores (labeled "remodeling sites") into cortical bone. Forces transmitted through the skeleton cause stresses within the bone, concentrated around these remodeling sites. These local concentrations may increase the risk of further damage to the bone material.

porosity is normal. However, when higher-than-usual amounts of damage accumulate within cortical bone, remodeling may introduce additional cortical porosity.[12] Pores within bone cause stress concentrations during loading, leading to additional localized damage (Figure 17.1). Furthermore, microdamage itself weakens the bone tissue by diminishing its material properties.

Bone remodeling is governed in part by loading rate, with moderately high loading rates stimulating additional bone remodeling, acquisition, and adaptation.[13,14] In young healthy adults, impact loads are known to initiate bone turnover.[15] Moderate amounts of impact loading are anabolic to bone, especially in growing children.[16,17] Similarly, when high impact loads from hopping and jogging are combined with resistance training, they can prevent bone loss in older women.[18]

Very high loading rates may be associated with an exaggerated bone remodeling response to microdamage, which could increase the risk of BSI. Peak VILR during rearfoot strike (RFS) running is significantly higher than when landing on the forefoot.[19] These high loading rates, combined with a high number of loading cycles (i.e., high running mileage), may be sufficient to initiate a BSI in some individuals. Extensive cortical remodeling has been observed in athletes with chronic anterior tibial BSI, although the loading rate was not quantified in these individuals.[9] In rabbits, high rate impact loads elicit more extensive cartilage damage and subchrondral bone remodeling than low rate impact loads.[20]

In summary, while moderate impact loads are associated with long-term benefits to bone strength, high impact rates may elicit a robust remodeling response in some individuals. This could initiate a BSI through mechanisms of increased cortical porosity, leading to stress concentrations that result in additional microdamage.

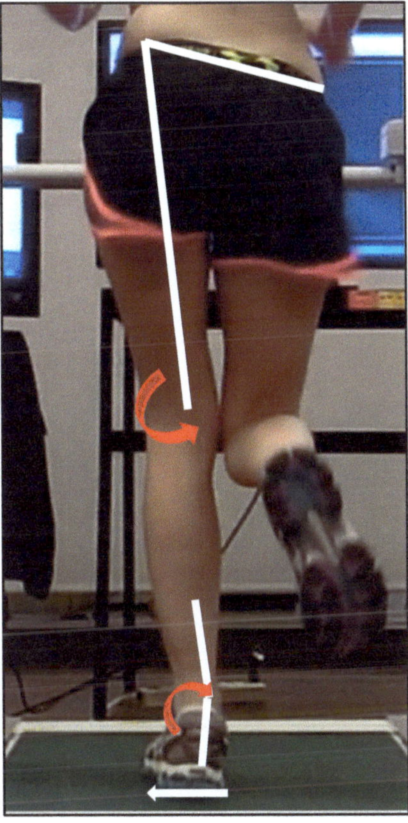

FIGURE 17.2 Runner with increased hip adduction and rearfoot eversion. These malalignments can alter the loads in the tibia by placing rotational forces at the proximal and distal ends of the tibia, creating a bending moment within the bone.

INFLUENCE OF FAULTY ALIGNMENT ON BONE STRESS INJURIES

Abnormal alignments of the lower extremity can influence the manner in which the skeleton is loaded. Only one study has examined the relationship between dynamic alignment and tibial stress fractures. Pohl et al. reported that individuals with a history of tibial stress fractures exhibited greater hip adduction as well as rearfoot eversion during running.[21] The combination of these movements results in a medialization of the lower extremity that can result in increased torques at the proximal and distal ends of the tibia (Figure 17.2). These torques applied under the compression load during stance have the potential to increase the bending moments on the tibia.

Strike pattern may also influence torques about the tibia. An RFS pattern is typically associated with a more extended knee at contact and a longer stride than a forefoot strike (FFS) pattern (Figure 17.3). This increases the inclination angle of the tibia likely resulting in a greater braking force than in an FFS pattern. Indeed, in unpublished data, we noted that peak braking force was 17% higher in 25 RFS versus 25 FFS runners (0.29 ± 0.04 vs. 0.24 ± 0.04) when running at similar speeds (2.55–2.60 m/s). These greater peak braking forces can contribute to greater bending loads about the tibia, which in turn may lead to greater bending moments in the tibia. In a recent prospective study by

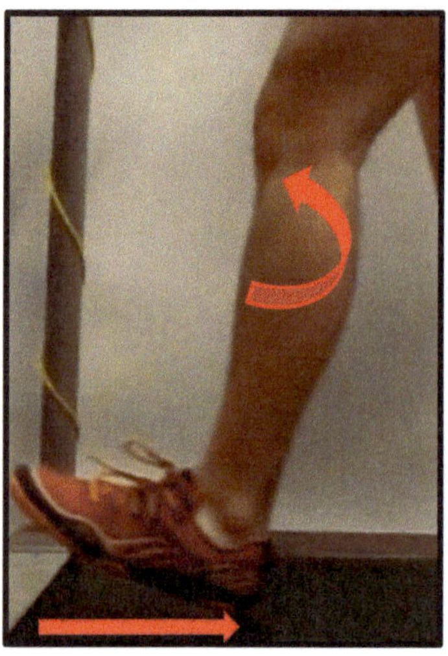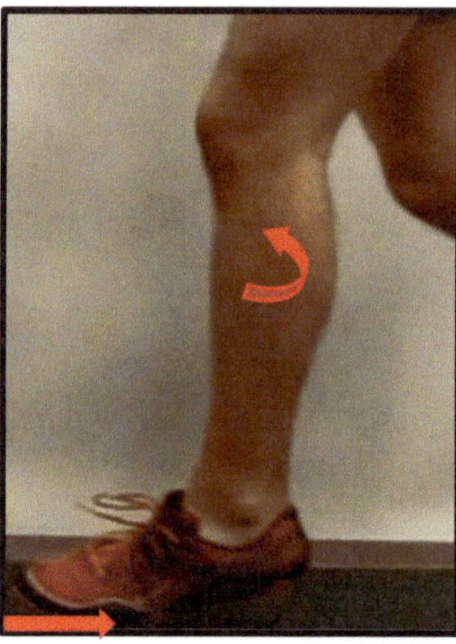

FIGURE 17.3 Rearfoot strike runner longer stride (left panel) has greater braking force than forefoot strike runner with shorter stride. This increased braking force can result in greater torques about the tibia.

Napier et al., higher peak braking forces were noted in runners who went on to sustain an injury.[22] Interestingly, 27% of these injuries were medial tibial stress syndrome, often considered a precursor to a tibial BSI.

Increased stride length may also increase the risk of a tibial BSI. In a probabilistic modelling study by Edwards et al., reducing stride length reduced the risk of developing a tibial stress fracture by 3% to 6%.[23] This was despite increasing the number of total steps that are associated with a shorter stride. In a prospective study, Luedke et al. related baseline cadence (which is inversely related to stride length) to the injuries sustained in 67 male and female high school cross-country runners.[24] They reported that longer strides were associated with a greater risk of developing anterior tibial pain than shorter stride lengths. It is unclear whether this pain was muscular or bony. However, the majority of these injuries resolved within 7 days, suggesting they were most likely related to the anterior tibialis strain.

Increased stride length has been associated with other stress fractures as well. An increase in pelvic stress fractures was noted in women following the implementation of mixed-sex marches in the military.[25,26] Hill et al. reported that, since reducing stride length from 30 inches to 27 inches during marching, there had been no other incidences of pelvic stress fractures.[25] Pope et al. implemented a multipronged study that included altering factors such as speed, surface, distances run, and stride length.[26] As a result, the incidence of pelvic fractures in female recruits was reduced from 11.2% to 0.6%. However, it is difficult to know which of the changes in Pope et al.'s study had the greatest effect. Reducing stride length may also influence metatarsal stress fracture risk. Using a musculoskeletal and finite element model, Firminger et al. reported a 4.2% reduction in the strain of the 4th metatarsal with a 10% reduction in stride length.[27]

While long strides can directly influence alignment, which can influence tissue loading, runners with long strides do not necessarily have higher impact loading than those with short strides. In a study of 169 runners, Futrell et al. reported that there was no relationship between habitual cadence and loadrate.[28] They noted that runners with habitually low cadences (longer strides) can have low load rates as well (and vice versa). Therefore, load rates cannot be accurately inferred from observing one's cadence.

GAIT RETRAINING FOR IMPACT LOADS AND FAULTY ALIGNMENT ASSOCIATED WITH TIBIAL BONE STRESS INJURIES

The decision to retrain a gait pattern should be predicated upon a thorough history and gait assessment of the runner. It is important to develop a clinical hypothesis upon which a retraining intervention can be based. Retraining should be targeted to an observed gait deviation. For example, if the cadence is already acceptable, increasing this further can result in an abnormal running gait pattern. Similarly, if a patient demonstrates normal hip adduction during running, there is no rationale for reducing it more. When a clinician is unable to identify a gait deviation that may be related to the BSI, then they should consider other potential causes. This may involve appropriate referrals for bone density tests, assessments of vitamin D levels, and endocrine function.

Principles of Motor Learning

Retraining involves the learning of a new motor pattern, and there are well-documented principles of motor learning that should be adhered to for optimal success.[29,30] The first involves the provision of feedback, which can be visual, auditory, or haptic in nature. Feedback provides for error detection that is critically needed for learning. Motor learning is facilitated first by an acquisition phase, where feedback is provided on a predetermined schedule. This helps to develop the kinesthetic awareness of what is right, based on the feedback, and what right feels like. During the second phase, the transfer phase, feedback is gradually removed so that the runner can learn to rely on what feels right. A faded feedback design gradually integrates these two phases.[29] Constant feedback will enhance performance but impede learning.[30] The faded feedback design optimizes learning, which is the goal of retraining.

Retraining for Faulty Alignment

In terms of alignment, both hip adduction and rearfoot eversion have been associated with tibial stress fractures.[21] There have been two studies in the literature aimed at reducing hip adduction, but they were not focused on tibial BSIs. These studies included patients with patellofemoral pain, as this has also been associated with increased hip adduction. However, this intervention could also be used for individuals with a tibial BSI and excessive hip adduction. In the first study, Noehren et al. provided hip adduction angular feedback on a screen using a real-time motion analysis system.[31] Runners were instructed to activate their gluteal muscles and maintain their hip adduction angle within a targeted range. Willy et al. repeated this study but simply used a mirror as feedback.[32] They asked the runners to activate their gluteal muscles in order to bring their knees apart as seen in the mirror. Both studies incorporated a faded feedback design that involved 8 sessions over 2 weeks. Runtime progressed from 15 to 30 minutes over the 8 sessions. Feedback was provided continuously for the first 4 sessions and then progressively removed for the last 4 sessions (Figure 17.4). Both studies demonstrated a significant reduction in hip adduction with persistence at 1 month. Willy et al demonstrated persistence at a 3 month follow-up as well.[32] Together, these studies demonstrate that retraining with a simple mirror can be as effective as using data from a motion analysis system. This is quite significant as most clinics have treadmills and mirrors, but few have motion analysis systems.

While increased rearfoot eversion has been related to tibial BSIs,[21] there have been no studies aimed at retraining rearfoot motion. Reducing adduction reduces the medialization of the leg and may indirectly reduce rearfoot eversion, but this has also not been tested. However, the recent advent of wearable sensors providing real-time

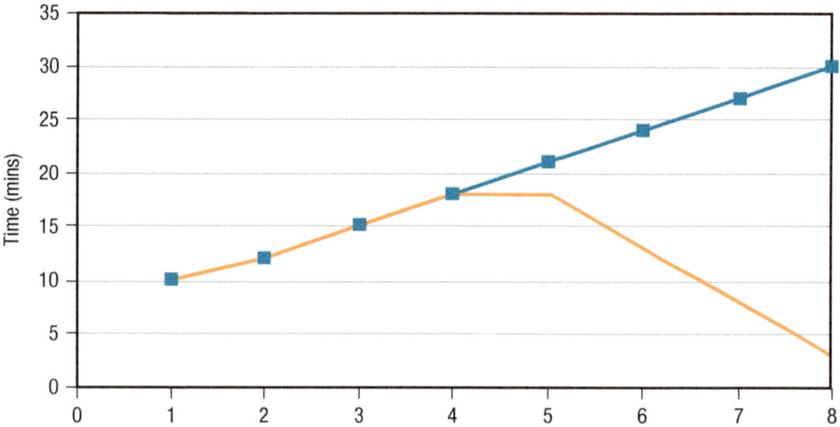

FIGURE 17.4 Faded feedback schedule during retraining. Runtime gradually increases from 10 to 30 minutes. Feedback is provided continually for the first 4 sessions and then gradually removed over the last 4 sessions.

feedback on rearfoot motion has great potential for directly reducing excessive rearfoot eversion in runners.

Retraining for Impact Loading

While impact loading has been related to tibial BSIs, there have been no retraining studies examining the effect of reducing impact loading on these injuries. The majority of retraining studies have utilized healthy individuals and can be classified into one of three groups. There are those that address running "softer," those that address increasing cadence, those that address transitioning to an FFS pattern, and finally others that compare between methods.

There are two studies that have retrained runners to land "softer." Bowser et al. recruited 20 recreational RFS runners exhibiting high tibial shock, a measure of impact loading associated with tibial BSIs.[7] These runners underwent 8 sessions of retraining, increasing from 15 to 30 minutes of running, using a faded feedback design similar to the studies of Noehren et al. and Willy et al.[31,32] They were provided with their tibial shock in real time and instructed to land "softer" and maintain the peak values under a threshold that was 50% of their baseline values (Figure 17.5). These runners served as their own controls and underwent a control period prior to their retraining, when they simply progressively increased their runtime from 15 to 30 minutes in 8 sessions over 2 weeks. Impact data, including both tibial shock and vertical load rates, were collected at baseline, post control period, post-retraining, and at 1-, 6-, and 12-month follow-ups. Tibial shock and vertical load rates were significantly reduced post-retraining and were maintained at each of the follow-ups.

In a related study, Chan et al. randomized 320 healthy RFS runners into a control and retraining group.[33] They also used a 2-week, 8-session, faded feedback design for the retraining group. Participants ran on an instrumented treadmill and were provided with their vertical ground reaction force curve in real time. They were instructed to land "softer" and to try to reduce or eliminate the impact peak of the vertical ground reaction force. Those in the control group followed the same treadmill running program; however, they did not receive feedback. Both groups were monitored for injuries for a period of 1 year. Significant reductions in vertical load rates were noted in the retraining group

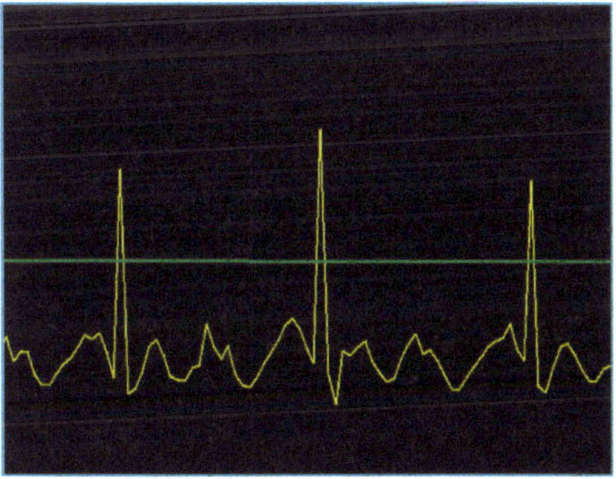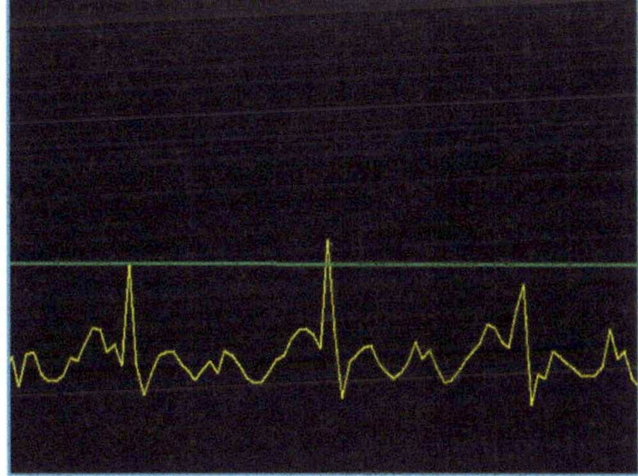

FIGURE 17.5 Reduction in tibial shock (right panel) with real-time feedback. Runners were asked to land softer, keeping their tibial shock values below the threshold line.

but not in the control group. More impressively, those in the retraining group had a 62% lower incidence of injuries. However, there were no BSIs in either group.

The influence of retraining cadence to reduce impact loading has also been studied. In a highly ecological study, Willy et al. recruited runners with high impact loading.[34] Following baseline testing, runners underwent 8 sessions of retraining to increase cadence by 7.5%. The retraining was conducted in the field with feedback being provided by a wearable sensor that transmitted the running cadence to a smartwatch. The feedback was provided on demand, as runners were free to look at their watches when they desired. They faded the feedback by only allowing feedback on certain runs across the 8 sessions. Following the retraining, these runners demonstrated a significant reduction in impact loading when measured in the lab. However, only 63% of the runners were able to maintain their increased cadence when monitored in the field at their 1-month follow-up. It is possible that a more structured faded feedback program may have yielded greater results. Along with reducing impact loading, increasing cadence leads to a reduction in hip adduction, which has been associated with tibial BSIs. A number of authors have demonstrated a 1.7° to 3.99° reduction in hip adduction with a 7.5% to 10% increase in cadence.[34–36]

Impact loading is markedly lower in FFS compared to RFS. Therefore, investigators have examined the effect of transitioning to an FFS pattern in order to reduce vertical load rates. Letafatkar et al. randomized 49 healthy male runners into an exercise group, an-exercise-with-retraining group, and a placebo exercise group.[37] The group did the retraining 3×/week for 8 weeks. Verbal feedback was provided by instructing the runner to land "softer" and on the ball of their foot. A mirror was used to provide feedback on the frontal plane alignment of the leg. Runtime was gradually increased over the 8 weeks. Feedback was faded over the last 2 weeks. Both the exercise and the exercise-plus-retraining group reduced their impact loading as well as their hip adduction; however, the exercise-plus-retraining group had a larger reduction. This group also had twice the reduction in injuries (64.5% vs. 32%) compared with the exercise alone group, evaluating injuries that occurred over a year (none of these were BSI). The placebo group reduced injuries by 15% but had no changes in any of the mechanics.

In a retraining study of healthy runners, Futrell et al. set out to compare the effect of increasing cadence and transitioning to an FFS pattern.[28] The authors reported that both the cadence and FFS groups increased their cadence, but load rates were reduced by 50%

in the FFS group compared with 12% in the cadence group. These results suggest that transitioning to an FFS pattern is more effective if reducing impact loading is the goal.

Most of the research on retraining, to date, has focused on impact loading and hip adduction, both of which have been associated with tibial stress fractures. However, as a practicing clinician, it is also important to consider other mechanics that may also need retraining for BSIs. As one example, increased toe-out is likely to increase the load to the medial foot and distal medial lower leg. With time, this may result in a BSI in either of these locations. This may provide a rationale for a retraining program focused on reducing the amount of toe-out the runner presents with. It is important to have a clinical hypothesis as to the etiology of the BSI. The retraining approach should be based on this hypothesis. Ultimately, the goal should be well-aligned, soft landings.

CLINICAL APPLICATION

Preparation for Retraining (1×/week for 4–6 weeks)

Very few studies in the literature address retraining preparation. This becomes more important when dealing with runners who are injured versus those who are healthy, as they may be more at risk for secondary injuries. Changing a motor pattern results in altering the demands on the musculoskeletal system. For example, transitioning to an FFS pattern requires greater activation of the foot and ankle musculature. Therefore, a progressive foot core program that includes both intrinsic and extrinsic muscle strengthening is advised. This program begins with learning how to abduct and adduct the toes (Figure 17.6). These dorsal and plantar interossei and especially abductor hallucis are important for overall foot stability.[38,39] Placing spreaders between the toes can initially

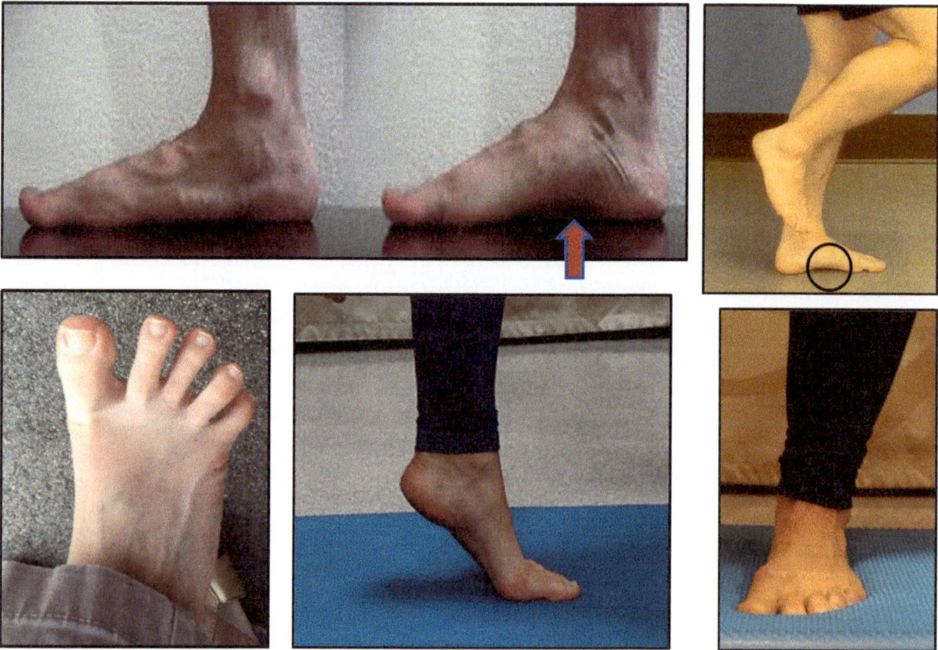

FIGURE 17.6 Examples of exercises to strengthen the foot core. Note that the foot remains in domed position during all of the weight-bearing activities.

assist these actions for those who have difficulty. Foot doming is considered a foundational exercise for strengthening the foot core. This is done by first stiffening the toes and then drawing the ball of the foot back toward the heel, thereby raising the arch (Figure 17.6). Foot doming is first done in standing on two feet and then one foot. This then progresses to doming and hopping on two feet and then one foot. These exercises are then advanced to more dynamic activities such as hopping in all four directions and hopping off of a step, all the time maintaining the foot dome and building endurance. Muscular fatigue has been associated with increased bone strain.[40] Therefore, strong arch muscles should be protective against the increased metatarsal strain that occurs when transitioning to an FFS pattern. Heel raises, with a focus on the eccentric phase, are also an important component of a foot strengthening program. They are begun as straight-kneed, double leg heel raises, progressing to single leg heel raises as well as single-leg isometric holds. These heel raises should also be done with the knee flexed to address the soleus muscle. Finally, jump roping and plyometric activities are added to develop muscular power. An example of an 8-week intrinsic foot-strengthening program is demonstrated in Exhibit 17.1.

When addressing faulty hip mechanics, such as increased hip adduction and internal rotation, a progressive hip strengthening program is also needed. For those who have difficulty activating their gluteal muscles, this may begin with the glute ladder exercise, whereby the patient lies prone and progressively modulates the gluteal activation. The patients begin by contracting their gluteal muscles 25% of their maximum, then 50%, 75%, and 100%, and then back down to 75%, 50%, and 25%. This is followed by

Exhibit 17.1 Example of an 8-Week Foot Intrinsic Muscle-Strengthening Program.

	Week 1	Week 2	Week 3	Week 4	Week 5	Week 6	Week 7	Week 8
Double leg heel raises - flat	3 sets of 10	3 sets of 20	3 sets of 30					
Double leg heel - off step			3 sets of 10	3 sets of 20	3 sets of 30			
Single leg heel raises - flat				3 sets of 10	3 sets of 20	3 sets of 30		
Single leg heel raises – off step					3 sets of 10	3 sets of 20	3 sets of 30	
Towel curls	3 sets of 10	3 sets of 20	3 sets of 30	3 sets of 30				
Toe Spread/Squeeze	3 sets of 10	3 sets of 20	3 sets of 30	3 sets of 30				
Doming	3 sets of 10	3 sets of 20	3 sets of 30	3 sets of 30				
Doming Hopping in place		3 sets of 10	3 sets of 20					
Doming Hopping Square			3 sets of 10 forward and back	3 sets of 20 forward and back	3 sets of 10 side to side	3 sets of 20 side to side	3 sets of 10 diagonal and back	3 sets of 20 diagonal and back
Doming Hopping off Step -2 ft					3 sets 10	3 sets of 20		
Doming Hopping off Step -1 ft							3 sets of 10	3 sets of 20

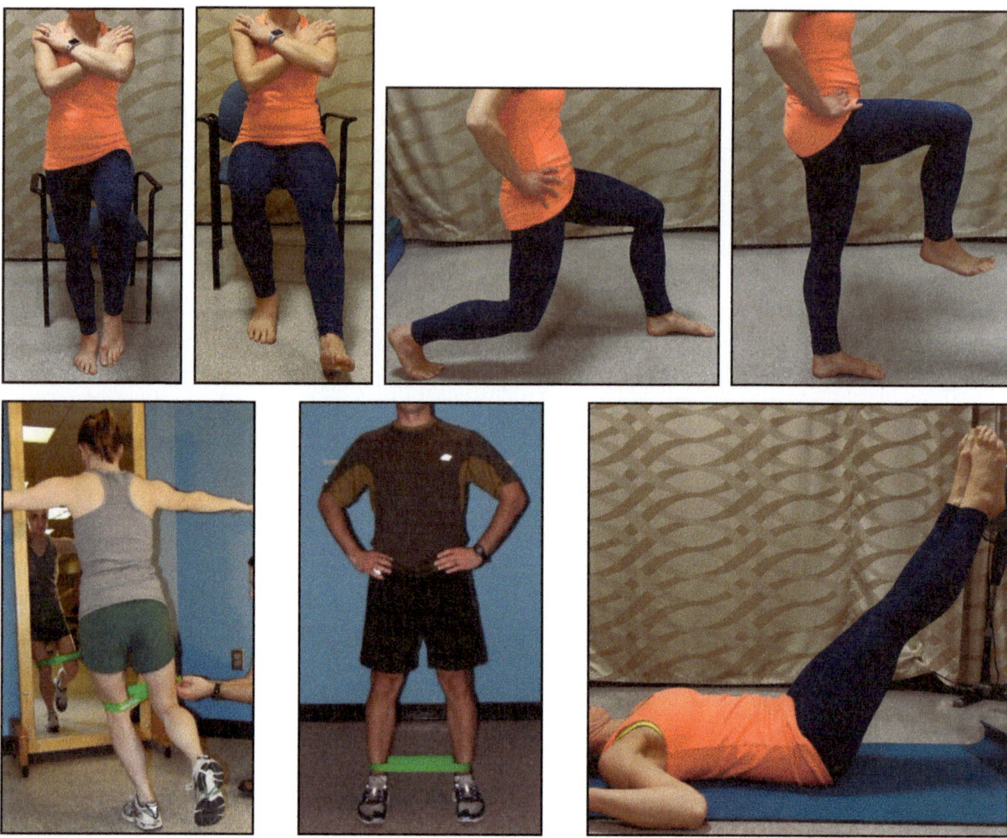

FIGURE 17.7 Examples of exercises to strengthen the hip core.

side-lying hip abduction exercises but quickly advances to weight-bearing exercises. These may begin with chair squat progressions (Figure 17.7), starting with double-leg squats and then single-leg squats. Additionally, standing lunges can be progressed to walking lunges. Abdominal strength should also be addressed with progressive planks, as well as leg lowering exercises while maintaining a neutral pelvis.

The foot and hip core training should be integrated into all of the functional training off of the treadmill. Attention should be paid to maintaining proper hip, knee, and foot/arch alignment during all single-leg landing activities. As running is a series of single-leg landings, this training off the treadmill will provide an excellent foundation for the retraining on the treadmill. Additionally, increasing the strength capacity of the lower extremity should reduce the risk of development of secondary injuries. It is recommended that the runner avoid additional outside impacting activities during this preparatory phase to avoid the risk of injury as they prepare for their retraining.

A Word About Footwear

Prior to the 1970s, all running footwear was minimal, lacking both arch support and a midsole.[41] However, over the past 50 years, running shoes have become increasingly more supportive and cushioned. These shoes are now considered the standard of running footwear.

Studies have shown that runners habituated to this standard running footwear land with an RFS pattern, while those habituated to barefoot running land with an FFS pattern.[42]

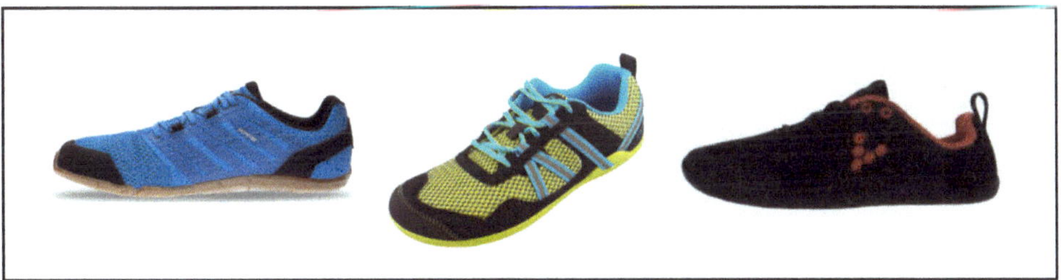

FIGURE 17.8 Examples of minimal running shoes. These shoes have no midsole, no arch support, no heel-to-toe drop, and have a flexible heel counter.

It has also been reported that running in minimal shoes, lacking a midsole (Figure 17.8), results in mechanics most closely to barefoot.[43] Landing impacts in all three directions (vertical, mediolateral, and anteroposterior) are lowest when running in minimal shoes compared to conventional shoes.[19] These studies together suggest that running in minimal shoes most closely replicates the natural mechanics of running barefoot.

Running in minimal shoes has other benefits. A number of studies have reported significant increases in the size of the intrinsic muscles of the arch in those who are habituated or have transitioned to minimal footwear.[44-46] This is due to the reduced support of a minimal shoe compared to a traditional shoe. Additionally, those habituated to minimal shoes have stronger, stiffer Achilles tendons.[47] Finally, it is easier to adopt an FFS pattern when running in shoes that lack elevated cushioned heels and medial and lateral sole flares.

For these reasons, minimal footwear is an important component of the retraining intervention. As a recent study by Ridge et al. reported that simply walking in minimal shoes significantly increases intrinsic foot muscle size, in our clinic runners begin walking in minimal shoes at the beginning of their pre-gait phase.[48] This, along with the foot core program they receive, helps to prepare the foot for the increased loads of running.

Retraining (3×/week for 4 weeks)

Prior to beginning the retraining on the treadmill, it is important that the runner be able to perform single-leg, well-aligned, soft landings. They must be able to generate a high rate of force development for propulsion. These qualities of movement should be demonstrated during functional activities off the treadmill prior to the beginning of the treadmill training. Therefore, criteria including the ability to perform repeated, well-aligned (foot and lower extremity) single-leg heel raise, squats, and single-leg hops should be required. Performance of repetitive, single-leg, explosive activities such as plyometrics should also be required.

If the retraining involves both transitioning to an FFS pattern and altering alignment such as hip adduction, this should be done in two phases. It is difficult for the runner to concentrate on two gait issues at the same time when first learning the new patterns. Therefore, it is suggested to begin with transitioning to the FFS pattern to provide the calves a head start on conditioning and endurance. Four sessions progressing from 10 to 20 minutes are usually adequate for the runner to learn to adopt the FFS pattern. While this pattern is typically associated with low impacts, the runner should still be cued to land as softly and quietly as possible. Feedback can be augmented with wearable technology, such as accelerometers strapped around the ankles. These devices can provide both visual and auditory cues regarding how hard the runner is landing (Figure 17.9). Patterns to avoid include excessive plantarflexion and inversion at footstrike. This may be a result of the runner overstriding. This phase is also the time to correct for excessive toe-in or toe-out that the runner may be exhibiting.

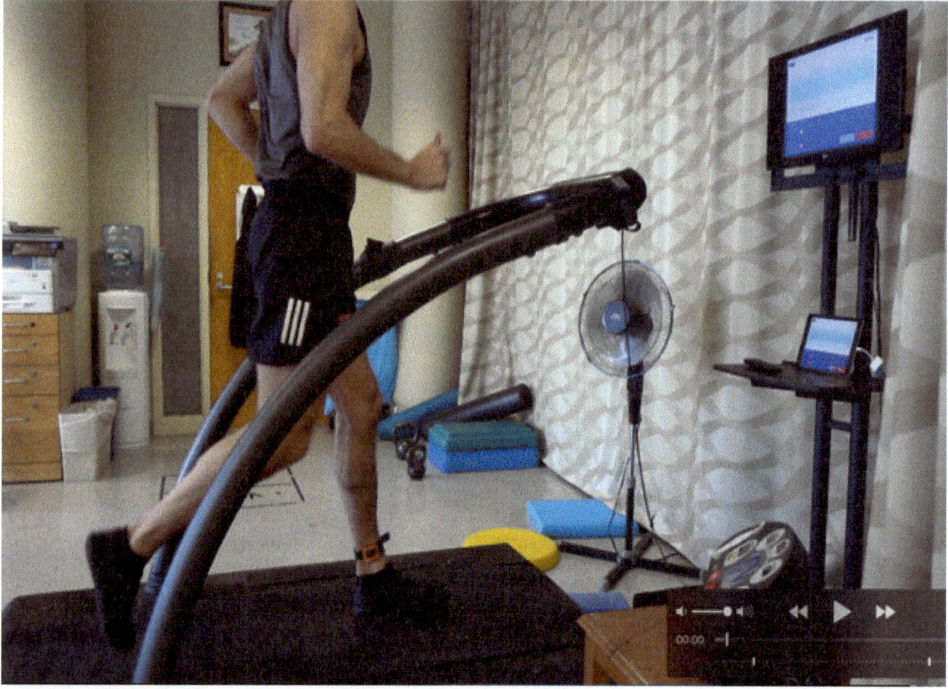

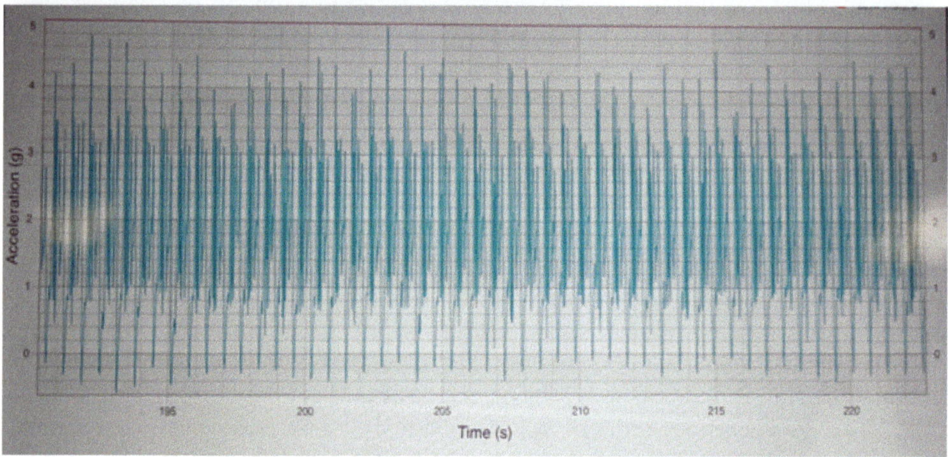

FIGURE 17.9 Runner retraining with an accelerometer attached to the left ankle while tibial shock feedback is provided to him on a monitor placed in front of him (top panel). The runner is asked to land softly on his forefoot keeping the peak tibial shock below 5 g's. The monitor is turned off during the fading of the feedback.

The next phase of the retraining is the realignment phase (while maintaining an FFS pattern). If the goal is to reduce hip adduction, the runner is instructed to activate their gluteal muscles such that their knees move apart and patellae point forward. This addresses both femoral adduction and internal rotation. During this phase, the treadmill runtime is increased from 10 to 30 minutes over 8 sessions. Feedback can be provided with a simple mirror providing a front view of the runner or with a video camera in the back of the runner projecting on a monitor in front of the runner. After the fourth session, feedback is removed from the beginning, middle, and end of each session. By the last session of this phase, the runner is only receiving 3 minutes of feedback during

Exhibit 17.2 10-Week Outdoor Running Schedule. Speed and intensity workouts can slowly be added once the runner has achieved their goal run time [original to author].

After your last gait retraining session, you will follow the running program listed below. If you experience any pain or soreness that lasts more than 48 hours, keep your running the same as the run before or take a day off. Only progress to the next running time if you are pain-free and calf soreness resolves by the time you start your next run.

**Expected PT appointments at end of these weeks

Warm up before, and cool down after each run

Week #	Day 1	Day 2	Day 3	Day 4	Day 5	Day 6	Day 7	Total Time
1	20 min. outdoors		20 min outdoors		20 min indoors		22 min outdoors	82 minutes
2**		25 min outdoors		25 min indoors		30 min outdoors		80 minutes
3	30 min outdoors		30 min outdoors		30 min indoors			90 minutes
4**		35 min outdoors		30 min outdoors		35 min outdoors		100 minutes
5	30 min outdoors		30 min indoors		20 min outdoors		35 min outdoors	115 minutes
6		40 min outdoors		30 min outdoors		40 min outdoors		110 minutes
7	30 min outdoors		30 min indoors		20 min outdoors		45 min outdoors	125 minutes
8		45 min outdoors		30 min outdoors		45 min outdoors		120 minutes
9	30 min outdoors		50 min outdoors				55 min outdoors	135 minutes
10		45 min outdoors		45 min outdoors		60 min outdoors		150 minutes

the 30-minute run. During the entire retraining phase, the runner should only be running during the clinic visits to assure that only the new pattern is being reinforced.

The final phase of the retraining is outdoor running. During this 10-week phase, the runner begins with 20 minutes of outdoor running at the speed at which they underwent their treadmill training on. Runtime is gradually increased, and frequency increases from 3 times per week to 4 times per week (Exhibit 17.2). The runner returns to the clinic at 2 weeks and 4 weeks into this phase. At each of these clinic visits, a video is taken to check the runner's mechanics, exercises are reviewed, and any other questions are addressed. During the last 6 weeks, the runner continues to gradually increase to their desired runtime. This 10-week period is needed to reinforce the runner's new mechanics and allow the musculoskeletal system time to adapt to the increasing mileage. Once the runner has reached their desired weekly mileage goal, then they can slowly increase their speed and intensity of workouts.

CONCLUSION

BSI are among the most serious that a runner can sustain as they can progress to an occult fracture and require periods of complete rest. The etiology of BSI is clearly multifactorial; however, mechanics have been shown to play a role. Gait retraining offers an approach to address the underlying mechanics to reduce the risk of recurrence, which is high in BSIs.[1] Gait retraining requires adequate time to build the capacity for new movement patterns as well as time to develop and reinforce this pattern. Therefore, the runner needs to commit to the process and have patience with the time that is needed. A gait retraining program needs to adhere to the motor control principles of appropriate practice and faded feedback in order for learning to occur. Guidance during the shift from treadmill to outdoor running is needed in order to make a safe transition into the runner's natural environment. Gait retraining requires a significant investment on the part of the clinician and the runner. However, this investment can pay great dividends if the runner is able to return to running with a reduced risk of sustaining another BSI.

KEY REFERENCES

Only key references appear in the print edition. The full reference list appears in the digital product found on http://connect.springerpub.com/content/book/978-0-8261-4424-9/part/sec04/chapter/ch17

1. Warden SJ, Davis IS, Fredericson M. Management and prevention of bone stress injuries in long-distance runners. *J Orthop Sports Phys Ther*. Oct 2014;44(10):749–765.

6. van der Worp H, Vrielink JW, Bredeweg SW. Do runners who suffer injuries have higher vertical ground reaction forces than those who remain injury-free? A systematic review and meta-analysis. *Br J Sports Med*. Apr 2016;50(8):450–457.

7. Bowser BJ, Fellin R, Milner CE, et al. Reducing impact loading in runners: a one-year follow-up. *Med Sci Sports Exerc*. Dec 2018;50(12):2500–2506.

20. Ewers BJ, Jayaraman VM, Banglmaier RF, et al. Rate of blunt impact loading affects changes in retropatellar cartilage and underlying bone in the rabbit patella. *J Biomech*. Jun 2002;35(6):747–755.

21. Pohl MB, Mullineaux DR, Milner CE, et al. Biomechanical predictors of retrospective tibial stress fractures in runners. *J Biomech*. 2008;41(6):1160–1165.

40. Milgrom C, Radeva-Petrova DR, Finestone A, et al. The effect of muscle fatigue on in vivo tibial strains. *J Biomech*. Jan 2007;40(4):845–850.

CHAPTER 18

Nutrition

Laura J. Moretti and Nicole M. Farnsworth

INTRODUCTION

Athletes place an incredible physical demand on their bodies through training and competition. Nutrition and adequate fueling are paramount in supporting optimal performance and recovery. Inadequacies in energy availability (EA), as well as specific macro and micronutrient deficiencies, can lead to myriad negative health and performance consequences. Specifically, low energy availability (LEA) and deficiencies in micronutrients can compromise bone turnover and increase susceptibility to bone stress injury (BSI).[1] In the adolescent athlete population, this can also impair normal bone growth and overall development, leading to long-term health complications. Determining an athlete's intake and outputs is a highly targeted area of study; however, there remains no validated protocol or method to accurately determine energy intake (EI) or exercise energy expenditure (EEE) without some margin of error.[2] This chapter aims to outline the importance of determining an athlete's EI and output in the setting of confounding variables and how to use this information to optimize bone health and overall athletic performance.

NUTRITION AND BONE HEALTH

One cannot discuss the correlation of nutrition and bone health without first addressing the idea of energy utilization in the body. Individuals are considered to have adequate EA when their caloric intake is adequate to support their caloric expenditures. This is generally the difference between EI and total energy expenditure (TEE) normalized to fat free mass (FFM).[3]

In terms of the athlete population, EA is considered paramount for assessing an athlete's energy status.[4,5] Loucks and Thuma determined that a level of 30 kcal/kg FFM/day is the threshold to maintain normal hormonal functioning in females; however, more recent studies have indicated that a level of 45 kcal/kg FFM/day is necessary to support performance and hormonal functioning in females.[6] Unfortunately, the EA threshold has been much less studied in the male population. A decrease in EI, increase in EEE, or a combination of the two can have a negative impact on an athlete's performance and overall health.[5] LEA is a relative state and is best diagnosed on an individual basis by evaluating all symptoms being presented; however, it is beyond the scope of this chapter to explore all such potential signs and symptoms of LEA. Both the female athlete triad (Triad) and relative energy deficiency in sports (RED-S) are based on the principle that a LEA state has negative impacts on a multitude of systems in the body. The triad explains the interrelationship between EA, menstrual function, and bone mineral density (BMD) in female athletes.[7] RED-S is a syndrome that encompasses the many negative health and performance effects of energy deficiency on both male and female athletes. The RED-S dual model system highlights the impact that LEA may have on bodily systems (e.g., gastrointestinal, immunological, endocrine, metabolic, hematological, cardiovascular, menstrual function, bone health, growth and development, and psychological) and on specific performance markers related to sport (e.g., decreased endurance performance, increased injury risk, decreased training response, impaired judgement, decreased coordination, decreased concentration, irritability, depression, decreased glycogen stores, and decreased muscle strength). RED-S can also have a psychological impact and cause a delay in growth and development in adolescent athletes.[8,9] It is beyond the scope of this chapter to discuss all components of LEA in detail; therefore, we will focus our discussion on its impact on bone health.

ASSESSING ENERGY AVAILABILITY IN ATHLETES

In order to assess EA, one must also have information on an individual's body composition, EI, and their EEE. However, there are challenges with assessing the input and output required to determine EA accurately. Assessing EA in athletes has proven to be a challenging undertaking mainly due to the fact that there is no standardized or validated protocol for this process. Dietary recalls are often inaccurate when obtained from self-reported sources, and the use of online software can also lead to reporting errors and discrepancies.[10] EEE can also be challenging to quantify given the high variability of training cycles and subsequent variations in energy output day to day and season to season.[9] Methods for assessing body composition and FFM are often inaccessible to the average person and are subject to variability in measurement due to technician skill. Predictive equations, including Harris–Benedict, Mifflin St. Jeor, Cunningham, or Schofield, can be utilized to help to estimate resting energy expenditure (REE).[11–14] However, it is important to note that many of these formulas are not validated in the adolescent population and are based on general guidelines for age, sex, height, and weight. Therefore, they may not accurately capture an athlete's needs, particularly if that individual has a suppressed metabolic rate, which can occur as a result of an energy deficit.[15] The measurement of EEE proves to be another barrier. Fitness trackers, MET calculations, GPS units, power meters, and heart rate monitors can provide some information but are limited in their ability to estimate energy cost of exercise in more complex activities.[16]

Given the list of limitations, it is important to take into consideration multiple methods of assessment as well as clinical judgment and observation. Although no one tool for assessment of intake or expenditure is perfect, a registered dietitian (RD) can help to identify an athlete's energy needs and identify any nutritional deficiencies by utilizing these available tools to create the best understanding for the individual athlete. Using clinical judgment and the resources available, an RD can estimate REE to determine whether or not assessed intake is adequate for performance. They can also educate the athlete on exercise metabolism and fueling strategies before, during, and after competition to optimize performance and meet elevated energy needs. An athlete's dietary intake may need to be adjusted throughout training cycles in order to prevent EA during different points in training.

POTENTIAL CAUSES OF LOW ENERGY AVAILABILITY IN THE ATHLETE POPULATION

The causes of LEA in an athlete are often multifaceted and can be inadvertent or intentional. This myriad of reasons for a LEA state contribute to the challenges of assessing it. LEA states may also be transient, or an athlete may not experience side effects concurrently with the caloric imbalance. Both male and female athletes often have a knowledge deficit about appropriate energy requirements to support their training loads or changes in training.[16,17] EI is made more complex by the known anorexigenic and appetite-suppressive effect of exercise across a range of intensities and durations.[18] For example, LEA states have been shown to either suppress or maintain levels of ghrelin (appetite-stimulating hormone) and leptin (appetite-suppressing hormone) after a bout of exercise, which can lead an athlete to under fuel for their training load.[19] Since body composition is a significant performative contributor to many sports, especially in weight class, endurance, and aesthetic sports, periods of weight loss and calorie restriction often contribute significantly to LEA.[20] Disordered eating (DE) and eating disorders (ED) are pertinent issues in athletes given they are at a significantly higher risk for these behaviors than the general population.[21] If the LEA state is a result of ED or DE, an interdisciplinary approach is recommended. An athlete's activity level, ability to participate in sport, and caloric intake will likely need to be addressed to improve EA. Food insecurity, lack of finances, and lack of nutrition knowledge are all major risk factors for the cause of LEA.[22] In collegiate athletes, lack of finances has been known to lead to poor nutrition choices; however, recent changes from the National Collegiate Athletic Association have resulted in increased access to healthy nutrition for collegiate athletes.[18]

These combined factors may lead an athlete who is already in LEA to consume fewer calories, thus further increasing the caloric deficit. The use of a skilled collaborative team including an RD and preferably one who is a certified specialist in sports dietetics (RD CSSD), a psychologist, a sports medicine physician, and an endocrinologist can help to properly assess the individual and understand how to intervene to obtain optimal clinical outcomes.

LOW ENERGY AVAILABILITY AND BONE HEALTH

In a LEA state, the human body adapts physiologically to promote survival. These changes, though helpful in preserving energy expenditure, can have harmful consequences, especially for the training athlete. LEA can lead to dysregulation of the hypothalamic–pituitary gonadal axis, thereby affecting reproductive, metabolic, and gastrointestinal functions. While low estrogen in particular is known to affect bone turnover via increased bone resorption, other hormonal and nutritional markers, such as suppressed insulin-like growth factor 1, increased cortisol, and decreased calcium and vitamin D status, also impair bone status.[1,23–25] These physiologic responses to LEA can affect bone turnover and result in a lack of or decrease in BMD accrual, which puts an athlete at risk for BSI.[2,26]

Perturbation of the hypothalamic–pituitary–ovarian (HPO) axis in female athletes often results in reproductive suppression and functional hypothalamic amenorrhea (FHA); therefore, the studies examining the long-term effects of LEA and bone health often include oligoamenorrheic or amenorrheic females.[5] A study of 175 female athletes found that oligoamenorrheic athletes reported more stress fractures and were found to have lower BMD and reduced bone strength when compared to eumenorrheic athletes and nonathlete controls.[27] Decreased BMD has been found in male athletes as well in association with LEA or markers of LEA such as body mass index (BMI) ≤17.5 kg/m², although further research is needed to examine the interrelatedness between LEA and bone health for males.[28–30]

NUTRIENTS NECESSARY FOR BONE HEALTH: CALCIUM AND VITAMIN D

While adequate EA supports optimal BMD development, calcium and vitamin D are key micronutrient players in bone health. The role of vitamin D in bone health includes optimizing calcium absorption and supporting the resorption of bone via osteoclasts.[31] Vitamin D is a fat-soluble vitamin and is synthesized by the body via sunlight exposure on the skin and hydroxylation in the liver and the kidney. Given the variability in sunlight exposure due to seasonal variability and lifestyle, among other factors, sun exposure has a variable effect on serum vitamin D levels.[32] Vitamin D is found in various dietary sources such as mushrooms and cold-water fish, and in the United States, it is fortified in a number of food products including milk and orange juice. Vitamin D is typically categorized into two forms: ergocalciferol (D_2), which comes from plant-based sources and fortified foods, and cholecalciferol (D_3), which comes from animal-based sources and is also the form synthesized in the body. Vitamin D_2 and vitamin D_3 are also available in supplemental form at varying dosages, and research has found vitamin D_3 to be more effective at improving serum vitamin D concentrations.[33]

With sunlight as a considerable source of vitamin D production, those living above the latitude of 37° north in the winter months as well as indoor athletes at any latitude (e.g., dance, basketball, ice hockey) are at a higher risk for development of vitamin D insufficiency (21–29 ng/mL) or deficiency (<20 ng/mL).[34–36] As such, greater care must be taken to monitor vitamin D levels and consume vitamin D–rich dietary sources for these athletes. Research suggests that vitamin D consumption and serum vitamin D levels at or above 30 ng/mL support bone health and are associated with a decreased risk of BSI.[37]

The recommended dietary allowance (RDA) for vitamin D for children and adults up to age 70 is 600 international units (IUs) of vitamin D per day (Table 18.1). In cases of vitamin D insufficiency or deficiency, supplementation protocol is dependent upon serum vitamin D levels. In cases of vitamin D insufficiency (25–30 ng/mL), supplementation of 2,000 IUs per day is indicated for restoration. In cases of lower serum vitamin D (<25 ng/mL), supplementation of 50,000 IUs vitamin D_2 once per week for 8 weeks followed up by a maintenance dose of 1,000 IUs of vitamin D_3 daily will promote improved vitamin D levels.[38]

Calcium, the most abundant mineral in the body, is necessary for bone development. Adequate calcium intake is associated with BMD development and decreased risk for

TABLE 18.1

RECOMMENDED DIETARY ALLOWANCES FOR VITAMIN D

AGE	MALE (IU)	FEMALE (IU)	PREGNANT OR LACTATING (IU)
0–12 months	400	400	
1–70 years	600	600	600
>70 years	800	800	

IU, international unit.

Source: Adapted from the National Institutes of Health. https://ods.od.nih.gov/factsheets/VitaminD-HealthProfessional

TABLE 18.2

RECOMMENDED DIETARY ALLOWANCES FOR CALCIUM

AGE	MALE (MG)	FEMALE (MG)	PREGNANT OR LACTATING (MG)
0–6 months	200	200	
7–12 months	260	260	
1–3 years	700	700	
4–8 years	1,000	1,000	
9–13 years	1,300	1,300	
14–18 years	1,300	1,300	1,300
19–50 years	1,000	1,000	1,000
51–70 years	1,000	1,200–1,500	
71+ years	1,200	1,200–1,500	

Source: From the National Institutes of Health. https://ods.od.nih.gov/factsheets/Calcium-HealthProfessional/#h2

osteoporosis.[39] Numerous studies have shown that milk and dairy consumption support BMD status.[40–45] Calcium is absorbed in the small intestine either actively or passively; its bioavailability depends on a few factors including the amount of calcium entering the small intestine, the acidity of the lumen, and the presence of other dietary components. Active calcium absorption is dependent on the status of vitamin D in the body; therefore, optimal vitamin D increases calcium absorption.[31] The RDA for calcium varies throughout the lifespan, with those in their growth and development years and postmenopausal women needing more than other groups (Table 18.2).

Dietary calcium is most notably found in dairy, such as milk, cheese, and yogurt. However, it can also be found in nondairy foods, such as broccoli, tofu, certain mushrooms, and almonds. While dietary calcium had a more positive effect on BMD than supplemental calcium, supplemental calcium can be used to improve body calcium status for those who cannot consume sufficient dietary calcium. The two predominant supplemental forms of calcium are citrate and carbonate, with citrate having a higher bioavailability and the ability to be taken with or without food. Calcium carbonate, on the other hand, is more readily absorbed in an acidic environment and should be taken with food; however, calcium's inhibitory properties as it relates to iron absorption suggest that calcium ingested at meal times could affect body iron status.[39,46] When consuming supplemental calcium, dosage should not exceed 500 mg at a time to maximize absorption; therefore, calcium may need to be taken 2 to 3 times per day to meet requirements of the athlete.[47]

Numerous studies have found that the ingestion of caffeine increases calcium excretion, however, research has found that individuals consuming moderate amounts of caffeine and adequate calcium do not have compromised bone health outcomes.[48–50] Individuals with malabsorption, such as those with celiac disease, also have a lower rate of absorption and lower BMD in comparison to controls without celiac disease, though increased calcium intake may offset the decreased absorption rate.[51] Dairy product consumption may be contraindicated in individuals with lactose intolerance or a dairy allergy; therefore, calcium and vitamin D supplementation may be warranted.

INJURY RECOVERY/BONE HEALING

For the injured athlete diagnosed with a BSI, nutrition can play a pivotal role in recovery and return to play. First and foremost, a full nutrition evaluation should be conducted by an appropriately qualified nutrition professional, ideally an RD with additional sports qualifications who has experience and expertise in working with this population.[4] A dietitian can assess EI and other relevant parts of an athlete's nutrition history to determine if LEA could have played a role in the injury, and if so ascertain what the cause of LEA is as this will dictate treatment. In cases of LEA, restoration of energy balance is critical for optimizing recovery time, impeding muscle loss, and preventing possible future BSI.[52]

With injury leading to decreased training and activity, the initial thought for many athletes is to decrease EI to prevent increases in body fat and body mass. However, research has demonstrated that the healing process may elevate energy needs depending on the severity of the injury and the additional effort required to move if and while immobilized. Therefore, EI may not need to be decreased significantly or at all. Estimating energy needs for the injured and nonexercising athlete should be done using one of the methods described earlier, with careful consideration given to the athlete's ability to ambulate and the stage of recovery that they are in. During times of injury, adequate caloric intake is essential to support adaptations in EA as a result of injury. Increased EI with the goal of weight gain may be indicated for those athletes determined to be too low in weight.[1] Consuming adequate calcium and vitamin D and correcting vitamin D deficiency if present can support general bone health and optimal bone building.

CONCLUSION

Nutrition and bone health are inextricably linked, with inadequate energy or nutrient intake increasing the risk of poor bone development and BSI, with appropriate nutrition playing an important role in healing from BSI. Given the limitations and challenges of EA assessment, a medical professional such as an RD CSSD can be pivotal in helping determine how to best utilize nutrition to foster optimal bone health by considering an athlete's EA and micronutrient status. Utilizing clinical judgment, coupled with one or more of the EA assessment methods when evaluating an athlete for BSI risk or to determine causation, can be helpful in determining the appropriate treatment approach to support optimal EA.

KEY REFERENCES

Only key references appear in the print edition. The full reference list appears in the digital product found on http://connect.springerpub.com/content/book/978-0-8261-4424-9/part/sec04/chapter/ch18

4. Thomas DT, Erdman KA, Burke LM. Position of the Academy of Nutrition and Dietetics, Dietitians of Canada, and the American College of Sports Medicine: nutrition and athletic performance. *J Acad Nutr Diet.* 2016 Mar;116(3):501–528.

5. Loucks AB, Verdun M, Heath EM. Low energy availability, not stress of exercise, alters LH pulsatility in exercising women. *Am Physiol Soc.* 1998;84(1):37–46.

8. Mountjoy M, Sundgot-Borgen J, Burke L, et al. The IOC consensus statement: beyond the Female Athlete Triad—relative energy deficiency in sport (RED-S). *Br J Sports Med.* 2014 Apr;48(7):491–497.

23. Elliott-Sale KJ, Tenforde AS, Parziale AL, et al. Endocrine effects of relative energy deficiency in sport. *Int J Sport Nutr Exerc Metab.* 2018 Jul 1;28(4):335–349.

27. Ackerman KE, Sokoloff NC, De Nardo Maffazioli G, et al. Fractures in relation to menstrual status and bone parameters in young athletes. *Med Sci Sports Exerc.* 2015 Aug;47(8): 1577–1586.

30. Papageorgiou M, Dolan E, Elliott-Sale KJ, et al. Reduced energy availability: implications for bone health in physically active populations. *Eur J Nutr.* 2018;57(3):847–859.

CHAPTER 19

Emerging Treatments

Brian W. Fullem and Amol Saxena

INTRODUCTION

Bone physiology may dictate the rate of bone stress injury (BSI) healing. A minimum of 3 to 4 weeks is typically required for athletes with low-grade injuries to return to sport, while some bones such as the navicular will take up to 3 to 4 months before a return to activity is possible.[1,2] This chapter explores the nonpharmacologic treatments that may aid, accelerate, or enhance bone healing for BSI. Extracorporeal shockwave therapy (ESWT), pulsed ultrasound, and pulse electromagnetic fields are several of the possible treatment options available that are explored in this chapter.

USE OF EXTRACORPOREAL SHOCKWAVE THERAPY FOR BONE INJURIES

ESWT has been utilized since 1980[3-5] with the original application of use being the destruction of kidney stones. The treatment was termed "lithotripsy" and within the decade following the treatment was broadened to initially include treatment of plantar fasciitis and since has been applied to treat tendinopathies and other soft tissue injuries as well as to help induce bone healing in delayed unions and nonunions.

In 1990, Haupt et al.[6] reported an observed interaction of ESWT with bone tissue demonstrated by x-ray findings of osseous thickening of the iliac bone 1 year following treatment of bladder or uretral stones. Subsequently, Valchanou and Michailov[7] used ESWT for the treatment of delayed unions and nonunions, and success was achieved without complications of bony union in 70 of 82 fractures. Additional studies have confirmed success in ESWT. Schmitz et al.[8] published an excellent review of ESWT randomized controlled trials (RCTs) from the physiotherapy evidence database (PEDro) in 2015. In addition to an excellent description of how ESWT works both clinically and in the actual delivery of the shockwaves, the study made several important points about the use of ESWT. ESWT is safe and effective. Local anesthesia will negatively affect the outcome. They noted from the current research at that time period that there was no scientific evidence in favor of radial extracorporeal shockwave therapy (rESWT) or focused

ESWT with respect to outcomes (regarding soft-tissue pathology). Their recommendation was that the terms "low energy" and "high energy" be replaced with "radial" and "focused." Their review of research also showed that higher total energy delivered also produces a better outcome, which can be achieved with a higher energy flux density and/or more shocks delivered.

ESWT for BSI has primarily utilized focused-type devices that produce a shockwave with an electrohydraulic or electromagnetic effect. Radial devices were developed later and have shown that they also enhance bone healing. Schaden et al.[9] reviewed the literature and cited Ingber[10] about a ESWT mechanotransduction theory: As a result of pressure, tensile and shearing forces delivered by shockwaves to the cells and to the extracellular matrix (ECM) messengers are liberated and activate different genes and groups of genes in the cell nucleus. This impact disposes the cells to produce spatial and temporal coordinated growth factors to stimulate healing processes.[10] Additional proposed mechanisms include upregulation of osteogenic and angiogenic growth factors with neovascularization and an upregulation of angiogenic and osteogenic growth factors.[11]

It has been shown that focused ESWT leads to the development of new blood vessels in the area of treatment and the stimulation of osteoblast differentiation from stem cells and inactive cells.[12,13] The periosteal cells are triggered, which contributes to cell migration and the development of callus in healing impaired bone. Focused ESWT applications in delayed bone fracture healing and in avascular necrosis has grown both experimentally and in clinical use in the past decade. Several studies have been performed starting in the late 1990s on the success of ESWT for delayed unions or nonunions.[14–16] Cacchio et al.[17] performed a prospective randomized controlled multicenter trial (evidence level I) comparing ESWT to "standard of care" surgery in the treatment of long bone nonunions. In all, 126 patients were randomized, and at 3 and 6 months post surgery or ESWT treatment, the ESWT group showed better healing. However at 12 and 24 months, the two groups showed equal healing.

Taki et al.[18] in a 2007 paper reviewed the use of ESWT for five cases of resistant stress fractures. The fractures were in the mid shaft of the anterior tibia cortex, 5th metatarsal, medial malleolus, and inferior pubic ramus. Two of the patients had prior surgery, and the others were treated conservatively on an average for 7.6 months prior to the use of ESWT. One focused ESWT treatment was performed under spinal anesthesia with 2,000 to 4,000 shocks at 22 to 28 kV (0.29 to 0.4 mJ/mm^2). Two of the fractures deemed unstable were immobilized for 4 weeks after treatment. Boney union, confirmed with CT or radiographs, was achieved on an average at 2.9 months in all five cases with return to sport on an average of 4 months.

Other authors reveal that stress fractures had enhanced healing with ESWT. Moretti et al.[19] followed 10 soccer players who had lower energy-focused ESWT performed for delayed unions of 5th metatarsal or anterior tibial cortex stress fractures. A focused ESWT device was used at a low energy level of 0.09 to 0.27 mJ/mm^2 for 4,000 shocks. The energy level was adjusted based on patient tolerance, and no anesthesia was required. The patients were treated with three (metatarsals) or four (Tibia) treatments spaced 48 to 72 hours apart, and most patients returned to activity within 3 months, with boney union achieved radiographically 6 to 14 weeks after ESWT treatment.

Wölfl et al.[20] concluded that ESWT may achieve bone turnover for patients with low bone mineral density (BMD) similar to those with normal BMD. Albisetti et al.[21] showed some benefit using ESWT for healing certain stress fractures such as proximal 2nd metatarsal stress fractures in dancers. Furia[22] in 2010 showed better results for the treatment of nonunions of 5th metatarsal fractures in a level 1 study with ESWT versus surgery.

Acute fractures can also receive benefit of faster healing, as noted in some recent studies. Griffin et al.[23] compared the evidence of using ESWT for acute fractures and found some benefit in their review. Gollwitzer et al.[24] showed that rESWT can produce bone formation in animals. They used rESWT at 0.16 mJ/mm^2 for 4,000 pulses and showed healing at 6 weeks, suggesting that at-risk fractures can be aided. As many ESWT devices in practice settings are radial units, practitioners may potentially use these devices to enhance bone healing.

Willems et al.[25] in a 2019 review article of the RCTs concluded, "ESWT seems to be effective for the treatment of delayed unions and non-unions. However, the quality of most studies is poor. Therefore, we strongly encourage conducting well-designed RCTs to prove the effectiveness of ESWT and potentially improve the treatment of non-unions because ESWT might be as effective as surgery but safer." The safety cannot be emphasized enough as there is virtually no downside or contraindication for the use of ESWT for lower extremity bone injuries.

USE OF PULSED ULTRASOUND FOR BONE INJURIES

Low-intensity pulsed ultrasound (LIPUS) has also been studied for bone healing with proof that it works for acute fractures.[26] Mechanisms for LIPUS include mechanical stimulation resulting in calcium turnover, promoting osteogenesis and healing through vascular endothelial growth factors, prostaglandin E, and alkaline phosphatase, and differentiation of chondrocyte to bone.

Most prior studies involved LIPUS for acute fractures. Gan et al.[27] published a 2014 double-blind study on the use of LIPUS for BSIs. The stress fractures were all identified via MRI using the Fredericson MRI grading scale for BSIs.[28] Ten patients in the treatment group and 13 patients in the placebo group (using a sham unit) treated the injured area daily with 20 minutes of LIPUS for 4 weeks for a total of 28 treatments. The authors concluded, "Low-intensity pulsed ultrasound was found not to be an effective treatment for the healing of lower limb BSIs in this study. However, this was measured over a relatively short duration of 4 weeks in a small, mostly female population."

Griffin et al.[26] published a review in 2014 of the RCTs of LIPUS for bone stress, concluding that "while a potential benefit of ultrasound for the treatment of acute fractures in adults cannot be ruled out, the currently available evidence from a set of clinically heterogeneous trials is insufficient to support the routine use of this intervention in clinical practice. Future trials should record functional outcomes and follow-up all trial participants." Ultrasound may influence angiogenesis and cell differentiation and accelerate bone ossification. Grivas et al.[29] presented a computational mechanobioregulation model that attempted to predict the ossification process in bone fracture healing after the use of LIPUS. The authors concluded that their model predicts a 22% reduction in bone fracture healing time.

While the use of LIPUS appears safe, the efficacy for use in BSIs is not supported by the evidence-based medical literature at the current time.

PULSED ELECTROMAGNETIC FIELDS/ ELECTRICAL STIMULATION

Pulsed electromagnetic fields (PEMF) are one of the first nonpharmacologic treatments for bone injuries and continue to be used via the use of an external bone stimulator. In a review article in 2019, Bhavsar et al.[30] reviewed 72 animal studies, which revealed positive outcomes in 77% of the subjects using direct current as the form of electrical-stimulation (E-Stim) on the tibial bone of dogs. In the 69 clinical studies that were reviewed, they reported a 73% success rate mainly examining nonunion or delayed union of the tibia using PEMF. Saxena et al.[31] found that implanted PEMF devices have an 86% success rate when used for foot and ankle fusions in high-risk patients, but it is invasive, requiring surgical implantation, which can sometimes necessitate a second surgery to remove the devices. At the current time, there are no studies on implanted devices in healthy athletic patients.

In a level 1 study, Beck et al.[32] treated all the participants with supplemental calcium and relative rest from training with the treatment group using a capacitively coupled electric field stimulation for 15 hours/day and the control group receiving a placebo treatment. Healing was measured via a hop test for 30 seconds without pain. The authors concluded that there was no difference in healing time.

Benazzo et al.[33] published a study in 1995 on the use of capacitive coupling on stress fractures in athletes. It was a level 4 study, and the authors stated that it would be too difficult to get athletes to agree to possibly receive placebo in order to achieve a higher level study. They found that difficult-to-heal stress fractures in the foot, such as the navicular and 5th metatarsal, were healed within 60 days after daily treatment of up to 15 hours.

In a 2000 retrospective study, Saxena[34] compared 46 various lower extremity BSIs not treated with PEMF with 25 similar BSIs that received PEMF. For metatarsal stress fractures (not including 5th metatarsals), the return to activity was 3 weeks for 8 athletes treated with PEMF versus 8.4 weeks for 11 athletes not treated with PEMF. The results in this case–control study were statistically significant, but further studies have not been performed. Insurance companies typically will not cover the cost of bone stimulation units until there is at least 3 months of lack of healing documented radiographically, by which time many BSIs are resolved. However, there are no reported complications in the use of this technology, so it is considered in the use of delayed union/nonunion.

OTHER MODALITIES: PHOTOBIOMODULATION—LOW-LEVEL LASER THERAPY

Low-level laser therapy (LLLT) is a form of photobiomodulation (PBM) that uses a light source to aid in healing and regeneration of tissue. The theory of the mechanism of action is that PBM works via the cell absorbing the light, producing an increase in adenosine triphosphate (ATP), modulation of calcium, and increase in nitric oxide, among other factors.[35] In a 2019 paper, Neto et al.[36] published the first review of the RCTs in the literature about PBM for bone injury treatment and found a low quality of evidence that the treatment provides some relief from pain and some improvement of function. The authors concluded that future studies need to be performed at a higher level of evidence.

PBM has been studied more extensively to help heal patients after rapid maxillary expansion (RME), which is an oral surgery to expand the palate. Skondra et al.[37] reviewed the RME literature in humans and reported an enhancement of bone regeneration and healing following midpalatal suture expansion. The authors cautioned that the existing literature provides a low level of evidence and further high-level studies are needed to prove that this treatment method is clinically applicable.

Animal studies have been much more promising in showing that LLLT can enhance bone healing. Aras et al.[38] studied RME in rats and found that the treatment stimulated bone regeneration but with a recurrence rate of up to 25% and no evidence as to whether LLLT can prevent relapse after RME surgery.

While there appears to be no negative side effects associated with this noninvasive treatment, the medical evidence does not support the treatment at the current time.

ELECTROMAGNETIC TRANSDUCTION

New types of shockwaves are emerging. Electromagnetic transduction (EMTT) is an electromagnetic field of 80 mT. Like ESWT, angiogenesis and bone production are enhanced. EMTT produces an electromagnetic field at a higher energy level than that of bone stimulators that use PEMF, which is typically <8 mT to enhance bone healing.[39] Wuschech et al.[40] performed a placebo-controlled study for osteoarthritis and found promising results. Current studies are limited to spine and tendinopathic conditions.[41,42] Combined with ESWT therapies, this new modality could enhance bone healing.

CONCLUSION

Nonpharmacological forms of bone stimulation are reviewed. Both forms of ESWT, radial and focused, have been shown to aid in bone healing, with high levels of evidence. PEMF has also been shown to assist for delayed unions, particularly when used directly. Other forms of bone stimulation such as LIPUS, LLLT, E-Stim, and EMTT have varying degrees of benefit or need further study.

KEY REFERENCES

Only key references appear in the print edition. The full reference list appears in the digital product found on http://connect.springerpub.com/content/book/978-0-8261-4424-9/part/sec04/chapter/ch19

8. Schmitz C, Császár NBM, Milz S, et al. Efficacy and safety of extracorporeal shock wave therapy for orthopedic conditions: a systematic review on studies listed in the PEDro database. *Br Med Bull.* 2015;116:115–138.

9. Schaden W, Mittermayr R, Haffner N, et al. Extracorporeal shockwave therapy (ESWT) – First choice treatment of fracture on-unions? *Int J Surg.* 2015;24(Part B):179–183.

12. Leal C, D'Agostino C, Gomez Garcia S, Fernandez A. Current concepts of shockwave therapy in stress fractures. *Int J Surg.* 2015;24:195–200.

15. Rompe JD, High-energy extracorporeal shock wave treatment of nonunions. *Clin Orthop Relat Res.* 2011;387:102–111.

24. Gollwitzer H, Gloeck T, Roessner M, et al. Radial extracorporeal shock wave therapy (rESWT) induces new bone formation in vivo: results of an animal study in rabbits. *Ultrasound Med Biol.* 2013;39(1):126–133.

CHAPTER 20

Orthobiologics and Injections in Bone Stress Injuries

Alexander Lloyd, Matthew C. Sherrier, and Kentaro Onishi

INTRODUCTION

Orthobiologics are compounds derived from human tissues that may provide benefits for treatment of orthopedic and musculoskeletal conditions.[1] They have generated interest for their possible healing properties leveraging innate repair mechanisms while avoiding side effects common to nonbiologic agents.[1-3] The most common orthobiologics are described in this chapter. Currently, all are considered experimental, and the U.S. Food and Drug Administration has yet to approve any of these agents for a bone stress injury (BSI) or fracture.

Platelet-Rich Plasma

Platelet-rich plasma (PRP) is derived from whole blood using centrifugation. It is broadly defined as autologous blood containing a higher concentration of platelets.[1,4] Once centrifuged, a portion of the blood is removed and used as a therapeutic injectate in the location of interest.[1,4,5] There are multiple proposed mechanisms for the efficacy of PRP, although the definitive pathways are largely unknown. One proposed mechanism is that alpha granules within platelets release multiple growth factors involved in healing to increase angiogenesis and facilitate allocation of blood supply to the area of injury.[1,6] PRP may also help with differentiation of local stem cells into lineages needed for repair of local tissues.[4,7] It has also been proposed that PRP modulates the local inflammatory response to attract cells involved in healing of the injured area.[8]

Bone Marrow Aspirate

Bone marrow aspirate (BMA)[9] is a derivative of bone marrow first used in orthopedic applications.[10-14] Bone marrow is harvested and either applied directly to fractures or concentrated through centrifugation to allow for isolation of progenitor cells and growth factors useful for bone regeneration. Iliac crest is the primary harvest site with at least one study showing posterior iliac crest to have a higher yield of progenitor cells than anterior iliac crest.[15-17] There are multiple proposed mechanisms behind the healing properties of BMA, including the activity of osteoprogenitor cells and paracrine activity, although the definitive mechanism has not been elucidated.[18-20]

Mesenchymal Stem Cells

Mesenchymal stem cells (MSCs) are a heterogeneous class of stromal cells found in many adult tissues that likely play a central role in the effect of BMA described earlier.[18] They can differentiate into multiple lineages (bone, muscle, cartilage, and fat) and modulate the immune system through paracrine effects.[1,21] Harvesting can occur at several sites including bone marrow, synovium, periosteum, adipose, blood, and umbilical cord tissues.[21–23] The mechanism of action for MSCs is unknown. Research has shown that these cells do not differentiate to directly replace damaged tissues in vivo, but rather may act through immunomodulation, suppression of inflammation, and paracrine modulation.[1,21,22,24–26] Methods for MSC derivation and delivery are variable. Commercial systems and labs often use unique methods of extraction from donor tissue, many of which are proprietary.[21,27,28]

BONE STRESS INJURY

BSI is the result of accumulated microdamage which is a form of injury common in athletes and affect children, adolescents, and adults at all levels of training.[29] Although there is a dearth of literature on the use of orthobiologics for BSI, their utilization for the treatment of bone marrow edema (BME) in the setting of knee osteoarthritis (OA) offers insight into ways these compounds may be helpful given the suspected similarity in pathogenesis as it relates to subchondral bone.[30]

Bone Marrow Edema in Knee Osteoarthritis

BME is a nonspecific term for an MRI pattern that can be observed in a variety of clinical entities.[31] BME manifests on MRI as high signal intensity on T2-weighted sequences and fat suppression with or without low T1 signal.[32] Histologic analysis of BME demonstrates reduced bone marrow volume replaced by dense fibrous connective tissue, fibrocartilage, hyaline cartilage, and presence of neovessels.[33,34] In the right clinical setting, BME can be associated with knee OA.[31] Similar to stress fractures, BME in knee OA results from repetitive trauma, altered biomechanics, and the subsequent development of microcracks, microedema, and microbleeding in the subchondral bone.[32,35] Enlargement of BME in the setting of OA has been shown to be predictive of increased cartilage loss, increased pain, and the need for arthroplasty.[36–38]

Intraosseous Use of Orthobiologics for the Treatment of Knee Osteoarthritis

The subchondral bone is a previously underappreciated component of the osteochondral unit, and an understanding of its characteristics is paramount to the development of targeted strategies for the treatment of knee OA.[30,35] Direct targeting of BME represents an area of ongoing research with respect to the use of orthobiologics for the treatment of knee OA. As there have been no published studies to date investigating the direct administration of BMA or MSCs to BME, we review the current literature on intraosseous (IO) administration of PRP for the treatment of knee OA.

Several studies have investigated intraarticular (IA) application of PRP for knee OA with conflicting results, which have been reviewed.[5] Limited consensus exists among several studies that showed decreased pain relief with IA PRP as severity of knee OA increases.[39] However, this application of PRP does not reach deeper components of the subchondral bone, which plays a pivotal role in the pathogenesis of knee OA.[35]

A combination of IA and IO injections of PRP has been proposed by Sanchez et al.[40] They found that IA injection of PRP combined with subchondral infiltration of PRP in patients with knee OA returned MSCs to a healthy concentration in the synovial fluid, whereas IA injection alone did not.[40] This combination of IA and IO PRP has been supported by pilot and observational studies that have shown this approach to be superior to IA alone.[41,42] Furthermore, in a recent randomized clinical trial ($n = 86$), patients with mild to moderate knee OA were randomized into three groups: the first group received two injections of IA + IO PRP separated by 2 weeks, the second group received two IA PRP injections separated by 2 weeks, and the third group received a series of five IA hyaluronic acid injections separated by 7 days. At 18-month follow-up, the group administered the combination of IA + IO PRP had significantly improved clinical outcome and quality-of-life measures compared to the other two treatment groups.[43]

ORTHOBIOLOGICS IN BONE STRESS INJURY

The use of biological materials for BSI or acute stress fracture is not supported by any current data. No systematic reports of its use have been published in the literature, although a cursory internet search will indicate that some practitioners may be using it informally for this purpose. In the absence of strong clinical data, this section describes the molecular principles and current orthopedic literature surrounding the use of orthobiologics to treat other types of fractures. While not perfectly analogous, the promising results of what is still an experimental treatment provide a rationale for similar use of orthobiologics in those with BSIs and fractures.

Molecular Rationale for the Use of Orthobiologics in Bone Stress Injury

In BSI, the molecular and biomechanical alterations induced by microfractures and bone edema interrupt homeostasis.[35,44] Extracellular matrix degradation triggers inflammatory pathways and upregulates proinflammatory signals, which have chemotactic effects on inflammatory cells and MSCs, further inducing platelet aggregation and initiating the repair cascade.[44-46] As the repair process proceeds, macrophages release a variety of growth factors, which further signal MSC migration, proliferation, and differentiation into angioblasts, chondroblasts, fibroblasts, and osteoblasts.[47,48] Vascular ingrowth to healing bone is regulated by fibroblast growth factor (FGF) and vascular endothelial growth factor (VEGF), among other factors.[48,49]

This inflammatory response is necessary to initiate bone healing; however, excessive inflammation can inhibit regeneration.[50] Moreover, it has been shown that high levels of proinflammatory cytokines in leukocyte-rich platelet-rich plasma (LR-PRP) may mitigate the beneficial effects of the growth factors on bone regeneration, as evidenced by the improved histological results of pure PRP when compared to LR-PRP in vitro.[51] IO administration of orthobiologics would theoretically increase the local concentrations of growth factors including transforming growth factor-β (TGF-β), platelet-derived growth factor, insulin-like growth factor, FGF, and VEGF, resulting in a modulatory effect on the TGF-β signaling pathway and thereby improving the joint biologic environment with regard to fracture healing.[5,52] As such, these therapeutics are used as a means of jump starting the acute inflammatory process in a way that—it is hoped—stimulates normal healing where abnormal healing has already occurred. The resulting ability to manipulate the local inflammatory environment to accelerate healing may offer a simple, less invasive, and more effective way to enhance bone formation and accelerate repair in the setting of BSIs.

Orthopedic Approach to Bone Regeneration

While not commonplace, cases of orthobiologic use for fracture management have been increasingly reported in the orthopedic literature. The choice of compound for treatment is based around three parameters: osteoconduction, osteoinduction, and osteogenesis.[17,18] Osteoconduction refers to a compound's ability to act as a scaffold on which new bone and supporting connective tissues can be built. Cancellous bone chips, which may be used in fracture repair, are an example of a grafting technique that provides a framework for new bone growth.[17] Osteoinduction refers to therapeutics that stimulate bone growth or repair, generally through growth factors or other paracrine compounds that stimulate cell differentiation into osteoblasts and chrondroblasts. Osteogenesis refers to a compound's ability to form new bone. In general, orthobiologic compounds are osteoinductive and, in some cases, osteogenic. Because orthobiologics are cell or growth factor based, they are generally not osteoconductive unless combined with other scaffolding elements.

Use of Bone Marrow Aspirate and Mesenchymal Stem Cells for Fracture Treatment

Connolly et al. were one of the first groups to demonstrate the effectiveness of using BMA for treating nonunion or delayed union fractures, particularly in tibial fractures.[10–12] A subsequent study reaffirmed good results with percutaneous treatment of nonunion sites.[13] Since these initial studies, BMA concentrate, which contains higher numbers of progenitor cells and MSCs, has become popular for treatment of fractures recalcitrant to healing.[18,19] However, these studies are limited to cases of delayed healing rather than application in acute fracture.

Several groups have examined the possibility of using MSCs for healing acute fractures, but most studies have been performed in animal models.[53] In an attempt to investigate the osteogenic potential of human cells, Jiang et al. recently examined adipose-derived stem cells harvested from a population of older patients with osteoporosis. They found good osteogenic properties of adipose-derived stem cells when cultured in hydrogel and implanted in nude mice with acute fractures; however, investigators did not expand their study to human applications.[54] At the time of publication, no formal studies using MSC have been performed in humans with acute fracture, although there are isolated reports of its use in the literature.[16]

Use of Platelet-Rich Plasma for Fracture Treatment

Significantly less research supports the use of PRP, and most of that research has also been performed in animal models.[5,55] Two recent systematic reviews of animal data found mostly supportive evidence for improved bone healing, although how applicable this is to humans remains to be determined.[53,55] Unfortunately, many of these studies suffer from the same lack of reporting regarding PRP preparation protocol and composition that has plagued PRP studies in other areas.[5,55] This further clouds conclusions about human fracture treatment that can be made from existing animal studies.

The clinical studies that have been performed largely focus on application of PRP during surgical procedures as an adjunct to surgical repair or stabilization.[56] A systematic review found that those clinical trials done outside of the initial surgical intervention were largely for treatment of delayed union or nonunion of fractures, although only a minority applied the PRP percutaneously rather than during a subsequent intervention.[56] Outcomes after PRP were favorable for bone healing, with 8 of the 10 examined suggesting a positive role for PRP, although it should be noted that this included only one RCT, which showed inferiority to the use of bone morphogenic protein-7.[56]

CONCLUSION

A foundation of basic science research exists for the use of orthobiologics in fracture healing, and increasing applications to humans continue to support theoretical effectiveness. However, work remains to be done in establishing any of these therapies for use in chronic or acute fractures, and no research currently addresses BSIs or fractures. Although the hypothetical benefit is promising, more research is needed before definitive conclusions can be made to support the clinical use of orthobiologics for the treatment of BSIs.

KEY REFERENCES

Only key references appear in the print edition. The full reference list appears in the digital product found on http://connect.springerpub.com/content/book/978-0-8261-4424-9/part/sec04/chapter/ch20

16. Schottel PC, Warner SJ. Role of bone marrow aspirate in orthopedic trauma. *Orthop Clin North Am*. 2017;48(3):311–321.

18. Calcei JG, Rodeo SA. Orthobiologics for bone healing. *Clin Sports Med*. 2019;38(1):79–95.

41. Sanchez M, Delgado D, Pompei O, et al. Treating severe knee osteoarthritis with combination of intra-osseous and intra-articular infiltrations of platelet-rich plasma: an observational study. *Cartilage*. 2019;10(2):245–253.

43. Su K, Bai Y, Wang J, et al. Comparison of hyaluronic acid and PRP intra-articular injection with combined intra-articular and intraosseous PRP injections to treat patients with knee osteoarthritis. *Clin Rheumatol*. 2018;37(5):1341–1350.

44. Delgado D, Garate A, Vincent H, et al. Current concepts in intraosseous Platelet-Rich Plasma injections for knee osteoarthritis. *J Clin Orthop Trauma*. 2019;10(1):36–41.

55. Marcazzan S, Weinstein RL, Del Fabbro M. Efficacy of platelets in bone healing: a systematic review on animal studies. *Platelets*. 2018;29(4):326–337.

56. Roffi A, Di Matteo B, Krishnakumar GS, et al. Platelet-rich plasma for the treatment of bone defects: from pre-clinical rational to evidence in the clinical practice. A systematic review. *Int Orthop*. 2017;41(2):221–237.

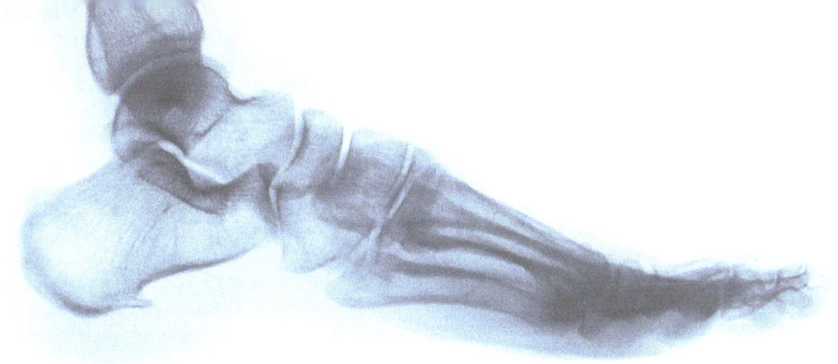

Index